Basic Radiology

Editors

Michael Y. M. Chen, MD
Associate Professor of Radiology
Department of Radiology
Wake Forest University School of Medicine
Winston-Salem, North Carolina

Thomas L. Pope, Jr., MD
Professor of Radiology
Department of Radiology
Medical University of South Carolina
Charleston, South Carolina

David J. Ott, MD
Professor of Radiology
Department of Radiology
Wake Forest University School of Medicine
Winston-Salem, North Carolina

Lange Medical Books/McGraw-Hill
Medical Publishing Division

New York Chicago San Francisco Lisbon London Madrid Mexico City
Milan New Delhi San Juan Seoul Singapore Sydney Toronto

The McGraw·Hill Companies

Basic Radiology

2 3 4 5 6 7 8 9 0 KGP/KGP 0 9 8 7 6 5 4

ISBN: 0-07-141026-0

Notice

Medicine is an ever-changing science. As new research and clinical experience broaden our knowledge, changes in treatment and drug therapy are required. The authors and the publisher of this work have checked with sources believed to be reliable in their efforts to provide information that is complete and generally in accord with the standards accepted at the time of publication. However, in view of the possibility of human error or changes in medical sciences, neither the authors nor the publisher nor any other party who has been involved in the preparation or publication of this work warrants that the information contained herein is in every respect accurate or complete, and they disclaim all responsibility for any errors or omissions or for the results obtained from use of the information contained in this work. Readers are encouraged to confirm the information contained herein with other sources. For example and in particular, readers are advised to check the product information sheet included in the package of each drug they plan to administer to be certain that the information contained in this work is accurate and that changes have not been made in the recommended dose or in the contraindications for administration. This recommendation is of particular importance in connection with new or infrequently used drugs.

This book was set in Garamond by GTS-PA.
The editors were Marc Strauss and Michelle Watt.
The production supervisor was Richard Ruzycka.
Project management was provided by GTS-PA.
Quebecor Kingsport was printer and binder.

This book is printed on acid-free paper.

Library of Congress Cataloging-in-Publication Data

Basic radiology: a Lange clinical book / editors, Michael Y. M. Chen, Thomas L. Pope,
    Jr., David J. Ott.
        p. ; cm.
    Includes bibliographical references and index.
    ISBN 0-07-141026-0
        1. Radiography, Medical. 2. Diagnostic imaging. I. Chen, Michael Y. M., 1941- II. Pope,
    Thomas Lee. III. Ott, David J. 1946-
        [DNLM: 1. Radiography. WN 180 B3114 2004]
    RC78.B34 2004
    616.07'572–dc22
                                                                2003059990

To the memory of my mother
M.Y.M.C.

To Lou, David, and Jason, to my mom, and to the memory of my dad
T.L.P., Jr.

To my family
D.J.O

Contents

Contributors

Sam T. Auringer, MD
Department of Radiology, Forsyth Medical Center, Winston-Salem, North Carolina

Robert E. Bechtold, MD
Professor, Department of Radiology, Wake Forest University School of Medicine, Winston-Salem, North Carolina

D. Matthew Bowen, MD
Department of Radiology, University of Tennessee at Knoxville, Knoxville, Tennessee

Michelle S. Bradbury, MD, PhD
Fellow, Department of Radiology, Wake Forest University School of Medicine, Winston-Salem, North Carolina

Michael Y. M. Chen, MD
Associate Professor of Radiology, Department of Radiology, Wake Forest University School of Medicine, Winston-Salem, North Carolina

Caroline Chiles, MD
Professor, Department of Radiology, Wake Forest University School of Medicine, Winston-Salem, North Carolina

Robert H. Choplin, MD
Professor, Department of Radiology, Indiana University School of Medicine, Indianapolis, Indiana

Robert L. Dixon, PhD
Professor, Department of Radiology, Wake Forest University School of Medicine, Winston-Salem, North Carolina

Rita I. Freimanis, MD
Associate Professor, Department of Radiology, Wake Forest University School of Medicine, Winston-Salem, North Carolina

Judson R. Gash, MD
Associate Professor, Department of Radiology, University of Tennessee at Knoxville, Knoxville, Tennessee

Lawrence E. Ginsberg, MD
Associate Professor, Department of Radiology, University of Texas, M.D. Anderson Cancer Center, Houston, Texas

Tamara Miner Haygood, MD
Department of Radiology, Fayette Memorial Hospital, La Grange, Texas

Johnny U. V. Monu, MD
Associate Professor, Department of Radiology, University of Rochester School of Medicine and Dentistry, Rochester, New York

David J. Ott, MD
Professor of Radiology, Department of Radiology, Wake Forest University School of Medicine, Winston-Salem, North Carolina

Thomas L. Pope, Jr., MD
Professor of Radiology, Department of Radiology, Medical University of South Carolina, Charleston, South Carolina

James G. Ravenel, MD
Assistant Professor, Department of Radiology, Medical University of South Carolina, Charleston, South Carolina

Daniel W. Williams III, MD
Professor, Department of Radiology, Wake Forest University School of Medicine, Winston-Salem, North Carolina

Preface

Our main goal in this book was the creation of a concise text on current radiologic imaging for medical students and residents interested in radiology. After two introductory chapters, an organ-system approach is followed. Applicable imaging techniques and their use and indications are discussed in each organ-related chapter. Question-oriented exercises targeting common diseases in each organ system are included.

The first chapter describes the various diagnostic imaging techniques that are available: conventional radiography, nuclear medicine, ultrasonography, computed tomography, and magnetic resonance imaging. In recent years, many new techniques such as CT angiography, CT colonography, MR angiography, and MR cholangiopancreatography have emerged as new generations of CT and MR equipment have been developed. The second chapter introduces the physics of radiation and its related biological effects and basic technical considerations for ultrasound and magnetic resonance imaging. The remaining chapters focus on individual organ systems, including the heart, lungs, breast, bones, joints, abdomen, urinary tract, alimentary tract, liver, biliary system, pancreas, brain, and spine. These organ-based chapters are similarly structured for consistency. Each chapter first briefly describes the relevant recent imaging developments within each organ system and then the imaging techniques that are applicable for evaluating each organ system are reviewed and the normal anatomy is illustrated. Commonly used radiologic techniques in all areas are described in the first chapter so that repetition is avoided. Then each chapter discusses the selection of appropriate techniques with an emphasis on the proper sequencing of imaging examinations. These choices are based on the clinical presentation, the need for patient preparation and potential conflicts between techniques. The final section of these chapters is the imaging exercises with questions. Each exercise consists of numerous images and specific questions focusing on common diseases or symptoms. One question per case is used in all exercises and the case and question numbers match for clarity. A short list of recent pertinent general readings and references is included at the end of each chapter.

We hope that this book will help medical students and residents not specializing in radiology to better understand and select the many imaging modalities now available for examining their patients. Our further hope is that the interactive exercises presented will familiarize our readers with the more common diseases that current radiologic imaging can most effectively evaluate.

We wish to thank Allen D. Elster, MD Director of the Division of Radiologic Sciences and Professor and Chairman of the Department of Radiology of the Wake Forest University School of Medicine, and C. Douglas Maynard, MD, now retired former Director of Division of Radiologic Sciences and Professor and Chairman of the Department of Radiology of the Wake Forest University School of Medicine, who have provided us with the supportive environment needed to complete this endeavor. This book would also not have been possible without the able support of Martin J. Wonsiewicz, Marc Strauss, Shelley Reinhardt, and their fine associates at Lange Medical Books/McGraw-Hill and Jackie Henry at Techbooks.

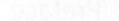

PART 1

Introduction

Michael Y. M. Chen & Michelle S. Bradbury

Conventional Radiography	**Ultrasonography**
Contrast Studies	**Magnetic Resonance Imaging**
Computed Tomography	**Nuclear Medicine**

The landmark discovery of x-rays by Roentgen in 1895 was made serendipitously following the fluorescence of a barium platinocyanide screen by an unknown radiation, after it had passed through a black cardboard-covered cathode-ray tube. By clever substitution of a photographic plate for the fluorescent screen, the existence of this radiation could be recorded. By placing a piece of platinum on the plate and exposing the plate to this radiation source, a light area appeared on the plate where the platinum absorbed the radiation. This unexpected finding was further confirmed after Roentgen placed his wife's hand on a cassette containing a photographic plate and made a 15-minute exposure! The bones appeared white on the developed plate, in contrast to the surrounding darker appearing flesh. Shortly thereafter, he prepared a short manuscript entitled "On a New Kind of Rays, a Preliminary Communication," which he presented to the Würzburg Physical Medical Society on December 28, 1895. In this document, he described the generation of these x-rays and discussed the relative transparency of almost all materials to this radiation, assuming the materials to be of equal thickness. Only the density of the material dictated the degree of transparency. He also noted that, in addition to barium platinocyanide, calcium compounds, uranium glass, ordinary glass, calcite, and rock salt fluoresced when exposed to x-rays. That photographic plates were sensitive to x-ray detection he felt was fortunate as "one is able to make a permanent record of many phenomena whereby deceptions are more easily avoided."

Since this discovery, the field of radiology has progressed rapidly, with successive advances made in the areas of catheter angiography (1950s), nuclear medicine (1960s), ultrasound and computed tomography (CT) (1970s), magnetic resonance imaging (MR imaging), positron emission tomography (PET), and interventional radiology (1980s), multidetector CT and ultrafast MR techniques (early to mid-1990s), and functional and molecular imaging (late 1990s to the present). The classification of radiologic subspecialties can be organ based, modality oriented, or organized according to subspecialty fields. Organ-based subspecialties include musculoskeletal, breast, neurologic, abdominal, thoracic, gastrointestinal, and genitourinary imaging. Ultrasound, PET, and MR imaging are classified as modality oriented. Subspecialty fields include pediatric imaging and women's imaging.

This chapter is intended to provide an overview of a variety of modalities in diagnostic radiology. The physics governing x-ray generation and image formation are described in Chapter 2. Subsequent chapters are organized using an organ-based approach, and are further subclassified in terms of specific imaging modalities. The proper selection of diagnostic studies is essential for ensuring the best possible patient care and for containing medical costs.

CONVENTIONAL RADIOGRAPHY

Conventional radiography remains a fundamental anatomic tool in the detection and diagnosis of disease presenting in the chest (Fig. 1–1), abdomen, pelvis, breasts, and bones, and continues to be utilized in the initial evaluation of the patient. Other modalities, including ultrasonography, CT, and MR imaging, have also been used to provide supplementary diagnostic information and, in some cases, have replaced plain radiograph examinations in the initial work-up of the patient.

Computed radiography (CR) or digital radiography has recently replaced conventional screen-film combination techniques. The most successful digital radiography method to date is photostimulable phosphor computed radiography (PPCR), initially developed in 1981. This technique uses a photostimulable phosphor plate within a cassette to capture and store transmitted x-rays in the form of trapped electrons. When the exposed cassette is scanned with a low-energy laser beam, electron release is stimulated, and the associated energy is used to encode the digital or gray-scale image. Advantages of this technique over conventional screen-film techniques include increased image quality, decreased patient dose, long plate lifetime, and a linear response of the storage phosphors over a wide range of exposures, permitting greater freedom in selecting exposure doses. Disadvantages include reduced spatial resolution due to optical scatter processes within the image plate during scanning. A newer technology that attempts to eliminate these signal losses employs materials such as amorphous selenium, a photoconductor that converts x-rays directly into electrical charges.

Fluoroscopy uses a continuous beam of x-rays to evaluate dynamic processes, such as bowel peristalsis and diaphragmatic excursion, and it is often employed for angiographic or other interventional procedures, including feeding tube or drainage catheter placement. It continues to be a frequently utilized modality in the evaluation of the upper and lower gastrointestinal tract (e.g., barium enema), joint spaces, and spinal cord in the case of a lumbar puncture or myelogram. The recently introduced digital detector systems, such as charged couple devices (CCDs), may begin to replace many of the fluoroscopic system components.

Conventional tomography produces an image in which the desired plane of interest is maintained in sharp focus, while structures located on either side of this plane are intentionally blurred. To achieve this end,

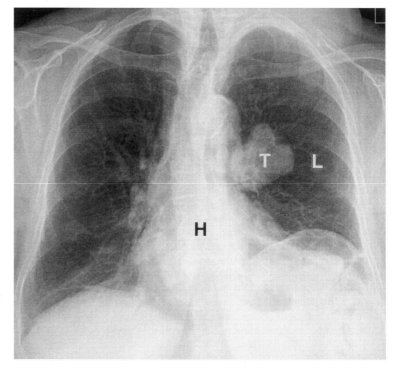

Fig. 1–1. Standard posteroanterior chest radiograph demonstrated the striking contrast between the heart (H) and lungs (L). A tumor (T) is seen at the left hilum.

the x-ray tube and film move in opposite directions concomitantly during the exposure. An 8- to 40-degree arc may be traversed during a tomographic exposure. The wider the arc used, the thinner the slice thickness obtained. Twenty-degree arcs are routinely used in renal studies (nephrotomograms). In addition to simple linear motions, the x-ray tube can perform more complex motions, which can increase blurring, thereby improving overall image quality. Although CT has replaced many conventional tomographic studies, particularly those relating to chest and musculoskeletal applications, it continues to be utilized for nephrotomograms.

The radiographs for screen-film mammography must have excellent resolution, contrast, and film density for optimal detection of breast lesions, particularly early breast carcinoma. A mammographic unit is installed with a special x-ray tube and a plastic breast compression device. Low voltages are utilized to enhance contrast resolution. Two views, craniocaudal (CC) and mediolateral oblique (MLO), are routinely obtained with the breasts maintained in compression. This permits reduced radiation exposure and improves overall image quality. Magnification views are typically acquired for further characterization of microcalcifications, whereas spot compression views are useful for resolving overlapping soft tissue structures, thus facilitating lesion detection. Ultrasonography (US) and, more recently, MR imaging have been used as complementary modalities for more detailed lesion characterization. Image-guided breast interventions are commonly performed and include preoperative needle localization, stereotactic core needle biopsy of microcalcifications, and US-guided procedures (core biopsy or fine-needle aspiration). Digital mammography units have recently been introduced for clinical use.

Contrast Studies

Decreased natural contrast between adjacent structures of roughly similar radiographic density mandates the use of contrast material. Contrast media are commonly utilized for the evaluation of the gastrointestinal tract, urinary tract, and vascular system; less frequent applications involve studies of the biliary tree for carcinoma or obstruction, spinal canal, joints for ligamentous or cartilaginous tears, potential fistulous tracts arising from abscesses, and the uterine cavity and fallopian tubes for uterine anomalies and tubal patency, respectively (hysterosalpingography). Interventional procedures involving catheter or percutaneous tube insertion (nephrostomy, gastrostomy, and biliary) are usually guided by administration of a small volume of contrast.

Barium suspensions, high-density compounds mixed with water, are commonly used in the examination of the gastrointestinal tract. The high radiographic density achieved using these agents is ideal for the standard upper gastrointestinal (UGI) series and for evaluation of the small bowel and colon. Both single- and double-contrast techniques can be performed in an UGI series after oral administration of a barium suspension or during a barium enema, following rectally administered barium (Fig. 1–2). In the single-contrast study, only a barium suspension is used, whereas double-contrast studies use both barium and air to delineate mucosal irregularities and superficially located lesions. Air can be introduced directly by inflating a rectal catheter during a barium enema study, or it can be intentionally generated after ingestion of an effervescent agent during a double-contrast UGI series. Small-bowel studies can be performed in several ways. A barium suspension can be administered orally and followed as it opacifies the small bowel (peroral approach). A second approach, enteroclysis, requires initial placement of a catheter in the proximal jejunum prior to barium infusion. Enteroclysis is preferred for evaluating focal small-bowel lesions or to determine the cause of a small-bowel obstruction. The small bowel

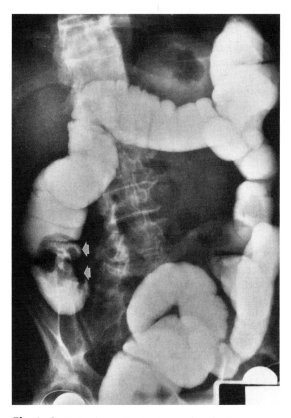

Fig. 1–2. A single-contrast retrograde colonic enema in the left posterior oblique view demonstrates an annular lesion representing a cecal carcinoma (*arrows*). Bilateral hip prostheses are an incidental observation.

can also be assessed via a retrograde approach, either secondary to reflux of barium during a barium enema or to direct infusion of contrast into an ileostomy.

Iodinated contrast agents are water soluble and can be classified in several ways, namely, whether the agent is ionic/nonionic, monomeric/dimeric, or hyperosmolar/hypo-osmolar in solution. First, contrast materials can be ionic or nonionic. An ionic compound dissociates into both anions and cations in water, while nonionic agents do not. The number of iodine atoms per milliliter of solution influences the degree of x-ray attenuation. High- and low-osmolality agents are defined in terms of both the number of iodine atoms in the molecule and the number of osmotically active particles generated in solution. Nonionic compounds were developed to decrease the osmolality of the agent while maintaining optimal contrast characteristics. Based on the above classifications, subcategories of agents can be identified, namely, hyperosmolar ionic (diatrizoate and its derivatives), low-osmolarity ionic (meglumine ioxaglate), nonionic monomers (iohexol, iopamidol, ioversol, iopromide), and nonionic dimers (iodixanol). Side effects, while uncommon, encompass a spectrum, ranging from mild reactions (flushing, tachycardia, and metallic taste in the mouth) to life-threatening effects (hypotension, severe bronchospasm, cardiac arrest). At the present time, the use of low-osmolality contrast agents is advocated, because these agents have a significantly lower incidence of drug reactions. However, because these agents cost considerably more than high-osmolality agents, criteria have been established for their use in more selective patient populations, such as patients who have had a previous reaction to contrast material.

Water-soluble contrast agents are used in the gastrointestinal tract for suspected perforation, prior to surgical procedures, for confirming the position of a percutaneously placed catheter, or for contraindications to barium suspensions. If these agents leak from the gastrointestinal tract, they may be absorbed by the peritoneum, unlike barium suspensions. The use of certain hyperosmolar agents in the gastrointestinal tract will cause fluid to enter the bowel lumen, thereby promoting a hypovolemic state. The likelihood of inducing these conditions with a lower osmolality agent is reduced. Because CT examinations utilize dilute water-soluble agents, the risks of hypovolemia are diminished.

Intravenous urography (IVU), the most common contrast study of the urinary tract, may utilize ionic or nonionic agents. After injection of contrast material into a peripheral vein, sequential filming of the kidneys is performed during the time the agent is concentrated by the kidneys (nephrographic phase, typically 1–3 minutes postinjection), as well as during contrast excretion into the renal collecting system and ureters (pyelographic phase, typically 3–10 minutes) (Fig. 1–3). Tomographic images are usually obtained prior to contrast administration to determine which images optimally depict the entire kidney. Primary indications for this study include hematuria, urinary tract calculi, ureteral obstruction, and evaluation of a suspected congenital anomaly. Nonenhanced helical CT is rapidly superceding the standard IVU examination in cases of stone disease and ureteral obstruction. However, IVU remains the procedure of choice for evaluation of suspected uroepithelial neoplasms, such as transitional cell carcinoma, because it more sensitively detects subtle mucosal irregularities. Retrograde studies of the renal collecting system (retrograde pyelography), ureter (retrograde ureterography), and bladder (cystography) can additionally be performed by direct instillation of water-soluble contrast material into the urinary bladder. These studies are typically performed for evaluation of vesicoureteral reflux, calculi, or tumor. Dynamic retrograde urethrography permits urethral assessment while the urethra is being distended by infusion of water-soluble contrast.

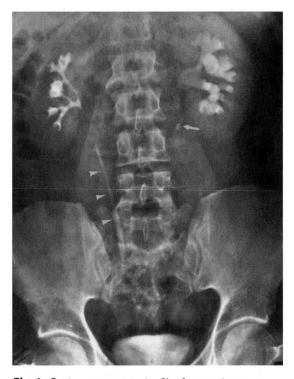

Fig. 1–3. An anteroposterior film from an intravenous urogram was taken at 10 minutes in a patient with a proximal left ureteral calculus (*arrow*) and associated left collecting system dilatation. The right collecting system is normal, and the right ureter (*arrowheads*) and bladder are visualized.

This study is typically performed for suspected urethral injury or stricture.

Hysterosalpingography is a radiographic method for evaluation of the endometrial cavity and the fallopian tubes following direct instillation of water-soluble contrast material (some institutions prefer oil-based iodinated contrast agents) into the cervical canal. This procedure is principally used as part of a primary or secondary infertility work-up, but other applications include detection of suspected uterine anomalies, assessment of tubal patency and morphology following tubal reconstructive surgery, or determination of the location of a uterine leiomyoma within the endometrial cavity. Two spot films are routinely taken during contrast opacification of the uterus and fallopian tubes, both before and after spillage into the peritoneal cavity. Transcervical recanalization of an obstructed fallopian tube has been introduced in recent years to improve the fertility rate.

Angiography, the study of the vascular system, is performed by injection of water-soluble contrast media intra-arterially (or intravenously, for venous studies) through a percutaneously placed catheter under fluoroscopic guidance. Pathologic processes involving both the vasculature and parenchyma can be characterized by fluoroscopic monitoring using either digital or conventional image recording. Specific diagnostic angiographic procedures can be performed, such as peripheral angiography, coronary angiography, thoracic/abdominal aortography, pulmonary angiography, cerebral angiography, and central venography or superior/inferior venocavography. Common applications include assessment of vascular disease (atherosclerosis, aneurysm, vasculitis), determination of vascular injury, vascular mapping for preoperative purposes (organ transplantation) or prior to therapeutic interventions (stent placement), characterization of tumor vascularity prior to endovascular procedures (embolization), and evaluation for pulmonary embolus.

Thoracic aortography is typically performed for the evaluation of suspected traumatic injury (Fig. 1–4),

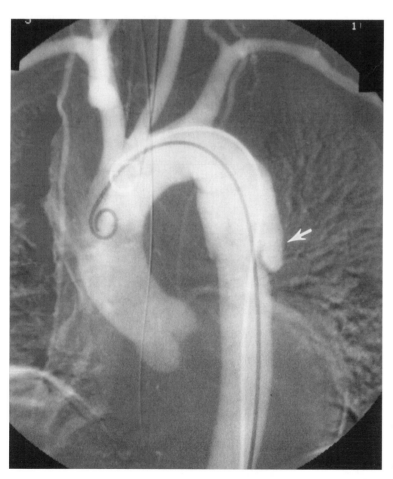

Fig. 1–4. An aortogram demonstrates transection (*arrow*) of the aortic arch at the aortic isthmus extending about 4 cm below.

dissection, aneurysm, vasculitis, thromboembolic disease, tumors, arteriovenous malformations (AVMs), or compression syndromes. This procedure is currently rivaled by both CT angiography and MR angiography, which have replaced conventional angiographic studies in various instances, such as in the determination of vessel dissection following blunt trauma. Coronary angiographic studies identify areas of stenosis or occlusion involving the coronary arteries, in addition to identifying aberrant vascularity. In patients suspected of having a pulmonary embolus, pulmonary angiography may be performed following cannulation of the femoral vein. This procedure is generally used when the results of a ventilation-perfusion (V/Q) scan or pulmonary CT angiography are equivocal, when a low-probability V/Q scan is obtained in the presence of continued high clinical suspicion, or when the performance of either of these studies is clinically impractical. Inferior venocavography is performed prior to filter placement for venous mapping and may additionally be used for evaluation of caval disease, including occlusion, obstruction, or extrinsic compression secondary to fibrosis or retroperitoneal lymphadenopathy.

Less commonly performed contrast studies include myelography for evaluation of spinal cord compression; fistulography for detection of epithelialized tracts arising from an inflammatory, infectious, or neoplastic process; sialography for the assessment of ductal obstruction or tumor involving the salivary glands; galactography for detection of masses within large breast ducts; and cholangiography for detection of biliary ductal masses or strictures. Lymphangiography, a rarely utilized procedure in which water-soluble contrast is injected into the lymphatic system, permits lymph nodes and lymph channels to be evaluated for the presence of malignancy.

Computed Tomography

Computed tomography, an axial tomographic technique, results in source images perpendicular to the long axis of the body (Fig. 1–5). Multiple generations of CT scanners have traditionally used a single-slice fan-beam system. In this system, x-ray photons are initially collimated into a thin fan-shaped beam that is attenuated by the patient being imaged. The attenuation profile of this fan-beam is recorded by a single row of detectors (array) roughly containing a 1000 detector elements. These attenuation values, which reflect the density and atomic number of various tissues, are usually expressed as relative attenuation coefficients, or Hounsfield units (HUs). By definition, the HU of water is zero, and that for air is −1000. Typically, the HU of soft tissues ranges from 10 to 50. Fat also has a negative HU, whereas bone is at least 1000 HU. The contrast resolution of vascular structures, organs, or hypervascular neoplasms can be enhanced following intravenous infusion of water-soluble contrast media. The type and amount of contrast

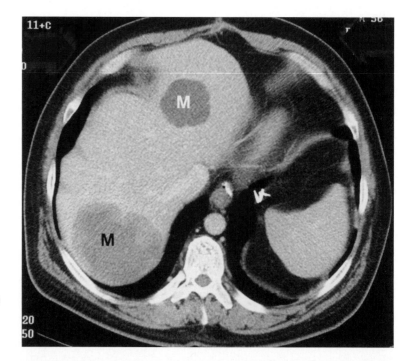

Fig. 1–5. Contrast-enhanced CT image of the upper abdomen demonstrates two low-attenuation areas (M) confirmed as multiple hepatic metastases from gastrointestinal stromal tumor.

agent used, the rate of administration, and the scan delay time will vary with the study indication. Additionally, oral contrast material, namely, water-soluble agents or barium suspensions, can be administered for improved bowel visualization. Artifacts may be produced by patient motion or high-density foreign bodies, such as surgical clips.

Conventional CT scanners have traditionally operated in a step-and-shoot mode, defined by data acquisition and patient positioning phases. During the data acquisition phase, the patient is kept in a stationary position, while the x-ray tube rotates around the patient. A complete set of projections is acquired at a prescribed scanning location, prior to the patient positioning phase. During this latter phase, the patient is transported to the next prescribed scanning location.

The first helical (spiral) CT scanner was introduced for clinical applications in the early 1990s. Helical CT is characterized by continuous patient transport through the gantry while a series of x-ray tube rotations simultaneously acquires volumetric data. These dynamic acquisitions are typically obtained during a single breath-hold of about 20 to 30 seconds. Currently available spiral scanners generally use a single-row detector array that acquires data from a tissue thickness prescribed by the width of the x-ray beam collimator (1–10 mm). Higher spatial resolutions can be achieved with narrower collimations. The advantages of helical CT technology include reduced scan times, improved speeds at which the volume of interest can be adequately imaged, increased ability to detect small lesions that may otherwise change position in non–breath-hold studies. In addition, gains in scan speed permit less contrast material to be administered for the same degree of vessel opacification.

The evolution of multidetector CT scanners (MDCTs) has resulted from the combination of helical scanning with multislice data acquisition. In this CT system, a multiple-row detector array is employed, as opposed to the single-row detector array utilized in single-slice helical scanners. Current state-of-the-art models are capable of acquiring 16, and soon 32, channels of helical data simultaneously. For a given length of anatomic coverage, MDCT can reduce scan time, permit imaging with thinner collimation, or both. The use of thinner collimation (1–2 mm), in conjunction with high-resolution reconstruction algorithms, yields images of higher spatial resolution (high-resolution CT), a technique commonly used for evaluation of diffuse interstitial lung disease or detection of pulmonary nodules. Multidetector CT offers the additional advantages of decreased contrast load, reduced respiratory and cardiac motion artifacts, and enhanced multiplanar reconstruction capabilities. Furthermore, these innovations have had a significant impact on the development of CT angiography.

CT ANGIOGRAPHY

CT angiography protocols combine high-resolution, volumetric helical CT acquisitions with intravenous bolus administration of iodinated contrast material. Using a MDCT scanner, images are acquired during a single breath-hold, ensuring that data acquisition will commence during times of peak vascular opacification. This has permitted successful imaging of entire vascular distributions, in addition to minimizing motion artifact and increasing longitudinal spatial resolution, potentially lowering administered contrast doses. The time between the start of contrast injection and the commencement of scanning can be tailored in response to a particular clinical question, permitting image acquisition during the arterial, venous, and/or equilibrium phases. Exquisite anatomic detail of both intra- and extraluminal structures is revealed using this technique, including detection of intimal calcification and mural thrombosis. CT angiography has become an important tool for assessment of the abdominal and iliac arteries and their branches, the thoracic aorta, the pulmonary arteries, and the extra- and intracranial carotid circulation.

CT COLONOGRAPHY

CT colonography (virtual colonoscopy), introduced in 1994, is a relatively new, noninvasive method of imaging the colon in which thin-section, helical CT data are used to generate two- or three-dimensional images of the colon. This technology has been used primarily in the detection and characterization of colonic polyps, rivaling traditional colonoscopic approaches and conventional barium enema examinations. These images display the mucosal surface of the colon and internal density of the detected lesions; they also directly demonstrate the bowel wall and extracolonic abdominal and pelvic structures.

ULTRASONOGRAPHY

Diagnostic ultrasound is a noninvasive imaging technique that uses high-frequency sound waves greater than 20 kilohertz (kHz). A device known as a *transducer* is used to emit and to receive sound waves from various tissues in the body. The transducer is placed against the patient's skin with a thin layer of coupling gel. This gel displaces the air that would otherwise reflect virtually all of the incident ultrasound beam. As sound travels into the patient, wave fronts spread out, diminishing the overall beam intensity. Beam attenuation also occurs secondary to partial tissue absorption with associated heat conversion. At tissue interfaces, the beam is partially reflected and transmitted. The reflected sound waves, or echoes, travel back to the transducer, are converted into electric signals, and then amplified. The amplitude of

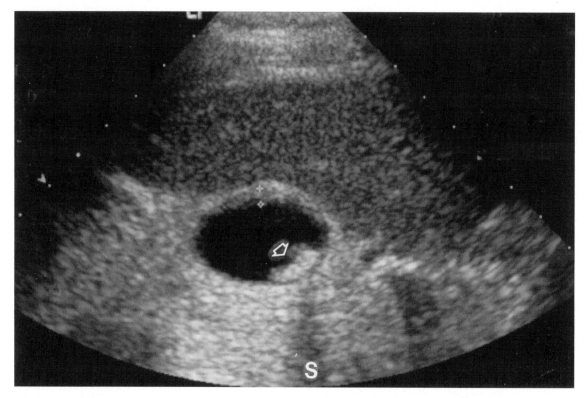

Fig. 1–6. A transverse ultrasound image of the gallbladder demonstrates a gallstone (*arrow*) with the characteristic distal acoustic shadowing (S) because sound waves cannot penetrate the gallstone.

the returning wave partially depends on the degree of beam absorption. A shade of gray is then assigned to each amplitude, with strong echoes being typically assigned a shade near the white end of the spectrum and weak echoes given a shade near the black end of the spectrum. In addition, the depth of the reflecting tissue can be calculated from the known total beam travel time and the average sound velocity in human tissue (1540 meters/second). Limitations of this modality are based on its operator-dependent nature, sensitivity of equipment to slow flow, variable visualization of midline abdominal organs (pancreas) or vasculature when obscured by overlying bowel gas, and inability of sound waves to penetrate gas or bone.

Ultrasonography has many common applications that involve imaging of the abdomen [liver, gallbladder (Fig. 1–6), pancreas, kidneys], pelvis (female reproductive organs), fetus (routine fetal surveys for detection of anomalies), vascular system (aneurysms, arteriovenous communications, deep-venous thrombosis), testicles (tumor, torsion, infection), pediatric brain (hemorrhage, congenital malformations), breast, and chest (size and location of pleural fluid collections). In addition,

ultrasound-guided interventions have been used for facilitating lesion biopsy, abscess drainage, and radiofrequency ablation.

Doppler ultrasound is used primarily to evaluate vascular flow by detecting frequency shifts in the reflected beam, utilizing a principle termed the *Doppler effect*. This effect occurs when a sound emitter or reflector is moving relative to the receiver of sound. Objects moving toward the detector appear to have a higher frequency and shorter wavelength, while objects moving away from the detector appear to have a lower frequency and longer wavelength. If the ultrasound beam strikes a reflector (vessel wall, heart) moving toward it, the reflected sound will have a higher frequency than the original beam. The reflected sound will be of lower frequency than the original beam if the reflector is moving away when the beam strikes it. The Doppler shift is the frequency difference between the original beam frequency and the reflected beam frequency. These frequency differences are used to calculate the corresponding flow velocities, from which a Doppler waveform, or tracing, can be generated. This tracing depicts the relationship between velocity and time and is unique to the flow pattern within the vessel. Color flow Doppler assigns colors (blue and red) to structures according to their motion toward or away from transducers. This information can be superimposed on a gray-scale image.

Endoluminal sonography uses a high-frequency catheter-based transducer (9–20 MHz) to image structures beyond the lumen of the hollow viscus. It is accurate in local staging of cancer and in detecting small lesions that may not be visualized with other imaging modalities. Limitations for optimal evaluation include inability to precisely position the transducer within an area of interest that may restrict full entry.

Endoluminal sonography has been applied in many fields. GI applications of endoluminal sonography include quantification of the size and wall thickness of esophageal carcinoma or varices. Transrectal ultrasound is performed for evaluation of the prostate. Genitourinary (GU) applications include guidance of collagen injections, examination of the severity and length of ureteral strictures, diagnosis of upper tract neoplasms and urethral diverticula, identification of submucosal calculi, and visualization of crossing vessels prior to endopyelotomy. The uterus, adnexa, and routine fetal examinations can be conducted using a transvaginal probe in the presence of an empty bladder. Sonohysterography, an ultrasound-guided procedure, requires instillation of a sterile saline solution into the uterine cavity following cannulation for evaluation of endometrial masses or other abnormalities. Transesophageal echocardiography is used for evaluating cardiovascular abnormalities after placement of a probe into the esophagus. More recently, intravascular applications of sonography have been promising for quantitating the degree of arterial stenosis and for monitoring the therapeutic effects of angioplasty in both peripheral and coronary arteries. Intravascular ultrasound (IVUS) has been applied to modeling plaque morphology, blood flow, and the geometry of the vessel lumen.

Three-dimensional ultrasound (3D-US) has developed during the last decade with advancements in computer processing power and has rapidly achieved widespread use with numerous clinical applications, including obstetrics and vascular imaging. 3D-US is used to quantify the volume of organs and pathology. It has been used predominantly in obstetrics for studying normal embryonic and/or fetal development and for detecting specific congenital anomalies in a fetus at risk given a known family history.

MAGNETIC RESONANCE IMAGING

In 1952, Felix Bloch and Edward Purcell were awarded the Nobel Prize in physics for their independent discovery of the magnetic resonance phenomenon in 1946. Between 1950 and 1970, nuclear magnetic resonance (NMR) was developed and used for chemical and physical molecular analysis. In 1971, Raymond Damadian showed that NMR may have utility in cancer diagnosis, based on observed prolonged relaxation times in pathologic tissue. The first 2D proton NMR image of a water sample was generated in 1972 by Paul Lauterbur using a back-projection technique, similar to that used in CT. In 1975, Richard Ernst used phase and frequency encoding, as well as Fourier transform analysis, to form the basis of current MR imaging techniques. All of these experiments used defined, nonuniform magnetic fields, or linear variations of field strength, along all coordinate axes. The application of these nonuniform fields (magnetic field gradients) permitted discrimination of various signals from different spatial locations. In MR imaging, a pulsed radio-frequency (rf) beam is used in the presence of a strong main magnetic field to generate high-quality images of the body. These images can be acquired in virtually any plane, although sagittal, coronal, and axial images are commonly obtained.

Hydrogen nuclei are favored for MR imaging. Once the patient is in place in an MR scanner, the randomly oriented hydrogen nuclei align with the static magnetic field. To detect a signal, a perturbing rf pulse is transiently applied to the patient, resulting in a net change in alignment of these nuclei. When the rf pulse is turned off, the spins return to their equilibrium state by dissipating energy to the surrounding molecules. The rate of energy loss is mediated by the intrinsic relaxation properties of the tissue, designated as the longitudinal (T_1) and transverse (T_2) relaxation times. T_1 represents the restoration of the longitudinal magnetization along the axis of the main magnetic field; T_2 represents the decay time of the magnetization in the transverse plane. Although a detailed explanation is beyond the scope of this chapter, substances (e.g., fluid) that have a long T_1 will appear dark on T_1-weighted images, whereas those with short T_1 (fat) will display high signal intensity. On T_2-weighted images, a long T_2 substance (fluid) will appear bright. Advantages of MR imaging include its superb contrast resolution, high spatial resolution, and lack of ionizing radiation.

The most commonly used, clinically approved contrast for MR imaging is a paramagnetic agent (atoms with unpaired electrons in their outer shells) containing gadolinium, termed *gadolinium dimeglumine* (or Gd-DTPA), a T_1-shortening agent. Tissue relaxation results from interactions between the unpaired electron of gadolinium and tissue hydrogen protons, which significantly decrease the T_1 of the blood relative to the surrounding tissues. Adverse reactions to this agent are far less frequent than those seen with iodinated compounds, with common reactions including nausea, vomiting, headache, paresthesias, or dizziness.

MR imaging is contraindicated for patients with metal implants or foreign bodies, such as intracranial aneurysm clips, intraorbital metallic foci, cardiac pacemakers, or specific types of cardiac valves. In these instances, these objects may be dislodged or damaged by the magnetic field. MR imaging may also be contraindicated for claustrophobic or uncooperative patients who may not respond to conscious sedation protocols.

Technical advances in gradient hardware, resulting in faster and stronger gradients, have permitted subsecond image scan times. Newer pulse sequences have been developed that currently augment the conventional MR pulse sequences (spin echo and gradient echo), increasing the sensitivity of clinical studies to disease detection. These rapid imaging techniques offer major advantages over conventional MR imaging, including decreased image acquisition times, minimized patient discomfort, and increased ability to image physiologic processes in the body.

Fast spin echo, fast gradient echo, diffusion imaging, perfusion imaging, and echo planar imaging are examples of fast imaging techniques that can be performed on clinical scanners. Diffusion-weighted imaging is exquisitely sensitive to the microscopic molecular motion of water, demonstrating areas of limited (restricted) intracellular diffusion following an acute ischemic event. This sequence is routinely utilized in clinical neuroimaging protocols, but is nonspecific for pathology; diffusion changes similar to that seen with acute ischemia can be observed with infection and some tumors. In conjunction with the results of diffusion-weighted imaging, areas of the brain at risk for further ischemia may be identified. Perfusion-weighted MR imaging, a less frequently used technique, provides information about the blood supply to a particular area of the brain following rapid bolus injection of Gd-DTPA. Echo planar imaging (EPI), introduced by Mansfield and Pykett in 1978, allows the collection of all data required for image reconstruction to occur within a fraction of a second, after a single rf pulse. This technology has resulted in significant clinical and scientific advances, such as in stroke evaluation and functional brain imaging, respectively. Functional MR imaging studies of the human brain using EPI techniques have allowed physiologic investigations of the functional organization of the brain.

Three-dimensional contrast-enhanced magnetic resonance angiography (MR angiography) is used for non-invasive assessment of many vascular abnormalities, including aneurysms, dissection, vessel anomalies, and coarctation. It has evolved from the use of fast scanning techniques on high gradient strength units, in combination with Gd-DTPA. Using this technique, volumetric acquisitions can be performed in a single breath-hold. In many cases, gadolinium-enhanced MR angiography has supplemented traditional noncontrast MR angiography (time-of-flight or phase contrast) techniques. Noncontrast MR angiography methods are partially hampered by longer acquisition times and motion artifacts. Single breath-hold, contrast-enhanced MR angiography techniques avoid many of these problems. Improvements in contrast resolution are achieved, regardless of the plane of acquisition. This has allowed reductions in the number of image sections needed to display a large vascular territory and in the overall imaging acquisition times. Multiphase dynamic imaging is usually performed after intravenous gadolinium administration, with the arteries best seen during the early phase and veins during the later phases.

MR imaging has traditionally been used for neurologic indications, including brain tumors (Fig. 1–7), acute ischemia, infection, and congenital abnormalities. More recently, MR imaging has been used for a number of non-neurologic indications, namely, spine, musculoskeletal, cardiac, hepatic, biliary, pancreatic, adrenal, renal, breast, and female pelvis applications. Spine MR studies are useful for evaluating degenerative changes, disk herniation, infection, metastatic disease, or congenital abnormalities. Common musculoskeletal applications involve the knee, shoulder, and hip. The primary indication for the knee is the assessment of the menisci and ligaments following internal derangement. Rotator cuff tear is the most typical shoulder indication. Cardiac studies are performed to identify congenital anomalies and complex malformations (malpositioning of great vessels and/or cardiac chambers). In the abdomen, hepatic MR imaging studies are often used to diagnose atypical presentations of liver lesions, metastatic diseases,

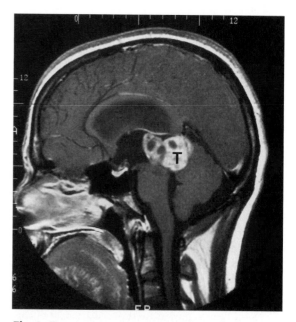

Fig. 1–7. A midline sagittal T_1-weighted contrast-enhanced MR image depicts a large tumor (T) in the region of the pineal gland. *(Courtesy of Daniel W. Williams, III, M.D., Winston-Salem, NC.)*

or hepatocellular carcinoma. Adrenal studies are performed primarily to distinguish adrenal adenomas from metastatic disease. Atypical renal masses, found incidentally on ultrasonography or CT, can often be better characterized on MR imaging. In addition, renal MR imaging is used to establish the presence and extent of tumor thrombus in cases of renal cell carcinoma for tumor staging purposes. Breast MR imaging is predominantly utilized for detection and evaluation of ruptured implants, and studies of the use of MR to detect and characterize heterogeneous cancers in the breast are promising. Finally, oncologic applications in the female pelvis have included the diagnosis and characterization of cervical and endometrial carcinomas, as well as adnexal lesions.

Magnetic resonance cholangiopancreatography (MRCP) is used to evaluate choledocholithiasis, retained gallstones, pancreatobiliary neoplasms, strictures, primary sclerosing cholangitis, and chronic pancreatitis. This noncontrast technique relies on the relatively stationary nature of the bile (compared with blood) to depict the predominantly fluid-filled pancreatic ducts and biliary tree. Rapid, heavily T_2-weighted, breath-hold sequences are utilized, resulting in high signal intensity ductal structures. In patients who have failed endoscopic retrograde cholangiopancreatography (ERCP) or who are unable to tolerate this procedure, MRCP has become a suitable alternative. MRCP is particularly useful in postoperative patients, patients with biliary system anomalies, and as a screening tool in patients with an otherwise low probability of a biliary abnormality. ERCP is generally reserved for therapeutic purposes, such as stent placement, stone extraction, or stricture dilatation.

Molecular MR imaging is a functional imaging strategy that probes biologic processes at a cellular or molecular level using targeted MR contrast agents. Applications include imaging gene expression and visualization of surface receptors.

NUCLEAR MEDICINE

Nuclear medicine studies are performed by administering a radiopharmaceutical to the patient and subsequently recording its distribution in the body over a defined period of time. In general, these studies are very sensitive, but relatively nonspecific, in the detection of pathophysiology. Correlation with pertinent clinical history, physical findings, laboratory data, and other diagnostic imaging procedures is, therefore, essential to rendering an accurate interpretation and for maximizing clinical benefits to both the patient and ordering physician.

Radiopharmaceuticals are radioactive compounds that typically do not elicit a physiologic response when administered for diagnostic or therapeutic purposes. Selective uptake of these compounds by various organs forms the basis for nuclear imaging. In addition, the radionuclide must be normally involved in the physiologic metabolism of the organ to be successfully imaged. These radiopharmaceuticals typically consist of two components: (1) the main component, which is the compound distributed to various organs by a number of physiologic mechanisms, and (2) the radionuclide tagged to this component, which emits gamma rays, permitting detection of the compound in the body. Mechanisms by which these radiopharmaceuticals localize in organ systems include active transport, phagocytosis, capillary blockade, cell sequestration, compartmental localization, exchange diffusion, chemisorption, antigen–antibody reactions, receptor binding, and metabolic trapping. Physiologic function can then be assessed, but spatial resolution is relatively poor.

Most nuclear medicine studies are performed with gamma cameras, which provide planar (two-dimensional) images. A gamma camera converts photons emitted by the ingested or injected radionuclide into a light pulse. This pulse is then converted into a voltage signal, which is used to produce an image of the radionuclide distribution. Gamma cameras may be analog or digital. An analog signal, used throughout the analog camera, is inherently noisy and can encompass an infinite array of values. A digital signal has a discrete number of values. Single photon emission computed tomography (SPECT) is a tomographic technique that utilizes a rotating gamma camera system. One advantage over two-dimensional planar images is the improved image contrast achieved by focusing on a thin slice of tissue, while eliminating the overlying and underlying confounding activity that may obscure lesions of interest.

Positron emission tomography is a molecular imaging modality that uses a positron emitter, 18F-fluorodeoxyglucose (18F-FDG), to create tomographic images by detecting gamma rays. Gamma rays are produced when the emitted positrons interact with electrons. This technique permits metabolic alterations in tumor cells to be detected and is used for diagnosing and staging. Advantages of both SPECT and PET include the ability to map the distribution of the radiopharmaceutical in three dimensions, with the added possibility of quantifying uptake, and the ability to generate cinematic displays of the organ imaged.

Common nuclear medicine procedures include (1) cardiac studies for evaluation of myocardial perfusion and/or ventricular function; (2) skeletal studies for detection of early bone metastases (Fig. 1–8), skeletal trauma, osteomyelitis, and primary bone neoplasms; (3) renograms and renal scans for assessment of renal function and morphologic defects (e.g., pyelonephritis); (4) ventilation–perfusion studies for identification of suspected pulmonary emboli; and (5) PET studies for tumor diagnosis and staging (e.g., lung, colorectal, breast, lymphoma, melanoma), as well as for evaluation of neurodegenerative disorders (dementia), brain tumor

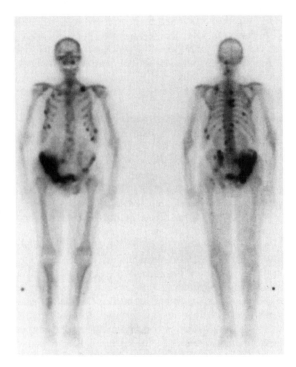

Fig. 1–8. A ^{99m}Tc-MDP bone scan in the anterior and posterior projections demonstrates multiple foci of increased radiopharmaceutical accumulation (spine, ribs, pelvis, and left clavicle) with the typical appearance of bone metastases. *(Courtesy of Robert J. Cowan, M.D., Winston-Salem, NC.)*

recurrence, and myocardial viability. A number of less commonly performed nuclear medicine studies include (1) diagnostic thyroid studies for evaluation of nodules and following iodine-131 therapy for hyperthyroidism and thyroid cancer, (2) hepatobiliary studies for determination of acute cholecystitis and bile duct patency, (3) brain imaging for assessment of brain death and dementia, (4) white blood cell studies for detection of infectious or inflammatory processes, (5) gastrointestinal bleeding studies for detection and localization of small bleeds, (6) lymphoscintigraphy to identify sentinel lymph nodes for surgery, and (7) parathyroid scans to identify adenomas and hyperplasia.

Relatively new developments in PET technology include the use of combined PET/CT imaging devices, synthesis of new tracers for targeting the biologic properties of cancer cells, *in vivo* imaging of cellular processes, and high-resolution PET instruments (microPET). Several advantages to using combined molecular and anatomic imaging (PET/CT scanners) include (1) the performance of physiologic and anatomic scanning in one examination; (2) limited patient motion; permitting accurate fusion of biologic and anatomic images; (3) greater ability to assign physiologic abnormalities to anatomical structures; and (4) improved diagnostic accuracy in the evaluation of hard-to-image regions of the body (e.g., head and neck), given the more precise assignment of metabolic alterations to anatomic landmarks. New molecular imaging probes may target and characterize the genetics and metabolic properties of *in vivo* tumor cells, allow monitoring of treatment responses, and yield prognostic information. MicroPET technology permits imaging of gene expression and assessment of cellular processes, such as metabolism.

BIBLIOGRAPHY

Dawn SK, Gotway MB, Webb WR. Multi-detector row spiral computed tomography in the diagnosis of thoracic diseases. *Respir Care.* 2001;46:912–921.

Di Salle F, Formisano E, Linden DE, et al. Exploring brain function with magnetic resonance imaging. *Eur J Radiol.* 1999;30:84–94.

Eisenberg RL. *Radiology: An Illustrated History.* St. Louis: Mosby–Year Book; 1992.

Elster AD, Burdette JH. *Questions and Answers in Magnetic Resonance Imaging.* 2nd ed. St. Louis: Mosby; 2001.

James JJ, Davies AG, Cowen AR, O'Conner PJ. Developments in digital radiography: an equipment update. *Eur Radiol.* 2001;11:2616–2626.

Mettler FA, Guiberteau MJ. *Essentials of Nuclear Medicine Imaging.* 4th ed. Philadelphia: Saunders; 1998.

Prince MR, Grist TM, Debatin JF. *3D Contrast MR Angiography.* 2nd ed. Berlin: Springer-Verlag; 1999.

Thrall JH. Directions in radiology for the next millennium. *AJR* 1998;171:1459–1462.

Webb WR, Brant WE, Helms CA. *Fundamentals of Body CT.* 2nd ed. Philadelphia: Saunders; 1998.

Williamson MR. *Essentials of Ultrasound.* Philadelphia: Saunders; 1996.

Winston CB, Schwartz LH. Advances in magnetic resonance imaging: applications in body imaging. *Cancer Invest.* 1998;16:413–420.

Zagoria RJ. *Genitourinary Radiology: The Requisites.* 2nd ed. St. Louis, Mosby, 2004.

The Physical Basis of Diagnostic Imaging

Robert L. Dixon

IMAGING WITH X-RAYS

What Is an X-Ray?

An x-ray is a discrete bundle of electromagnetic energy called a *photon*. In that regard, it is similar to other forms of electromagnetic energy such as light, infrared, ultraviolet, radio waves, or gamma rays. The associated electromagnetic energy can be thought of as oscillating electric and magnetic fields propagating through space at the "speed of light." The various forms of electromagnetic energy differ only in frequency (or wavelength). However, because the energy carried by each photon is proportional to the frequency (the proportionality constant is called *Planck's constant*), the higher frequency x-ray or gamma-ray photons are much more energetic than, for example, light photons and can readily ionize the atoms in materials on which they impinge. The energy of a light photon is of the order of 1 electron volt (eV), whereas the average energy of an x-ray photon in a diagnostic x-ray beam is of the order of 30 kiloelectron volts (keV) and its wavelength is smaller than the diameter of an atom (10^{-8} cm).

In summary, an x-ray beam can be thought of as a swarm of photons traveling at the speed of light, each photon representing a bundle of electromagnetic energy.

Production of X-Rays

Electromagnetic radiation can be produced in a variety of ways. One method makes use of the acceleration or deceleration of electrons. For example, a radio transmitter is merely a source of high-frequency alternating current that causes electrons in an antenna wire to which it is connected to oscillate (accelerate and decelerate), thereby producing radio waves (photons) at the transmitter frequency. In an x-ray tube, electrons boiled off from a hot filament (Fig. 2–1) are accelerated toward a tungsten anode by a high voltage on the order of 100 kilovolts (kV). Just before hitting the anode, the electrons will have a kinetic energy in kiloelectron volts equal in magnitude to the kilovoltage (e.g., if the voltage across the x-ray tube is 100 kV, the electron energy is 100 keV). When the electrons smash into the tungsten anode, most of them hit other electrons, and their energy is dissipated in the form of heat. In fact, the anode may become white-hot during an x-ray exposure, which is one reason for choosing an anode with a very high melting point, such as tungsten. The electrons penetrate the anode to a depth less than 0.1 mm. A small fraction of the electrons, however, may have a close encounter with a tungsten nucleus, which, due to its large positive charge, exerts a large attractive force on the electron, giving the electron a hard jerk (acceleration) of sufficient

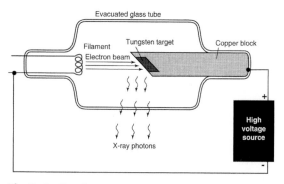

Fig. 2–1. Simple x-ray tube.

magnitude to produce an x-ray photon. The energy of the x-ray photon, which is derived from the energy of the incident electron, depends on the magnitude of the acceleration imparted to the electron. The magnitude of the acceleration, in turn, depends on how close the electron passes by the nucleus. If one imagines a target consisting of a series of concentric circles, such as a dart board, with the bull's-eye centered on the nucleus, more electrons clearly will impinge at larger distances than in the bull's-eye; hence, a variety of x-ray photon energies will be produced at a given tube voltage (kV) up to a maximum equal to the tube voltage (a hit in the bull's-eye), where the electron gives up all of its energy to the x-ray photon. Increasing the voltage will shift the x-ray photon spectrum to higher energies, and higher energy photons are more penetrating. The radiation produced in this manner is called *Bremsstrahlung* (braking radiation) and represents only about 1% of the electron energy dumped into the anode by the electron beam; the other 99% goes into heat. The other reason for using tungsten is that it is a heavy element with a large positive charge in the nucleus that can provide enough acceleration to the electron to produce an x-ray photon.

The electron current from filament to anode in the x-ray tube is called the *mA*, because it is measured in milliamperes. The mA is simply a measure of the number of electrons per second making the trip across the x-ray tube from filament to anode. The rate of x-ray production (number of x-rays produced per second) is proportional to the product of milliamperage and kilovoltage squared. The quantity of x-rays produced in an exposure of duration s (in seconds) is proportional to the product of mA and time. This quantity is called the *mAs*. The quantity of x-rays at a given point is generally measured in terms of the amount of ionization per cubic centimeter of air produced at that point by the x-rays and is measured in roentgens (R) or in coulombs per kilogram of air. This quantity is called *exposure,* and

1 R of exposure results in 2×10^9 ionizations per cubic centimeter of air.

The electron beam is made to impinge on a small area (of the order of 1 mm in diameter) on the anode to approximate a point source of x-rays. Because a radiograph is a shadow picture, the smaller the focal spot, the sharper the image. By analogy, a shadow picture on the wall (such as a rabbit made with one's hand), will be much sharper if a point source of light such as a candle is used rather than an extended light source such as a fluorescent tube. The *penumbra* (or lack of sharpness) of the shadow will depend not only on the source size, but also on the magnification, as can be illustrated by making a shadow of one's hand on a piece of paper using a small light source such as a single light bulb. The closer your hand is brought to the paper (the smaller the magnification), the sharper the edges of the shadow. Similarly, the magnification of the x-ray image produced by the point source is lower the closer the patient is to the film and the further the source is from the film. The *magnification factor* (M) is defined as the ratio of image size to object size and is equal to the ratio of the focal-to-film distance divided by the focal-to-object distance ($M \geq 1$, and $M = 1$ means no magnification is produced; i.e., either the object is right against the film or the focal spot is infinitely far away). The penumbra, blurring, or lack of sharpness (Δx) produced on an otherwise perfectly sharp edge of an object and due to the finite focal spot size of dimension a is expressed by the equation

$$\Delta x = a(M - 1)$$

Unfortunately, the smaller the focal spot, the more likely the anode will melt. The power (energy per second) dumped into the anode is equal to the product of the kilovoltage and milliamperage; i.e., at 100 kV and 500 mA, 50,000 watts (W) of heat energy is deposited into an area of the order of a few square millimeters. (Imagine a 50,000-W light bulb to get an idea of the heat generated.)

Interaction of X-Rays with Matter

X-rays primarily interact with matter through interaction of their oscillating electric field with the atomic electrons in the material. Having no electrical charge, x-rays are more penetrating than other types of ionizing radiation (such as alpha or beta particles) and are therefore useful for imaging the human body. The x-rays may be absorbed or scattered by the atomic electrons. In the absorption process (photoelectric absorption), the x-ray is completely absorbed, giving all of its energy to an inner shell atomic electron, which is then ejected from the atom and goes on to ionize other atoms in the immediate vicinity of the initial interaction. In the scattering process (compton scattering), the x-ray ricochets off an atomic electron, losing some of its energy and changing its direction. The recoiling electron also goes on to ionize hundreds of atoms in the vicinity. Electrons from both processes go on to ionize many other atoms, and are responsible for the biological damage produced by x-rays.

The attenuation of the x-ray intensity with thickness of material follows an exponential law due to the random hit-or-miss nature of the interaction. The process is similar to firing a volley of rifle bullets into a forest, where the bullets may either stick in a tree (be absorbed) or ricochet off a tree (scatter). The deeper you go into the forest, the fewer bullets there are; however, a bullet still has a chance of traveling through the forest without hitting a tree. Likewise, an x-ray can make it all the way through a patient's body without touching anything and remain unchanged, as if it had passed through a vacuum instead. These are called *primary x-rays.* Typically, only about 1% of the incident x-rays penetrate the patient, and only about a third of these are primary x-rays; the rest are *scattered x-rays* that do not contribute to the anatomic image. An x-ray image is a shadow or projection image, which assumes that x-rays reaching the film have traveled in a straight line from the source, but this is true only for the primary x-rays. As Figure 2–2A shows, the film density (blackness) at point *P* on the film is related to the anatomy along line *FP*. The scattered photon reaches the film along the path *FSP* and is relaying information about the anatomy at the random point *S* to point *P* on the film. Scatter simply produces a uniform gray background; it does not contribute to the image. Because scatter reduces image contrast, it is desirable that the scatter be removed. This task is accomplished by use of an antiscatter grid (Fig. 2–2B). This grid consists of a series of narrow lead strips with radiolucent (low-attenuation) interspace material to remove some of the scatter. With the grid, the scattered photon shown in the figure can no longer reach the film, but the primary x-rays can. More of the scatter than primary x-rays are eliminated by the grid, hence, image contrast increases but at the cost of an increase of a factor of 2 to 3 in patient dose. This increase occurs because the scatter, which was previously blackening the film, has been reduced, and therefore, higher x-ray exposure to the front of the patient is necessary to get the requisite number of x-rays through the grid to blacken the film. The grid is usually made to move a few interspaces during the exposure by a motor drive in order to wash out the grid lines.

The absorption process is more prevalent at lower kilovoltages and in materials with higher atomic numbers. Bones appear white on an x-ray film because photoelectric absorption of x-rays is greater in bone

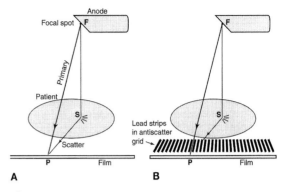

Fig. 2–2. **A** Scattered and primary x-ray photons reaching the same point *P* on film. **B** Scattered photon is removed by antiscatter grid, while primary photon gets through.

than in soft tissue due to the higher atomic number of bone. Lead is a useful shielding material for x-rays due to its high atomic number. The probability of the absorption process decreases rapidly with photon energy (as $1/E^3$) and the scattering process decreases slowly (as $1/E$); hence, the x-ray beam becomes more penetrating as kilovoltage increases. The scattering process is roughly independent of the atomic number of the attenuating material (all electrons look alike to the photon for the scattering process), whereas the absorption process is more probable for tightly bound electrons such as the inner electrons in heavier elements.

Increasing the kilovoltage is therefore beneficial to the patient in that it reduces the radiation dose; i.e., fewer x-rays into the front side of the patient are needed to get the requisite number out of the backside to blacken the film. An increase in kilovoltage, however, will reduce image contrast since the absorption process, which is sensitive to atomic number, will decrease and the scattering process is independent of the atomic number of the materials. Even with materials of the same atomic number, contrast improves at lower kilovoltage settings due to higher attenuation, which results in greater differential attenuation between different thicknesses of the same material. Thus, a trade-off exists between image quality (contrast) and patient dose that must be weighed in the selection of kilovoltage.

The Radiographic Image

For production of radiographic images, the x-ray film is placed in a cassette and sandwiched between two fluorescent screens that glow under x-ray exposure, and it is primarily the light from these fluorescent screens that blackens the film. Although x-ray film, which is quite similar to ordinary photographic film, can be blackened by direct x-ray exposure, the film does not absorb the penetrating x-rays very efficiently, because the emulsion consists of silver halide crystals embedded in a low-atomic-number gelatin base. The fluorescent screens, called *intensifying screens,* are made of high-atomic-number materials, which therefore absorb x-rays very efficiently and also emit hundreds of light photons per x-ray absorbed. These light photons, in turn, are efficiently absorbed by the film. As a result, x-ray exposure to the patient is reduced by a factor of the order of 100 compared to direct x-ray exposure of the film. The screens do produce a loss of sharpness of the image due to the spreading of the light from the point of x-ray absorption before the light reaches the film. This effect can be reduced by making the screen thinner; however, it then absorbs a smaller fraction of the incident x-rays and therefore results in a "slower" system (more patient exposure is required). In recent years digital image receptors have come into use. One type, called *computed radiography,* utilizes a cassette with a photostimulable phosphor material that stores the x-ray image in the form of trapped electrons for later readout by a scanned laser beam that releases the electrons from their traps. On release, these electrons cause the emission of light from the phosphor, which has a shorter wavelength than that of the laser beam. This light signal is read out and digitized, thereby forming a digital image. Another type, called *direct radiography,* consists of a flat-panel digital detector plate that is built into the x-ray unit itself. In these the x-ray image is converted to an electrical signal from a fine matrix of thin-film transistor elements, which creates a digital image having a pixel size of 0.2 mm or less. These digital images, which consist of an array of numbers in a matrix, can be processed to improve image quality, displayed and manipulated on a viewing monitor, and then printed onto film using a laser film printer. The advantage of these digital systems is that the image can be processed to improve contrast and to provide edge enhancement, and the film can be printed to the appropriate darkness regardless of the x-ray exposure.

Recall that the quantity of x-rays produced during an exposure is proportional to

$$mAs \cdot kV^2$$

However, because the beam is more penetrating at high kilovoltage, the x-ray exposure that reaches the film through a patient is roughly proportional to

$$mAs \cdot kV^4$$

That is, it depends very strongly on kilovoltage. The exposure time required to blacken the film is thus proportional to

$$s \approx \frac{1}{mA \cdot kV^4}$$

The heat deposited in the anode is proportional to the product of kilovolts and mAs.

Choice of an exposure technique is generally made by first selecting the kilovoltage. A lower kilovoltage gives greater image contrast but also higher patient exposure and requires a longer exposure time at a given milliampere setting because the x-ray beam is less penetrating and x-ray production is lower at the lower kilovoltages. Thus, for thick body parts, care must be taken not to choose too low a kilovoltage.

Generally, x-ray tubes have two focal spot sizes produced by two different (selectable) filament sizes. That is, they have a large and a small focal spot (e.g., 1.25 and 0.6 mm). With the small focal spot, however, the electron energy is deposited in a smaller area, thereby creating a higher anode temperature. Hence, at a given kilovoltage, the maximum milliamperage that can be used without melting the anode is limited to a lower value, thereby resulting in a longer exposure time. The small focal spot will result in a sharper image, however, if the longer exposure time required by its selection does not "stop" patient motion; then motion of the patient during the exposure may blur any sharpness gain realized by use of the small focal spot. In any case, the small focal spot is useful only for looking at fine detail, such as bony detail, and its use does not significantly improve, for instance, an abdominal radiograph in which soft-tissue contrast is the objective. The small focal spot might be used for radiographs of the skull or extremities. The exposure time selected should be short enough to stop the motion of the anatomic part being radiographed. A very short time would be required for the heart and somewhat longer times for the abdomen or chest. Exposure time is less critical for the head or extremities, which are not subject to motion in most cases.

Having selected the kilovoltage and exposure time, one must then select the milliamperage so that the milliampere-seconds (the product of milliamperage and time) is large enough to blacken the film suitably. If the milliamperage required is above 200 to 300 mA, a small focal spot generally cannot be used, because it will not allow this high a value of milliamperage without melting the anode.

On many x-ray units, a phototimer sensor (automatic exposure control) is used to automatically terminate the x-ray exposure when a given x-ray exposure has been accumulated at the cassette position. In this way, the film is blackened sufficiently regardless of patient thickness and kilovoltage selection. When using this feature, however, the operator loses control of the exposure time, and choosing the highest milliamperage allowable by the tube will ensure the minimum exposure time.

Fluoroscopy

If, instead of using the light from a fluorescent screen to blacken a film, one viewed the fluorescent screen directly with the naked eye, then one would be performing fluoroscopy as it was done in the early days of medical x-ray use. Unfortunately, the image made in this fashion was very dim, even at a high exposure rate to the patient, so modern fluoroscopy uses an image intensifier that amplifies the light from a fluorescent screen. A typical fluoroscopic imaging system is shown in Fig. 2–3. The image intensifier tube is an evacuated glass or metal tube with a fluorescent screen (input phosphor) that glows with the image produced by the x-ray pattern that exits the patient. The light from the input phosphor causes ejection of electrons from a photoelectric material adjacent to the input phosphor. These electrons are accelerated via a high voltage (30 kV) and are also focused to preserve the image onto a small (1-in.-diameter) screen (the output phosphor), which glows with the image due to the energy deposited by the impact of the accelerated electrons. The output phosphor glows much brighter than the input phosphor (about 3000 times brighter) due to the energy gain provided by the acceleration of the electrons and also due to minification of the image on the output phosphor. The image on the output phosphor can be viewed with the naked eye, usually with a series of lenses and mirrors, but the image is more commonly viewed by focusing a video camera onto the output phosphor and viewing the image on a TV monitor via a closed-circuit TV system. The fluoroscopic image generally has less contrast and less resolution of fine detail than a radiographic image; however, it is clearly convenient to view the image in real time—particularly when observing the flow of radiopaque contrast agents ingested or injected into the body. (These contrast materials, such as iodine or barium compounds, have a higher atomic number than soft tissue and hence absorb more x-rays.) During fluoroscopic examinations, the x-ray tube is typically operated below 100 kV and below a 3-mA tube current. Even so, entrance exposure rates (at the point where the x-ray beam enters the patient) are about 2 to 5 R/min, depending on patient thickness; hence, fluoroscopic examinations generally result in significantly higher patient exposures than do radiographic examinations.

Fluoroscopic systems generally have an automatic brightness control in which the brightness of the output phosphor is sensed by using a light detector. The brightness signal from this detector is compared to a reference level, and the difference signal is used to instruct the x-ray generator to vary milliamperage or kilovoltage (or both) in order to maintain a constant brightness at the output phosphor. For example, after ingestion of barium in a barium-swallow examination, the barium absorbs significantly more x-rays, and the image would tend to go dark without such a system. As the brightness falls below the reference level, however, the automatic brightness control causes the x-ray generator to increase the milliamperage or kilovoltage to maintain a constant brightness on the monitor.

Recording of Fluoroscopic Images

Fluoroscopic images can be recorded for later viewing by several methods. The TV image can be recorded using a videotape recorder or a videodisc recorder, the latter having the advantage of being able to view one frame at a time as well as providing random access rather than the sequential viewing required by videotape.

In addition, some systems have the capability of digitizing the electric signal from a TV frame and storing it in computer memory chips. These systems often have a "last image hold" capability that holds the last TV frame on the monitor. This method is also used in digital subtraction angiography (DSA); that is, the analog signal from the TV camera is digitized and stored frame by frame in a computer memory in a 512 × 512 or 1024 × 1024 image matrix. A short radiographic x-ray pulse is usually used for making the image. Images made just before and after injection of contrast material into the arteries can be subtracted digitally, so that only the vascular system appears in the subtracted image.

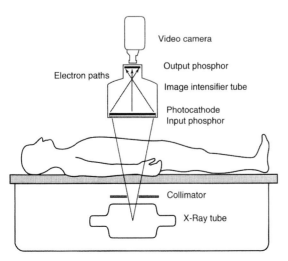

Fig. 2–3. Fluoroscopic imaging system.

Spot Film Devices

The aforementioned image recording methods merely store the image recorded by the TV camera, which is of lower quality than a radiographic image and has even poorer resolution than the image appearing on the output phosphor of the image-intensifier tube due to the limitations of the TV imaging process. To record higher quality images during a fluoroscopic examination, spot film devices are used. The most common device transports a conventional radiographic screen-film cassette to a position in front of the image intensifier at the push of a button on the fluoroscopic carriage. The x-ray tube is then switched into a radiographic mode (i.e., the milliamperage is increased from low milliamperes to 200 to 400 mA to shorten exposure time), and a conventional radiographic image is obtained on film. Digital spot films can be obtained by digitizing a TV frame from the image intensifier acquired with a short exposure burst at a higher exposure value than that of a single continuous fluoroscopic frame. These produce an image of higher quality (lower noise) than that obtained from the fluoroscopic image.

Computed Tomography

In radiography or fluoroscopy, one is creating a shadow picture or a projection of the attenuation properties of the human body onto a plane. Thus each ray from the source to a given point on the film, such as ray *FP* in Fig. 2–2, conveys information about the sum of the attenuation along a line in the body; i.e., anatomic structures are piled on top of each other and flattened into the radiographic image. In an attempt to give a different perspective, one can obtain projections from two different directions (e.g., a lateral and an anteroposterior radiograph), so that the structures that are piled on top of each other differ in each projection. In the late 1960s, a British engineer, Goeffry Hounsfield, concluded that if one obtained projection data from a sufficient number of different angles, one could reconstruct the attenuation properties of each volume element in the body and display these as a cross-sectional image. This required the computational power of a computer to accomplish, and the basic idea is illustrated in Fig. 2–4. The x-rays from a source are detected by a series of individual detectors (rather than film) after penetrating the body, and each detector defines a ray from the source through the body, thereby creating a projection. The width of the x-ray beam in the dimension perpendicular to the page is only about 10 mm; hence, only one slice of the body in the longitudinal direction is imaged at a time.

The x-ray tube and the detector bank are rotated 360 degrees about the patient to obtain, for example, 720 projections at 0.5-degree intervals. The computer is then able to reconstruct a cross-sectional image of the slice of the

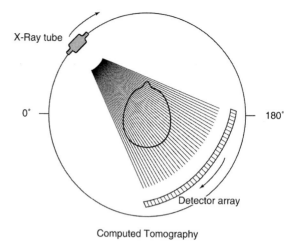

Fig. 2–4. Computed tomographic (CT) scanning geometry. A single projection of the head is illustrated.

body by dividing the slice into an imaginary matrix. In a matrix of 512×512 pixels in the transverse plane, each pixel represents an area of about 0.5×0.5 mm in a 25-cm-diameter body. The computer assigns a numerical value to each pixel, which represents the amount of attenuation contributed by the volume element of the body represented by that pixel. These numbers are converted into a gray-scale image for viewing. In an axial scan series, after one slice is completed, the patient is advanced via a motorized couch by 10 mm in order to image the adjacent slice, and up to 30 slices (images) may be done to reconstruct the anatomy over a 30-cm length of the patient. Newer scanners, called *helical* (or *spiral*) *CT scanners,* use a continuous advance of the patient through the scan beam rather than the stepping couch motion utilized in axial scans, and axial slices are reconstructed by interpolation of data into the slice from a complete rotation. Also multislice helical scanners with subsecond rotation times have been developed that collect data for reconstruction of several slices in each rotation, thus a 30-cm length of patient anatomy can be imaged in 15 seconds or less.

MAGNETIC RESONANCE IMAGING

The technique called *nuclear magnetic resonance,* developed by physicists in the 1940s, was first utilized for imaging the human body in the late 1970s. The nuclei of some atoms (notably hydrogen nuclei in the body) have a fundamental angular momentum called *spin,* which causes them to behave like tiny spinning magnets. When placed in a uniform external magnetic field and excited by a radio pulse tuned to a resonant frequency that is proportional to the externally applied magnetic field strength (Larmor frequency), the axis of rotation of the nuclei will precess around the applied magnetic field direction in a similar fashion to the precession of a leaning gyroscope or top about the gravitational field direction (Fig. 2–5). This precession can be detected because the collection of processing magnets (protons in the body) induces an oscillatory voltage in a pickup or receiver coil. This oscillation at the Larmor frequency can be detected by connect-

ing the pickup coil to a radio receiver. In effect, one could hear the protons "singing" in unison into the coil at the Larmor frequency. This provides no imaging information; however, if the external magnetic field is made nonuniform in space in a known fashion (i.e., a magnetic field gradient is utilized), then protons at different locations will precess at different frequencies, thereby creating a relationship between location in the body and precessional frequency. With application of such a gradient, the protons no longer sing in unison, but at different frequencies depending on their location, as in a chorus; i.e., the sopranos would be located where the magnetic field was largest and the baritones where it was smallest. By listening to different frequencies, one can deduce from the signal strength at a given frequency how many protons are present at the location corresponding to that frequency. This method of imaging allows one to map the density of protons in the body in three dimensions; however, most images are obtained and displayed as planar cross-sectional images similar to those in CT scans and having a slice thickness of 10 mm and a typical matrix size of 128×256. For greater contrast, the proton density images may also be weighted by the relaxation times (T_1, T_2) which are measures of the realignment times of protons with respect to the magnetic field direction. This weighing is typically accomplished by varying the radio-frequency pulse durations and spacings in a variety of pulse sequences, the spin-echo pulse sequence being the most commonly used.

The hardware of a (nuclear) magnetic resonance imaging machine (Fig. 2–6) consists typically of a cylindrical superconducting coil surrounding the patient to generate a large, static magnetic field; auxiliary coils for generating the magnetic field gradients; radio transmitter/receiver coils in proximity to the patient; electronics for radio-frequency transmitting and receiving; and a computer to orchestrate the events and to reconstruct the spatial image from the frequency spectra.

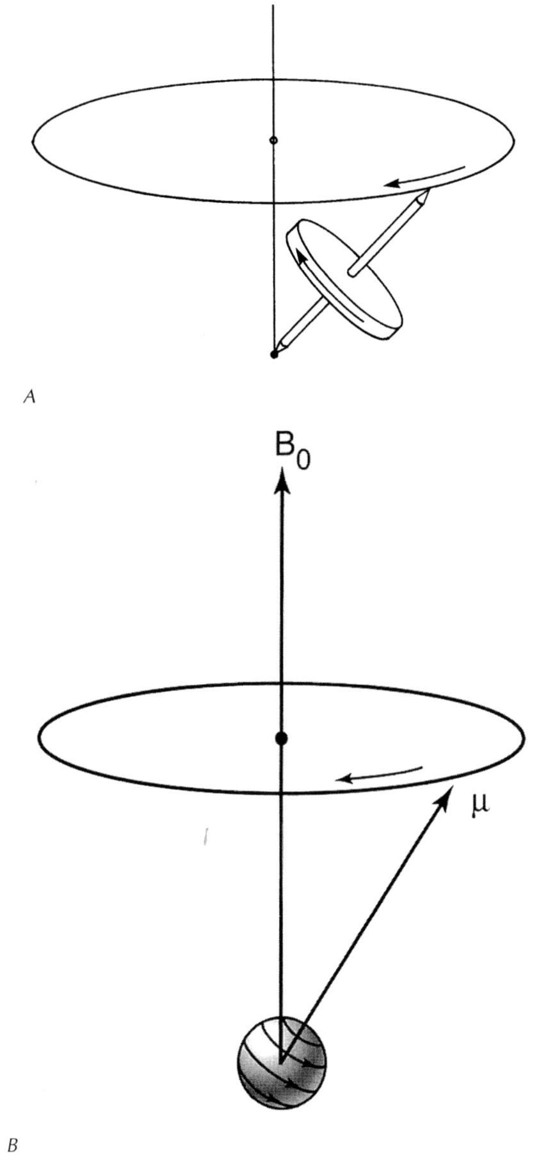

A

B_0

μ

B

Fig. 2–5. A Precession of a gyroscope about the earth's gravitational field. **B** Precession of the spin axis of a proton of magnetic moment μ about an applied magnetic field B_0.

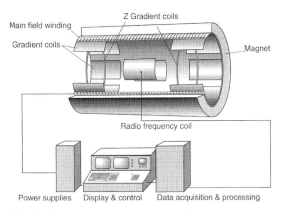

Fig. 2–6. Magnetic resonance imaging hardware.

ULTRASOUND IMAGING

Sound (or pressure) waves in the 3- to 10-MHz frequency range are used for imaging the body by detecting the intensity of the reflected waves from various organs and displaying this reflected intensity as a gray-scale (or color) image. The sound waves are generated by applying an electrical pulse to a piezoelectric crystal. This crystal also acts as a receiver of the reflected waves after the transmitter pulse is terminated. A typical ultrasound transducer contains a linear array of such crystals, which can be fired in sequence or operated as a phased array to cause the ultrasound beam to rapidly scan across an area 5 to 10 cm in width for real-time imaging. The useful imaging depth is determined by the frequency; the higher frequencies (shorter wavelengths) have less penetrability. For example, at 10 MHz the imaging depth is limited to a few centimeters. Unfortunately, the lower the frequency, the poorer the axial resolution, because objects that are closer together than a wavelength cannot be separated. Hence, there is a trade-off between axial resolution and penetration depth. Because ultrasound radiation is nonionizing, no adverse biologic effects have been observed at diagnostic power levels.

BIOLOGIC EFFECTS OF X-RAYS

The biologic effects of x-irradiation are due to the recoiling electrons produced by the absorption or scattering of the incident x-rays, these electrons having enough kinetic energy to ionize hundreds of atoms along their trajectory. These electrons may damage DNA molecules directly or produce free radicals that can chemically damage genetic material; either effect may result in cell death or mutation. Magnetic resonance imaging and ultrasonic imaging do not utilize ionizing radiation, and there is no significant evidence that any biologic damage results from these imaging modalities.

Effect on the Patient

The primary risk to patients undergoing medical x-ray examinations is radiation-induced cancer, primarily leukemia, thyroid, breast, lung, and gastrointestinal cancer. These relative risks are considered to be related to radiation dose and effective dose, which is essentially the exposure to various critical organs multiplied by an organ-weighing factor. (The units of radiation dose or exposure—a rem, a rad, and a roentgen—are essentially equivalent for x- and gamma-ray irradiation.) Table 2–1 lists typical effective doses in millirems for various examinations and the resulting relative increase in cancer risk per million persons. For example, if 1 million persons received lumbar spine examinations, 51 additional, randomly occurring cases of cancer (above that occurring naturally) would occur in this population over its lifetime.

Table 2–1. Typical Effective Doses and Resulting Increased Risk of Fatal Cancer for Various X-Ray Examinations

X-Ray examination	Typical effective dose (mrem) (1 mrem = 0.01 mSv)	Lifetime risk of fatal cancer per million persons
Lumbar spine	127	51
Upper gastro-intestinal tract	244	98
Abdomen (KUB)	56	22
Pelvis	44	18
Chest	8	3

The Pregnant Patient

The fetus consists of rapidly dividing cells and hence is more sensitive to radiation, particularly in the first trimester. The principal risks to the fetus from *in utero* irradiation are cancer induction, malformation (e.g., small head size), or mental retardation.

Every fertile female patient should be asked if she might be pregnant; if so, the relative risks of the diagnostic x-ray procedure versus the expected benefit should be weighed before the procedure is performed, or alternate imaging procedures such as MR imaging or ultrasound should be considered. Note, however, that the added risk from diagnostic x-ray procedures is generally negligible compared to the normal risks of pregnancy, because fetal doses are typically below 5 rad in these procedures.

The National Council on Radiation Protection (NCRP) in its report NCRP No. 54 states:

The risk (to the fetus) is considered to be negligible at 5 rad or less when compared to the other risks of pregnancy, and the risk of malformations is significantly increased above control levels only at doses above 15 rad. Therefore, exposure to the fetus to radiation arising from diagnostic procedures would rarely be cause, by itself, for terminating a pregnancy.

If the x-ray examination involves the abdomen in such a way that the fetus is in the direct x-ray beam, then fetal doses are typically in the 1 to 4 rad (1 rad = 1 cGy) range depending on the number of films and fluoroscopic time (if any). If the examination does not involve the abdomen, and the fetus receives only scatter radiation, the fetal dose is generally small (typically, well below 1 rad).

BIBLIOGRAPHY

National Council on Radiation Protection and Measurements. *Medical Radiation Exposure of Pregnant and Potentially Pregnant Women.* NCRP Report No. 54. Bethesda, Md: National Council on Radiation Protection and Measurement; 1989.

PART 2

Chest

Imaging of the Heart and Great Vessels

3

James G. Ravenel & Thomas L. Pope, Jr.

INTRODUCTION

The heart and great vessels are complex structures that are critically important to human function. They serve as the "pump" and major proximal "pipes" distributing blood and nutrients to the body. This chapter describes the normal radiographic appearance of the heart, pericardium, and great vessels (aorta and pulmonary vessels) and briefly outlines some of the more common pathologic entities in this organ system. Critical evaluation of the findings on the imaging examinations of this region is not possible without paying attention to the lungs, because these two organ systems mirror changes in each other. The most common abnormalities encountered in the cardiovascular system are hypertension, pulmonary arterial hypertension (usually secondary to chronic pulmonary disease), congestive heart failure, atherosclerotic disease, and valvular disease. Less common cardiac and great vessel diseases such as congenital heart disease, neoplasms, and diseases of the pericardium are described in less detail. The last topic of monitoring devices and postoperative changes is one with which students should be familiar.

We are assuming that the student understands the basic normal anatomy of the cardiovascular system from the basic science and clinical years. At the completion of this chapter the student should have an understanding of the wide range of imaging modalities used, an appreciation for the potential yield from these examinations, a basic knowledge of the normal imaging anatomy on the conventional radiograph, and a familiarity with more common postoperative alterations and the various monitoring devices that may be present in the intensive care unit.

TECHNIQUES AND NORMAL ANATOMY

A variety of techniques have been developed to evaluate the heart and great vessels (Table 3–1). In this section, we briefly describe the major tests used in imaging this system.

Conventional Radiographs

The most common imaging test for evaluating the heart and great vessels is the chest radiograph, which consists of an upright posterior-to-anterior (PA) and left lateral (LAT) projections. The terms *PA* and *left lateral* refer to the direction the x-ray beam takes through the body before it reaches the radiographic cassette. Chest radiographs are usually obtained with high kilovoltage and milliamperage to minimize exposure time and cardiac motion. When possible, the distance between the x-ray tube source and the film is at least 6 feet to minimize magnification and distortion.

The examination is ideally performed with the patient at maximal inspiration. A good rule of thumb for estimating adequate inspiration is to be able to count 9 to 10 posterior ribs or 5 to 6 anterior ribs from the lung apices to the hemidiaphragms through the aerated lungs (Fig. 3–1). When a chest radiograph is taken in the expiratory phase of respiration, the patient may appear to have cardiomegaly, vascular congestion, and even pulmonary edema. This appearance,

Table 3–1. Imaging Tests for Heart, Great Vessels, and Pericardium

Conventional radiographs
Posteroanterior and lateral
Oblique
Portable AP
Echocardiography
Transthoracic
Transesophageal
Radionuclide imaging
Positron emission tomography
Computed tomography
Magnetic resonance imaging
Angiography
Coronary arteriography
Aortography
Pulmonary arteriography

however, is merely artifactual and caused by poor inspiration (Fig. 3–2).

Severely ill, debilitated patients or patients who cannot be transported to the radiology department can have their chest radiographs obtained with a portable x-ray machine. Patients in the intensive care unit (ICU) who have intravascular catheters or who are undergoing mechanical ventilation frequently have chest radiographs performed as a survey for complications that may not be revealed by physical examination or laboratory data. These examinations are done with the cassette placed behind the patient in bed and are therefore anterior-to-posterior (AP) projections. The technical factors, which are controlled by the technologist at the time of the examination, vary with the size of the patient and the distance of the radiographic plate from the x-ray source (or machine). An attempt is still made to obtain the examination during maximum inspiration but this objective may be difficult to achieve in some patients, especially those who have dyspnea.

With the patient in the supine position, there is normally a redistribution of blood flow to the upper lobe pulmonary veins (cephalization), and the heart may appear enlarged relative to its appearance on the upright PA radiograph, because of magnification (Fig. 3–3). Some patients are able to sit for their examinations, while others are radiographed in a semi-upright position. Ideally, the technologist should mark the exact position of the patient when the radiograph is obtained, and the date and time of the examination should be recorded in all cases. Changes in patient positioning and ventilator settings can have substantial effects on the radiographic appearance and must be taken into account when evaluating any change in the radiograph from a previous study.

The chest radiograph, whether it is obtained in the upright, semi-upright, sitting, or supine position, should always be the initial screening examination in the evaluation of the cardiovascular system. Because it is essentially a screening study, the chest x-ray must be correlated with the clinical symptoms and physical examination to determine the overall significance of the radiographic findings. This information is also used to decide if other imaging tests are appropriate and which ones will potentially result in the highest diagnostic yield. Decisions regarding further imaging also depend on the impact on the clinical management of the patient, the potential for treatment of any abnormality that may be discovered, the cost and availability of the technique, and the expertise of the interpreting radiologist.

The conventional radiograph is an excellent screening test for the patient suspected of having disease involving the heart and great vessels because the overall anatomy of these areas is demonstrated well. Whenever possible, all radiographs should be reviewed with all prior relevant imaging studies. Even when a prior chest radiograph is

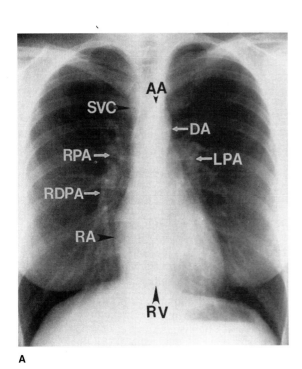

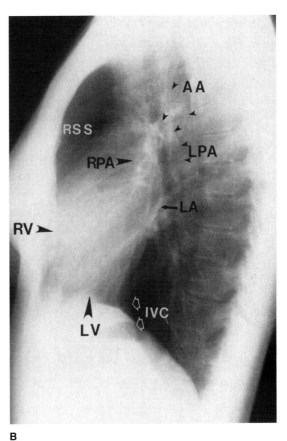

A

B

Fig. 3–1. **A** PA view of normal chest. RA = right atrium, RDPA = right descending pulmonary artery, RPA = right main pulmonary artery, SVC = superior vena cava, AA = aortic arch, DA = proximal descending thoracic aorta, LPA = left pulmonary artery, RV = right ventricle. **B** Lateral view of normal chest. RV = right ventricle, RSS = retrosternal clear space, AA = ascending aorta, LPA = left pulmonary artery, RPA = right pulmonary artery en face, IVC = inferior vena cava, LA = left atrium, and LV = left ventricle.

not available, additional information may be ascertained by reviewing other prior images such as thoracic spine or rib-detail image when available. Advanced imaging studies such as computed tomography (CT) and magnetic resonance (MR) imaging can also be used to help clarify complex findings on chest radiographs.

The normal cardiac silhouette size may be determined by the cardiothoracic ratio (CT ratio), a measurement obtained from the PA view. This ratio is calculated by dividing the transverse cardiac diameter (measured from each side) by the widest diameter of the chest (measured from the inner aspect of the right and left lung fields near the hemidiaphragms). The average normal value for this ratio in adults is 0.50, although up to 60% may be normal (Fig. 3–4). Any measurement greater than 50% is usually considered abnormal in an

upright inspiratory-phase PA film. This CT ratio cannot be reliably used for the AP projection of the chest since the heart is magnified (Fig. 3–3). The size of the patient and the degree of lung expansion also should be considered. For instance, in a small person with a petite frame and a small thoracic cage, the heart size may be normal, but the cardiothoracic ratio may measure more than 50%. Similarly, if the patient has pulmonary disease such as emphysema, the heart may be enlarged, but because of the overinflation of the lungs, the cardiothoracic ratio may still be normal. In practice, most radiologists do not perform this measurement and instead rely on experience and "gestalt" to evaluate heart size.

The contours of the heart, mediastinum, and great vessels on the PA view should be evaluated on each chest film (Fig. 3–1*A*). A reasonable approach is to begin in the

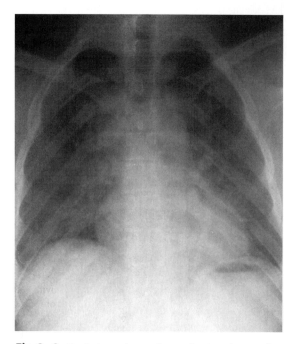

Fig. 3–2. Expiratory phase of a respiration chest radiograph shows low lung volumes, crowded bronchovascular markings, and apparent increased heart size. If the degree of inspiration is not noted, the interpreter may incorrectly diagnose disease. *(Courtesy of Robert H. Choplin, M.D., Indianapolis, IN.)*

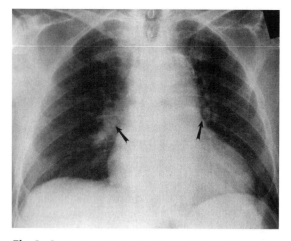

Fig. 3–3. Supine AP chest radiograph showing apparent increase in heart size and prominent bronchovascular markings *(arrows)*.

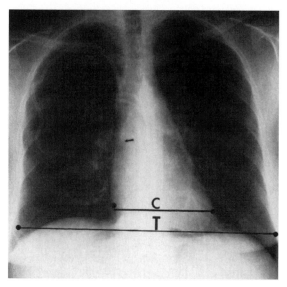

Fig. 3–4. Upright PA chest radiograph in a patient with leukemia shows normal cardio- (C) thoracic (T) ratio and how it is measured. Incidentally noted is the tip of an internal jugular triple-lumen catheter in the superior vena cava *(arrow)*.

upper right side of the mediastinum just lateral to the spine and below the right clavicle. The curved soft-tissue shadow represents the right border of the superior vena cava (SVC). Below the SVC is the right cardiac border formed by the right atrium. The inferior heart border, or base of the heart, is the area just above the diaphragm and is comprised primarily of the right ventricle, although there is some contribution from the left ventricular shadow. The left ventricle makes up the majority of the apex of the heart, which points to the left of the spine. The origins of the right and left pulmonary arteries are generally well demarcated on the normal PA film as they emerge from the mediastinum. The most prominent and recognizable component of the right pulmonary artery, the right descending pulmonary artery (RDPA) is seen just to the right of the superior cardiac border and descends inferiorly. It can usually be easily followed until it branches. The left main pulmonary artery is less well defined, but its origin can usually be seen above and lateral to the left atrial appendage just before it branches. The aorta originates posterior and to the right of the main pulmonary artery and the border of the ascending portion of the aorta can usually be seen superimposed on the inferior portion of the SVC. The transverse arch is not outlined by air and therefore cannot be seen as it crosses the mediastinum. However, the descending aorta can be seen to the left of the mediastinum as it turns inferiorly. The left border of the descending thoracic aorta should be followed down to the aortic hiatus. Any loss of this contour or any contour abnormality may indicate pathology and should be investigated. Dilation or ectasia, localized bulges, and calcification may occur within the aorta as a normal part of the aging process, but should be viewed as abnormal in younger individuals. Of course, the spine, ribs, adjacent soft tissues, and upper abdominal contents should all be scrutinized. The left atrium lies just inferior to the tracheal carina, but it is usually not visualized as a discrete structure on the normal PA view. Signs of left atrial enlargement, which can be seen on the PA examination, are discussed later.

The lateral view of the chest also reveals important information regarding the cardiac contour (Fig. 3–1*B*). Just behind the sternum there is normally a radiolucent area called the *retrosternal clear space* (RSS). This region represents lung interposed between the chest wall and the anterior margin of the ascending aorta. Any density present within the RSS may be due to anterior mediastinal mass or postsurgical changes. The anterior border of the cardiac shadow is composed primarily of the anterior wall of the right ventricle. Right ventricular enlargement may also encroach into the RSS. The posterior margin of the cardiac silhouette is formed by the left atrium and left ventricle. Just posterior and inferior to the left ventricle is a linear soft-tissue shadow leading into the heart formed by the inferior vena cava (IVC). The left ventricular shadow should not project more than 2 cm posterior to the posterior border of the IVC. The transverse aortic arch can usually be discerned on the normal lateral chest film as a smooth curving shadow originating anteriorly, crossing the mediastinum in a semilunar fashion, and then descending posteriorly as a linear shadow superimposed over the vertebral bodies. The left pulmonary artery (LPA) produces a similar curvilinear shadow just below the aortic arch before it branches. Just below the LPA, the left main/left upper lobe bronchus can be seen (projected end-on) as a round lucency. The right pulmonary artery (RPA) is seen en face down its lumen as an oval soft-tissue structure anterior to the bronchus intermedius and below and anterior to the left pulmonary artery.

Echocardiography

Echocardiography uses high-frequency ultrasound to evaluate the heart and great vessels. The major indications for the technique are listed in Table 3–2. The examination provides a dynamic rendition of cardiac great vessel anatomy and, when combined with the Doppler technique, yields information regarding cardiac and great vessel blood flow (hemodynamics) as well. Because of the high frame rates inherent in ultrasonography, echocardiography can image the heart in a dynamic real-time fashion, so that the motion of cardiac structures can be reliably

Table 3–2. Major Indications for Echocardiography

Ventricular function
Congenital heart disease
Valvular heart disease
Cardiomyopathy
Pericardial effusion
Suspected cardiac masses
Aortic disease (proximally)

evaluated. Echocardiography is useful in assessing ventricular function, valvular heart disease, myocardial disease, pericardial disease, intracardiac masses, and aortic abnormalities (Figs. 3–5 and 3–6). With Doppler technology the cardiac chamber function, valvular function, and intracardiac shunts frequently seen in congenital heart disease can be assessed. Combined Doppler echocardiography is a commonly performed procedure because it is relatively inexpensive and widely available, provides a wealth of information, is noninvasive, has no risk of ionizing radiation, and can also be performed at the bedside of critically ill patients. Furthermore, the results are immediately available because no special postexamination image processing is required. However, this technique is technically challenging and requires a great deal of operator expertise. Also, a small percentage of patients have poor acoustic windows that can severely degrade image quality. This disadvantage can be obviated by placing the sonographic probe in the esophagus, a procedure called *transesophageal echocardiography* (TEE). TEE yields consistently excellent images of the heart and great vessels, but involves a small amount of discomfort and risk to the patient. More recently, echocardiography has been combined with stress-testing modalities to assess inducible myocardial ischemia using wall motion analysis of left ventricular function.

Radionuclide Imaging (Nuclear Medicine)

Cardiac radionuclide imaging, primarily used for the patient with suspected myocardial ischemia or infarction, requires an intravenous injection of radioactively labeled compounds that have an affinity for the myocardium. These compounds localize within the myocardium in diseased or damaged areas, and a radioactivity detector such as a gamma camera can image their distribution. These tests are most commonly used in the evaluation of patients with angina and atypical chest pain (Fig. 3–7). Positron emission tomography (PET) is an investigational tool that has shown promise in assessing myocardial viability in patients with known coronary artery disease who represent a therapeutic dilemma after they are evaluated with other imaging modalities (Fig. 3–8). This technique, however, has tremendous clinical potential and will likely become a valuable technique in the future.

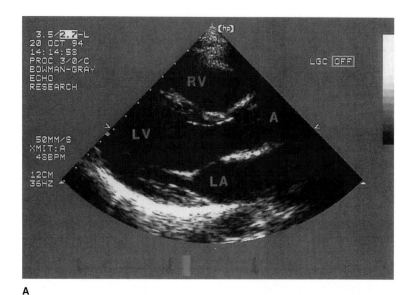

A

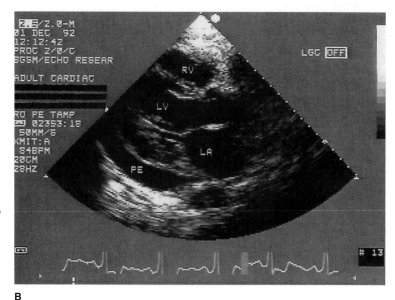

Fig. 3–5. **A** Normal transthoracic echocardiogram from a healthy subject. Views are taken from the left midparasternal region through an intercostal space. The structure closest to the apex of the screen is the chest wall. The mitral valve, separating the left atrium and left ventricle, is partially open in this image from early systole. A = aorta, LA = left atrium, LV = left ventricle, and RV = right ventricle. **B** Transthoracic echocardiogram, left parasternal view, from a patient with a moderate-sized posterior pericardial effusion (PE), visualized as a sonolucent space between the epicardium and pericardium. RV = right ventricle, LV = left ventricle, and LA = left atrium.

B

Computed Tomography

Current helical and multislice CT scanners provide static axial images of the heart and great vessels (Fig. 3–9) and can be reformatted into coronal, sagittal, and oblique views. Coupled with ECG gating, motion of the heart can be greatly diminished. The major indications for CT are to characterize or confirm a suspected mediastinal or pulmonary mass seen on PA and lateral chest radiographs, to evaluate patients suspected of having an aortic abnormality, or to assess for pulmonary embolism. It is hoped that as it becomes feasible to rotate the CT gantry faster, noninvasive imaging of the coronary arteries will become a reality. At the present time, some physicians use the measurement of calcium in the coronary arteries detected at CT to stratify the risk of future cardiovascular events (Fig. 3–10). Contrast administration is mandatory when questions arise that are related to intrinsic cardiac anatomy or abnormalities of the thoracic aorta such as dissection or for evaluation of the pulmonary arteries for pulmonary

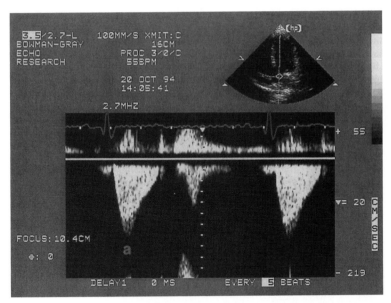

Fig. 3–6. Transthoracic spectral Doppler tracing taken from an intercostal space over the cardiac apex. The Doppler sample is placed in line with the left ventricular outflow and aorta (shown in miniature echocardiogram image at top right). Velocity of flow is denoted along the left edge of the tracing in centimeters per second. The Doppler tracing shows that aortic peak velocity (a) is normal (140 cm/sec). This technique can reliably assess the presence of and quantitate the severity of aortic stenosis.

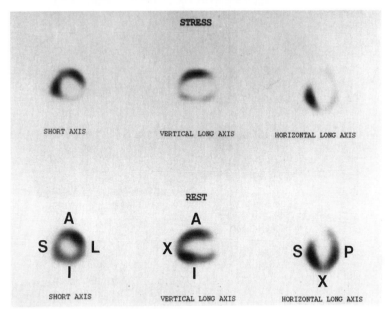

Fig. 3–7. Thallium myocardial perfusion images. Images obtained with the patient at peak stress (on top row) are compared with those obtained during rest (bottom row). The wall segments are labeled on the resting images (bottom row). Seen in the short-axis views (on left) are the anterior wall segment (A), lateral wall (L), inferior wall (I), and septum (S). In the vertical long-axis views (in the middle) the anterior wall, inferior wall, and apex (X) can be seen. Seen in the horizontal long-axis views are the posterolateral wall (P), septum, and apex. In normal persons, perfusion is homogeneous in all segments, and stress and resting images appear similar. In patients with obstructive coronary artery disease, relative lack of perfusion is seen during stress in wall segments supplied by the obstructed arteries. The rest perfusion images in this patient are normal. However in the stress images, the inferior, lateral, and posterolateral walls show "dropout," consistent with reduced perfusion in these wall segments, relative to adjacent normal segments. The patient subsequently underwent coronary arteriography, which showed a high-grade obstruction in the left circumflex coronary artery. *(Courtesy of Robert J. Cowan, M.D., Winston-Salem, NC.)*

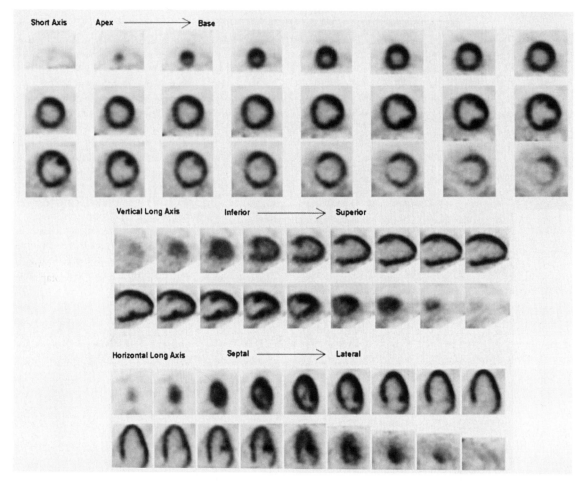

Short Axis   Apex ⟶ Base

Vertical Long Axis   Inferior ⟶ Superior

Horizontal Long Axis   Septal ⟶ Lateral

Fig. 3–8. 18-flouro-deoxyglucose FDG-PET myocardial viability study shows normal perfusion to the entire left ventricle. This shows that tissue is metabolically active; i.e., myocardial infarct is not present. *(Courtesy of Leonie Gordon, M.D., Charleston, SC.)*

embolism. For many of these applications rapid administration of contrast is necessary (up to 4–5 cc/sec) and a well-functioning large-bore (at least 18- to 20-gauge) IV catheter must be present to ensure a high-quality study.

Magnetic Resonance Imaging

MR imaging has also gained rapid acceptance for cardiac evaluation because it does not use ionizing radiation, can provide morphologic and physiologic data, and can be performed to give cine-loop images. Using high-field-strength magnets to generate images by radio-frequency pulse manipulation of hydrogen atoms, MR imaging offers superb soft-tissue differentiation, is noninvasive, and usually requires no contrast material administration (Fig. 3–11). Unfortunately, the time and effort needed to perform this examination makes MR imaging largely a problem-solving tool, rather than a screening study. The major indications for MR imaging are congenital heart disease and suspected intracardiac masses, valvular dysfunction, and aortic abnormality (in particular, aortic dissection). MR imaging has also shown some promise in diagnosing pulmonary embolism, measuring the degree of damage from coronary artery atherosclerosis, and evaluating the composition of atherosclerotic plaque.

Angiography

Coronary angiography is one of the most commonly performed imaging tests for evaluating the heart and great vessels. After the introduction of a catheter into a catheter, and then injects larger amounts of contrast material for diagnostic purposes. This injection of contrast material can be videotaped, recorded as standard or digital radiographs, or digitally stored for later review. The four major types of angiography are *angiocardiography* (heart), *coronary arteriography* (coronary arteries), *aortography* (aorta), and *pulmonary angiography* (pulmonary arteries and lungs). Developed by radiologists, angiocardiography and coronary arteriography are now almost exclusively performed by cardiologists.

Angiocardiography is used primarily to evaluate ventricular contractility and wall motion and cardiac output in patients with suspected myocardial dysfunction. It is also used to evaluate cardiac valvular function in patients who have murmurs detected at physical examination. The purpose of coronary arteriography is to define the degree of coronary artery obstruction, usually caused by atherosclerosis. In this procedure a catheter is generally placed into the origin of each coronary artery orifice and contrast material is injected into the arteries and videotaped or

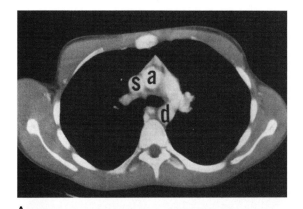

A

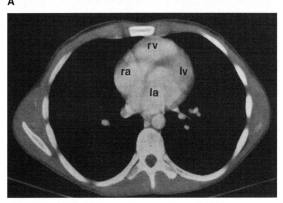

B

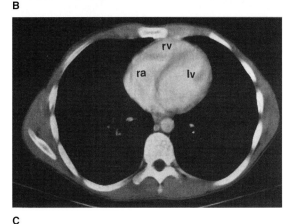

C

Fig. 3–9. Axial CT images **A, B, C** in the superior-to-inferior direction show the superior vena cava (s), ascending aorta (a), descending aorta (d), right ventricle (rv), right atrium (ra), left atrium (la), and left ventricle (lv).

peripheral vessel (usually the femoral or axillary vein or artery), the angiographer, under fluoroscopic visualization, positions the catheter in the region of interest, injects contrast material to confirm the location of the

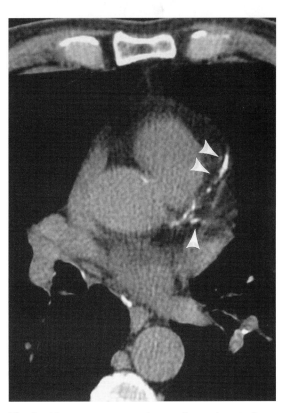

Fig. 3–10. Axial CT image shows atherosclerotic disease in the left anterior descending and left circumflex arteries (*arrowheads*) as evidenced by the presence of calcium.

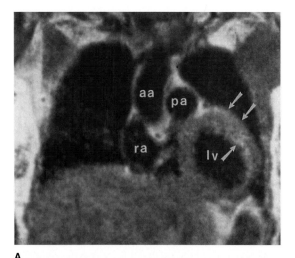

A

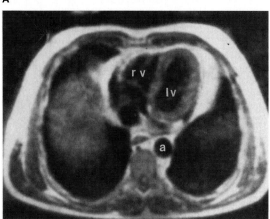

B

Fig. 3–11. **A** Normal coronal MR image shows the right atrium (ra), ascending aorta (aa), pulmonary artery (pa), and left ventricle (lv). Note how well the thickness of the myocardium in the left ventricle is depicted with MR imaging (*arrows*). **B** Normal axial MR image shows the right ventricle (rv), left ventricle (lv), and descending aorta (a). MR imaging is an excellent way to noninvasively visualize the cardiac and great vessel structures.

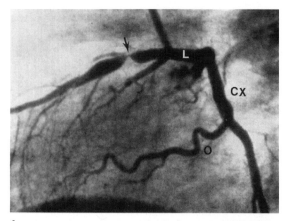

A

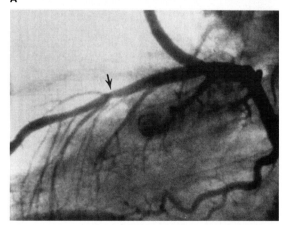

B

Fig. 3–12. **A** Coronary arteriogram. Images were obtained from the left lateral projection with contrast injection into the left main coronary artery. The left anterior descending (L), left circumflex (CX), and first obtuse marginal (O) branches are visualized. Severe stenosis is seen in the midportion of the left anterior descending artery (*arrow*) in this patient, who had unstable angina pectoris. *(Courtesy of Gregory Braden, M.D., Winston-Salem, NC.)* **B** Coronary arteriogram, same projection and patient as in *A*, obtained 1 day later. The stenosis in the left anterior descending coronary artery (*arrow*) has been reduced after percutaneous balloon angioplasty. *(Courtesy of Gregory Braden, M.D., Winston-Salem, NC.)*

filmed, as described earlier (Fig. 3–12). Coronary angiography can also be performed in the acute setting of suspected coronary occlusion, and a balloon catheter or thrombolytic agent can be placed through the catheter in an attempt to relieve the coronary artery obstruction.

Aortography is used primarily to evaluate suspected aortic disease (Fig. 3–13*A*). Although aortography remains the standard for traumatic injury (Fig. 3–13*B*), CT has largely replaced aortography. Pulmonary angiog-

raphy is also declining in interest and use due to improvements in helical CT. Today one of the more common uses of pulmonary angiography is to treat massive pulmonary embolism with thrombolytic therapy or treat arteriovenous malformations. Pulmonary artery catheterization is also used to measure the pulmonary

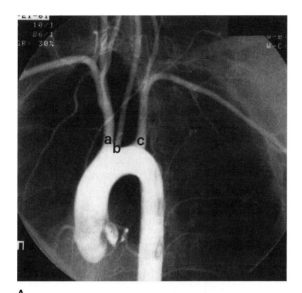

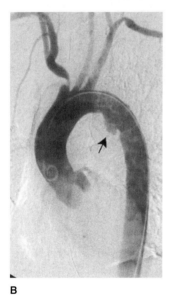

Fig. 3–13. **A** Normal aortogram in patient suspected of having traumatic aortic injury. Note the normal origins of "take-offs" of the right brachiocephalic artery (a), left common carotid artery (b), and left subclavian artery (c) from the arch of the aorta. *(Courtesy of William D. Routh, M.D., Jackson, MS.)* **B** Aortogram in a patient with acute traumatic aortic injury. The site of injury is the focal outpouching at the insertion of the ductus arteriosus *(arrow)*.

artery pressures in patients suspected of having pulmonary arterial hypertension.

TECHNIQUE SELECTION

A wide array of imaging tests can be used to evaluate the cardiovascular system (Table 3–1). After a thorough history and physical examination, the initial screening study should always be a chest radiograph. Ideally the PA and lateral views should be obtained with maximum inspiration. This study gives important information about the cardiac contour and the status of the lungs and is a good examination for excluding disorders that would require immediate treatment, such as pneumothorax. Furthermore, evaluation of the chest radiograph can often lead to a specific diagnosis and treatment or can help determine the need for another imaging study.

Depending on the history and physical examination findings, echocardiography and cardiac angiography are probably the most commonly performed secondary imaging examinations. Echocardiography is a good screening test to assess cardiac and great vessel valvular motion and structural abnormalities, cardiac chamber morphology, and flow. Angiography delineates the structural status of the coronary arteries and can give information on blood flow through the cardiac chambers, valves, and proximal great vessels, mainly in patients with suspected atherosclerosis. It is also used to guide interventions such as stent placement in the coronary arteries. Because of its inherent risks, coronary arteriography is usually reserved for patients with signs and symptoms of myocardial ischemia or infarction either on the basis of history or results of electrocardiography, echocardiography, or radionuclide myocardial imaging.

In patients with suspected pulmonary emboli, helical CT is the most appropriate test in the setting of an abnormal chest x-ray (Fig. 3–14). The ventilation-perfusion (V/Q) scan can be performed if the chest radiograph is normal. It is also the preferred examination in young females due to the radiation dose to the breast by CT. Both of these tests can confirm the clinically suspected diagnosis of pulmonary embolic disease and often provides a useful "map" of the most suspicious regions of the lung for the angiographer if an angiogram is required for the definitive diagnosis of pulmonary embolism. CT can also detect alternative important diagnoses not detected by either V/Q scan or pulmonary angiography.

Echocardiography, MR imaging, or cardiac angiography may be selected for patients with suspected congenital heart disease. The advantages of MR imaging in this setting is that it is noninvasive, generally needs no contrast material administration, and uses no ionizing radiation, an important consideration in the pediatric patient. For

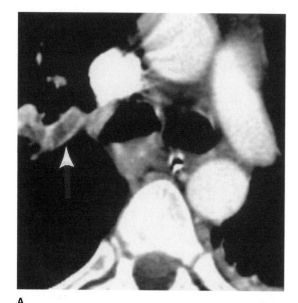

A

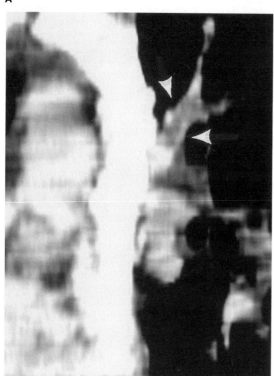

B

Fig. 3–14. Axial **A** and coronal **B** CT images show filling defect (*arrowheads*) in right upper lobe artery from pulmonary embolism.

these reasons, MR imaging has become the preferred imaging test in the pediatric population.

Suspected aortic dissection (either atherosclerotic or traumatic in origin) can be evaluated by helical CT, TEE, aortography, or MR imaging. Helical CT is the imaging modality of choice for acute dissection due to its accuracy and availability (Fig. 3–15). With multislice technology, CT angiography can provide images in multiple planes to show the relation of the dissection to key branch vessels. TEE has the advantages of being quick and noninvasive, and the examination can be performed expediently at the bedside. MR imaging is noninvasive,

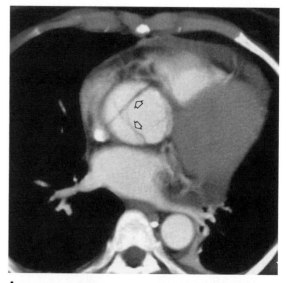

A

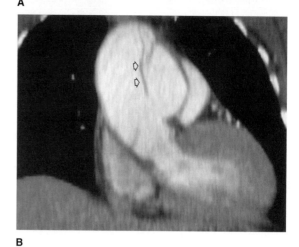

B

Fig. 3–15. Axial **A** and coronal **B** CT images show intimal flap of type A dissection (*arrows*).

uses no ionizing radiation, is less operator dependent, and can be performed in multiple planes. It is limited by availability, imaging time, and because it cannot be used in patients with certain implanted devices, particularly pacemakers. Angiography has mostly been relegated to minimally invasive treatments such as stent-graft placement. Because survival rates often depend on early surgical intervention, the availability and timeliness of the examinations are important.

In patients whose chest radiographs suggest intrinsic pulmonary or mediastinal processes, chest CT is currently the preferred modality. The use of contrast depends on the indication, preference of the radiologist, and any possible contraindications to administration of intravenous contrast for individual patients. MR imaging may become more important in this situation if it becomes less costly and, at the present time, PET plays a critical role in the staging of patients with lung cancer and lymphoma.

Finally, regardless of the situation, it is reasonable for the clinician and radiologist to decide together which imaging tests are most appropriate. In many instances the next most efficacious and least costly imaging examination is not always clear-cut. In fact, in some circumstances, it is not necessary to perform another test because of the limited potential yield from the examination or because there is no adequate therapy for the suspected abnormality. It is hoped that future recommendations for test selection will be determined by well-designed prospective unbiased outcome studies comparing all of these modalities in various clinical scenarios. In the meantime, a commonsense approach, taking into consideration the history and physical examination findings, the information gleaned from the conventional radiograph, and the potential yield from the array of other available imaging tests, is the most appropriate tact. In all instances, communication between the clinician and radiologist is critical for the best patient care.

Monitoring Devices

In clinical hospital practice, particularly in the ICU setting, a variety of catheters and tubes are used to monitor various parameters in patients (Fig. 3–16). The student should be familiar with the normal routes and positions of these devices, as well as inappropriate positions and complications. Table 3–3 lists the most common monitoring devices.

The basic venous anatomy of the upper mediastinum should be reviewed and kept in mind when evaluating catheter placement. The most common routes of catheter insertion in the chest include the internal jugular and subclavian veins. Radiographs obtained after insertion show the catheter following either the course of the internal jugular or subclavian vein and passing through the brachiocephalic vein. It then curves gently

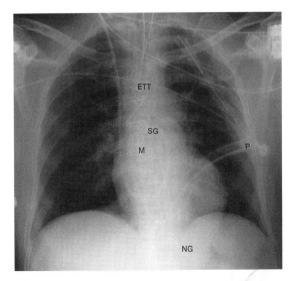

Fig. 3–16. Frontal radiograph immediately after coronary artery bypass surgery shows typical lines and tubes encountered in the ICU. Endotracheal tube (ETT), nasogastric tube (NG), Swan-Ganz catheter (SG), mediastinal drain (M), and left pleural drain (P) are present.

downward to terminate in the superior vena cava proximal to the right atrium (Fig. 3–17). One normal variation of venous anatomy is the persistent left superior vena cava. In this situation the catheter descends down the left mediastinum terminating in the left SVC (Fig. 3–18). The left SVC ultimately drains into the coronary sinus, which then enters the right atrium.

Intrathoracic central venous catheters are used mainly for monitoring central venous pressure (CVP), maintaining proper nutrition, delivering medication, and conducting hemodialysis. It is standard practice to request a chest radiograph after catheter placement to verify its location and to check for potential complications, such as pneumothorax (Fig. 3–19) or hemothorax. Measurement of CVP is optimally obtained when the tip of the catheter is proximal to the right atrium and distal to the most proximal valves of the large veins. A catheter tip proximal to the veins gives an inaccurate reading of CVP, and a tip too close to the right atrium may cause arrhythmias from

Table 3–3. Common Monitoring Devices

Central venous catheters
Flow-directed arterial catheters (Swan-Ganz catheters)
Intra-aortic counterpulsation balloon
Cardiac pacemakers

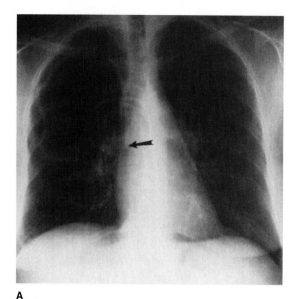

A

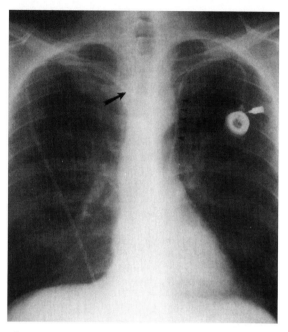

Fig. 3–18. Upright PA chest radiograph in a patient with leukemia shows two central venous catheters. The right subclavian catheter terminates in the superior vena cava (*arrow*). The left subclavian catheter extends into the mediastinum along a persistent left superior vena cava (*arrowheads*).

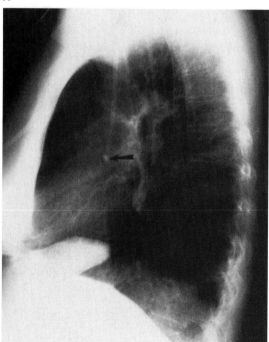

B

Fig. 3–17. PA **A** and lateral **B** views of a patient whose subclavian catheter placement is normal with its tip in the superior vena cava above the right atrium (*arrows*).

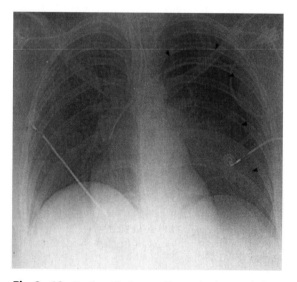

Fig. 3–19. Supine AP chest radiograph obtained after placement of left subclavian catheter shows a large left pneumothorax (*arrowheads*).

Table 3–4. Potential Complications of Catheters

Malposition
Catheter knotting/fragmentation
Pneumothorax
Vascular injury
Thrombosis (venous)
Infarction (arterial)
Infection/septic emboli/endocarditis
Air embolism
Cardiac arrhythmias
Nerve injury
    Brachial plexus
    Phrenic
    Recurrent laryngeal
Fistulae
    Arteriovenous
    Venobronchial
    Arteriobronchial

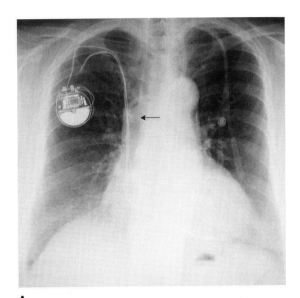

A

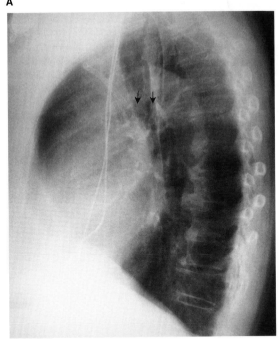

B

Fig. 3–20. PA **A** and lateral **B** views show central venous catheter with tip in azygous vein (*arrows*).

irritation of the right atrial myocardium. Knowing why a catheter has been inserted is of critical importance to the radiologist in determining if the catheter has been appropriately positioned. For instance, if it has been placed just for fluids and/or medications, a termination in the brachiocephalic vein is satisfactory. Conversely, a plasmapheresis catheter should never be located in the right atrium due to the risk of complications. More frequently, central venous catheters are being placed centrally via a peripheral vein. These catheters have minimal risk, can remain in place for longer periods of time without being exchanged, and are primarily used for the delivery of fluids and long-term antibiotics.

The major potential complications from catheter placement are outlined in Table 3–4. A malpositioned central venous catheter may result in inaccurate CVP measurement, thrombosis, catheter knotting, and infusion of substances into the mediastinum or pleura. Catheter tips against the wall of the SVC may erode into the mediastinum or may extend retrograde into tributary veins, particularly the azygous vein (Fig. 3–20).

Flow-directed arterial catheters are also regularly used in cardiac and ICU patients to monitor cardiac output. The most common flow-directed catheter is the Swan-Ganz (SG) catheter (Fig. 3–16). It is usually inserted percutaneously into the left or right subclavian vein and threaded through the brachiocephalic vein, superior vena cava, right atrium, tricuspid valve, right ventricle, and pulmonic valve, and then directed out into the main pulmonary artery. Usually terminating in the right or left pulmonary arteries, the SG tip should be distal to the pulmonary valve and proximal to the smaller pulmonary arterial vessels so it will not cause occlusion and, potentially, thrombosis. A simple rule of thumb is that the catheter should not extend past the mediastinal bor-

ders. It may then be intermittently "wedged" into a distal pulmonary artery branch to obtain a pulmonary capillary wedge pressure.

Complications of SG catheter placement are similar to other central venous catheters. The tip may be positioned in a number of inappropriate vessels or locations, and a chest radiograph should be obtained after catheter insertion to confirm its position (Fig. 3–21). Introduction of any catheter into the subclavian vein, because of its proximity to the lung apex, can cause pneumothorax (Fig. 3–19). A catheter tip positioned in the right ventricle can lead to ventricular arrhythmias, and leaving the catheter tip too distal may result in a pulmonary artery pseudoaneurysm or pulmonary infarct.

An intra-aortic counterpulsation balloon pump (IABP) is occasionally used in patients with cardiogenic shock. This catheter measures approximately 26 cm in length and is surrounded by a balloon, which inflates with helium or carbon dioxide gas during diastole and deflates during systole. Deflation during systole decreases afterload and results in diminished left ventricular work and oxygen requirements, while the inflation of the balloon during diastole increases cardiac pressure to help ensure adequate perfusion of the coronary arteries. The catheter, introduced percutaneously into the thoracic aorta via the common femoral artery or placed into the ascending aorta at the time of surgery, should be positioned so that its tip is just distal to the origin of the left subclavian artery. The tip of the catheter has a small radiopaque marker so that this position can be ascertained on the chest radiograph (Fig. 3–22). The major complications of the IAPB result from positioning of its tip proximal to the left subclavian artery, which may cause occlusion of the left subclavian vessel orifice,

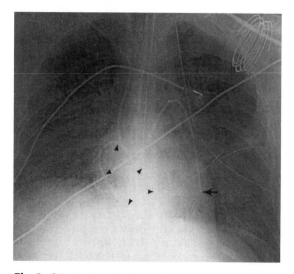

Fig. 3–21. Supine AP chest radiograph of a patient in the ICU in congestive failure shows a Swan-Ganz catheter tip positioned too far distally within the left lower lobe pulmonary artery (*arrow*). Notice the coiled catheter in the right atrium (*arrowheads*).

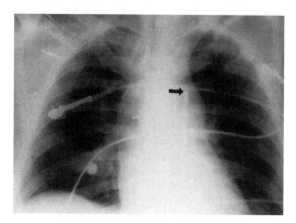

Fig. 3–22. Supine AP radiograph of patient 6 hours following coronary artery bypass surgery shows an IABP in normal position distal to the origin of the left subclavian artery (*arrow*).

cerebral artery embolization, or aortic tear. If positioned too low, the balloon may occlude the celiac, superior mesenteric, and renal arteries.

The three major types of cardiac pacemakers are *epicardial*, *subxiphoid*, and *transvenous*. There is wide variation in their use in clinical practice today. Unipolar or bipolar pacemakers are most common and usually implanted in the chest wall with leads inserted into the subclavian vein. The unipolar pacemaker tip is normally situated at the apex of the right ventricle. The bipolar pacemaker has a proximal lead that terminates in the right atrium and a distal lead that terminates within the right ventricle (similar to the unipolar pacemaker position). Occasionally, a third lead will be present in the coronary sinus, appearing superior to the right ventricular lead (Fig. 3–23). Its posterior position can be confirmed on the lateral view. Transvenous placement of cardiac pacemakers carries the same potential complications, as does placement of any other catheter. The purpose of the chest radiograph after the pacemaker insertion is to document the appropriate placement of these leads, to check for complications from placement, and to establish a baseline examination to compare with future chest radiographs.

EXERCISES

EXERCISE 3-1: INCREASED HEART SIZE

Clinical Histories:

Case 3-1. A 20-year-old uncooperative man with minimal chest pain (Fig. 3–24)

Case 3-2. A 70-year-old man with uremia (Fig. 3–25)

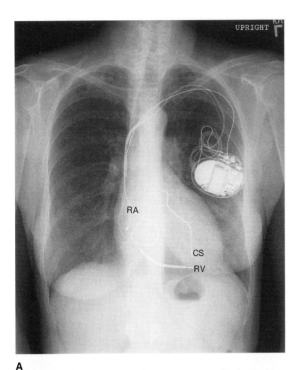

A

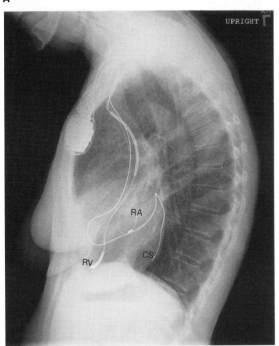

B

Fig. 3–23. PA **A** and lateral **B** views show the most common locations of pacing leads: right atrium (RA), right ventricle (RV), and coronary sinus (CS).

Case 3-3. A 60-year-old alcoholic man with shortness of breath (Fig. 3–26)

Case 3-4. A 28-year-old woman with a loud systolic murmur and without cyanosis (Fig. 3–27)

Case 3-5. A 55-year-old woman with an acute shortness of breath (Fig. 3–28*A*); Fig. 3–28*B* obtained 1 month prior

Questions:

3-1. The most likely diagnosis in Case 3-1 (Fig. 3–24) is
  A. congestive heart failure.
  B. pericardial effusion.
  C. intracardiac shunt.
  D. expiratory phase of respiration.
  E. pulmonic stenosis.

3-2. The most likely diagnosis in Case 3-2 (Fig. 3–25) is
  A. mediastinal masses.
  B. intracardiac shunts (ASD and VSD).
  C. pericardial effusion or cardiomyopathy.
  D. combined aortic and pulmonary arterial disease.
  E. technical aberrations.

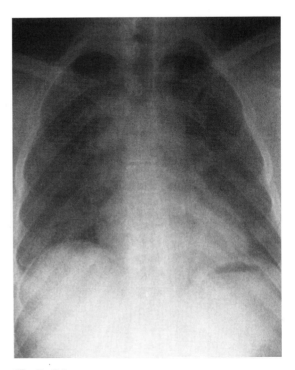

Fig. 3–24.

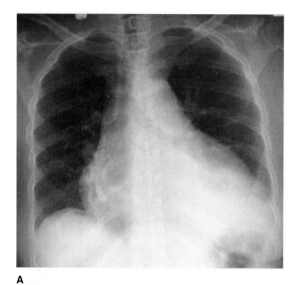

A

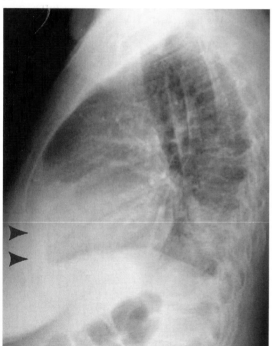

B

Fig. 3–25.

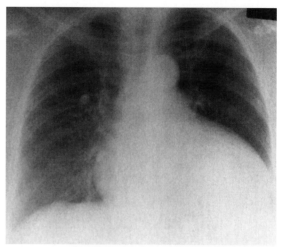

Fig. 3–26.

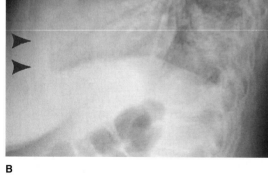

Fig. 3–27.

D. combined aortic and pulmonary arterial disease.

E. technical aberrations.

3-3. The most likely diagnosis in Case 3-3 (Fig. 3–26) is

A. mediastinal masses.
B. intracardiac shunts (ASD and VSD).
C. pericardial effusion or cadiomyopathy.

3-4. The most likely diagnosis in Case 3-4 (Fig. 3–27) is

A. Ebstein's anomaly.
B. mediastinal mass.

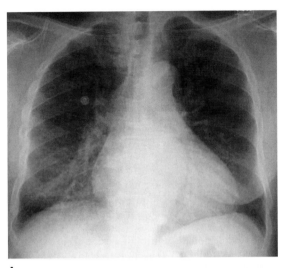

A

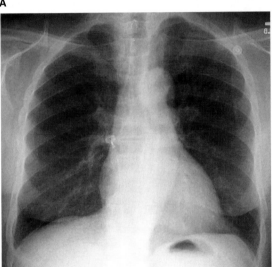

B

Fig. 3–28.

Radiologic Findings:

3-1. This case (Fig. 3–24) represents an apparent "enlarged heart" due to an expiratory phase of respiration in an uncooperative patient. (*D* is the correct answer to Question 3-1.) Note the decreased lung volumes and the elevation of the hemidiaphragms. The resultant crowding of vessels obscures much of the cardiac border. The technique of inspiratory PA and radiographs is preferred to avoid "diagnosing" diseases that a patient does not have.

3-2. This case (Fig. 3–25) is an example of pericardial effusion. (*C* is the correct answer to Question 3-2.) The conventional radiograph finding on the frontal view is a so-called "globular" or "water-bottle" configuration of the heart.

3-3. This case (Fig. 3–26) shows a radiographic finding similar to that of in Case 3-2. This is the case of cardiomyopathy. (C is the correct answer to Question 3-3.)

3-4. This patient (Fig. 3–27) has cardiomegaly, increased pulmonary vascularity, and prominent pulmonary arteries, findings suggestive of an intracardiac shunt, which in this case was an atrial septal defect (ASD). (C is the correct answer to Question 3-4.) The lateral radiograph (Fig. 3–29) shows the enlarged central

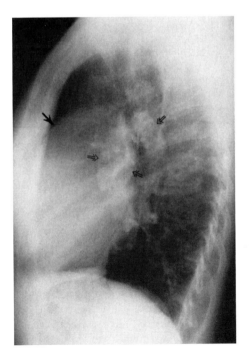

Fig. 3–29. Lateral view of patient in Case 3-4 shows filling in of the retrosternal space by the enlarged right ventricle (*arrow*) and large right and left pulmonary arteries from the pulmonary arterial hypertension (*open arrows*).

C. intracardiac shunt.
D. pericardial effusion.
E. mitral and aortic stenosis.

3-5. The most likely diagnosis in Case 3-5 (Figs. 3–28*A* and *B*) is
A. cardiomyopathy.
B. pulmonary edema and congestive heart failure.
C. pericardial effusion.
D. acute pneumonia.
E. aortic dissection.

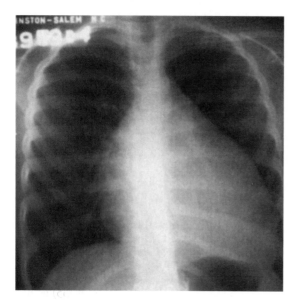

Fig. 3–30. Upright PA view of a young child with Ebstein's anomaly shows the globular-shaped heart characteristic of this disorder. *(Courtesy of Thomas E. Sumner, M.D., Winston-Salem, NC.)*

pulmonary arteries and right ventricular prominence due to increased flow.

3-5. This case (Fig. 3–28*A*) illustrates cardiomegaly, increased pulmonary vascularity, redistribution of blood flow to the upper lobes, and Kerley B lines typical of pulmonary edema. (*B* is the correct answer to Question 3-5.) Note the normal radiograph 1 month prior (Fig. 3–28*B*).

Discussion:

Pericardial effusion and cardiomyopathy have similar appearances on PA chest radiographs (Cases 3-2 and 3-3). This appearance is often referred to as a globular shape or a water-bottle heart. When this appearance is observed, an echocardiogram is the next best imaging test to differentiate between these two entities. However, this diagnosis may be suggested on the lateral radiograph by a separation of the pericardial and epicardial fat by pericardial fluid, as exhibited in Fig. 3–25*B* (*arrowheads*). Mediastinal masses may occur in a location or a distribution that makes the heart appear enlarged on the chest radiograph. CT is the next best test to confirm a clinical suspicion of a mass and to evaluate mediastinal adenopathy.

Ebstein's anomaly, mentioned in Question 3-4, is an uncommon type of congenital heart disease that may also result in a globular-shaped appearance of the heart on the chest radiograph (Fig. 3–30). In these patients, the tricuspid valve is displaced downward, resulting in tricuspid regurgitation. There is usually an associated ASD. The

tricuspid insufficiency results in a massively enlarged right atrium, and the pulmonary vascularity is usually diminished due to decreased flow through the pulmonary arteries. These patients often present with congestive failure early in life, and echocardiography, MR imaging, or cardiac angiography is necessary to make this diagnosis.

Increased heart size is a common clinical problem that may be caused by a variety of abnormalities. Cardiac enlargement may be diagnosed if the cardiothoracic ratio is greater than 60%. Often the lateral view is helpful for confirming left atrial and left ventricular enlargement. The most common cause of enlargement is atherosclerotic disease, although a number of other entities may cause an increased cardiac silhouette. In congestive heart failure (CHF) hydrostatic forces result in fluid collection in the interlobular septa, those connective tissue sheaths, veins, and lymphatics surrounding the secondary pulmonary lobule (Fig. 3–31, *arrows*). As hydrostatic pressures increase, fluid can accumulate in the alveoli, giving an air-space pattern of disease. Intracardiac shunts, especially ventricular septal defect, can also cause cardiac enlargement because of the increased flow from the internal shunting. VSD is the most common congenital cardiac anomaly, and the intracardiac shunt must be at least 2 to 1 for the radiograph to show recognizable changes.

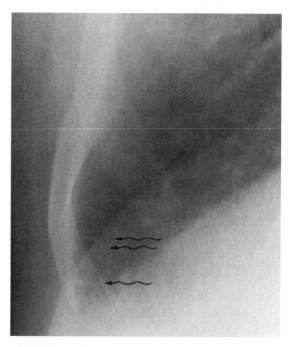

Fig. 3–31. Coned-down view of right costophrenic angle region shows thin, linear radiopaque lines extending to the pleural surface. These are Kerley B lines (thickened interlobular septae) (*arrows*).

EXERCISE 3-2: ALTERATIONS IN CARDIAC CONTOUR

Clinical Histories:

Case 3-6. A 65-year-old man with a long history of an abnormality seen on his electrocardiogram (Fig. 3–32)

Case 3-7. A 30-year-old woman with systolic and diastolic murmurs and a history of rheumatic fever as a child (Fig. 3–33) (Courtesy of Caroline Chiles, M.D., Winston-Salem, NC).

Case 3-8. A 75-year-old man with a history of a myocardial infarction 10 years earlier had this study done as a routine screening examination (Fig. 3–34)

Case 3-9. A 24-year-old man with recurrent pulmonary infections (Fig. 3–35)

Case 3-10. A 3-year-old child with a history of cardiac complications since birth (Fig. 3–36)

Questions:

3-6. In Case 3-6 (Fig. 3–32), the most likely cause of the radiographic abnormality is

  A. tetralogy of Fallot.
  B. malingering.
  C. long-standing hypertension.
  D. congenital heart disease.
  E. drug abuse.

3-7. In Case 3-7 (Fig. 3–33), the contour abnormality is

  A. left atrial enlargement.
  B. left ventricular hypertrophy.
  C. pulmonic stenosis.
  D. right atrial enlargement.
  E. right ventricular hypertrophy.

3-8. In Case 3-8 (Fig. 3–34), the cardiac contour abnormality is

  A. left atrial enlargement.
  B. left ventricular enlargement.
  C. right atrial enlargement.
  D. left ventricular aneurysm.
  E. right ventricular aneurysm.

3-9. The diagnosis in Case 3-9 (Fig. 3–35) is

  A. situs inversus.
  B. dextrocardia.
  C. technical aberration.
  D. tetralogy of Fallot.
  E. pulmonary atresia.

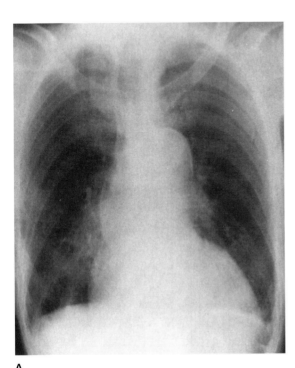

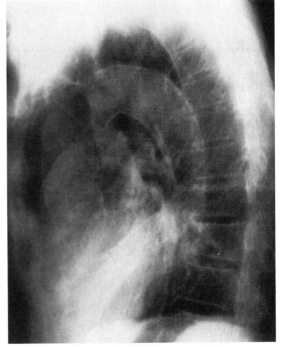

A   B

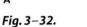

Fig. 3–32.

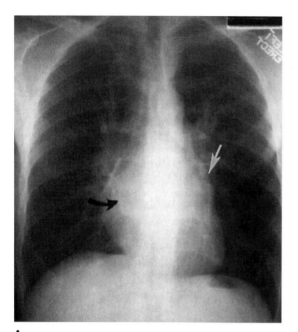
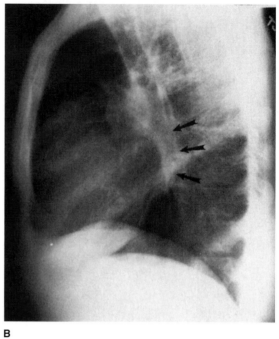

A   B

Fig. 3–33.

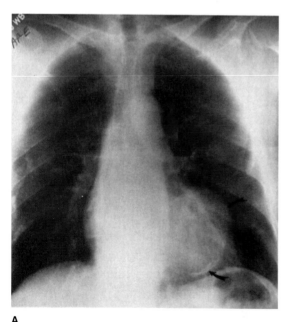

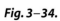

A   B

Fig. 3–34.

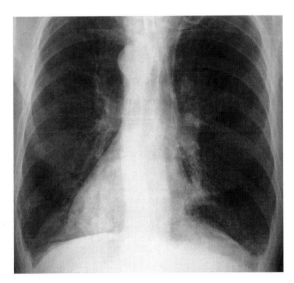

Fig. 3–35.

3-10. The configuration of the heart in Case 3-10 (Fig. 3–36) has been called the

    A.   boot-shaped heart.

    B.   third mogul of the heart.

    C.   snowman appearance.

    D.   double contour sign.

    E.   water-bottle heart.

Radiographic Findings:

3-6. In this case (Fig. 3–32), the classical findings of enlargement of the left ventricle, characteristic of left ventricular hypertrophy, are seen on both the PA and the lateral radiograph. Extensive aortic calcification and ectasia are also present. The most common cause of left ventricular hypertrophy is long-standing hypertension. (*C* is the correct answer to Question 3-6.)

3-7. In this case (Fig. 3–33), a double contour to the right side of the heart is seen on the PA radiograph (*black arrow*). There is also an enlarged left atrial appendage (*white arrow*). The lateral radiograph shows enlargement of the left atrial shadow, the superior and posterior region of the cardiac contour (*arrows*) and posterior displacement of the left main bronchus. (*A* is the correct answer to Question 3-7.) Along with increased pulmonary vascularity, the constellation of findings is characteristic of left atrial enlargement due to mitral valve insufficiency.

3-8. The PA and lateral radiographs in this case (Fig. 3–34) show an enlargement of the left ventricular contour with a focal bulge containing calcification within its wall (*arrows*). The lateral radiograph confirms the calcification (*curved arrows*). Given the history of myocardial infarction

10 years earlier, the most likely diagnosis is a left ventricular aneurysm. (*D* is the correct answer to Question 3-8.)

3-9. The patient in this case (Fig. 3–35) shows the apex of the heart to be on the right side of the chest and the descending aorta to be in its correct position on the left. These findings are diagnostic of dextrocardia, which in this case is secondary to Kartagener's syndrome. (*B* is the correct answer to Question 3-9.)

3-10. In this case (Fig. 3–36), tetralogy of Fallot, the apex of the left ventricle is elevated by right ventricular hypertrophy. These findings are sometimes referred to as a boot-shaped heart. (*A* is the correct answer to Question 3-10.)

Discussion:

Alterations of the normal cardiac contour are common clinical scenarios. The most common contour abnormality is probably enlargement of the left ventricle from long-standing hypertension, as exhibited by the 65-year-old man in Case 3-6 (Fig. 3–32). Cardiac enlargement is first suggested on the PA view by an increase in the CT ratio to greater than 50%. Left ventricular enlargement is suggested by prominence of the apex of the cardiac contour. On the lateral projection, the left ventricle should not project more than 2 cm posterior to the IVC measured 2 cm above the diaphragm. If the left ventricle projects more than 2 cm behind this landmark, left ventricular enlargement should be suspected.

Left atrial enlargement (LAE), as shown in Case 3-7 (Fig. 3–33), occurs mainly with left-sided obstructive lesions such as mitral stenosis or mitral regurgitation, often the result of rheumatic heart disease. The major sign of LAE on the PA view is a double density centrally caused by the dilated left atrium extending to the right of the

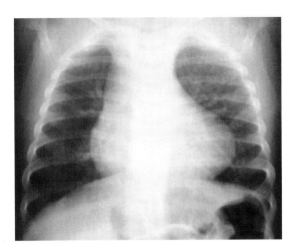

Fig. 3–36.

spine projected behind the right atrium (Fig. 3–33A, black arrow). Another sign of LAE is enlargement of the left atrial appendage. The left atrial appendage is immediately adjacent and inferior to the left main bronchus. When enlarged, there is an extra bump along the left heart border, the so-called third mogul of the left cardiac border (Fig. 3–33A, white arrow). LAE also causes a separation and widening of the carinal angle that can be seen on the PA chest radiograph, although this is a late sign of LAE. The carinal angle normally measures between 60 and 120 degrees. Widening of this angle may occasionally be caused by subcarinal adenopathy and therefore should be correlated with other signs of LAE.

The left atrium makes up the posterior cardiac shadow just above the left ventricle (LA in Fig. 3–1). Left atrial enlargement is recognized on the lateral film by enlargement and posterior displacement of the left atrial shadow (Fig. 3–33B, arrows). As further enlargement occurs, the left atrium displaces the left main and left lower lobe bronchus posteriorly.

Right ventricular enlargement (RVE) or hypertrophy (RVH) results most commonly from right-sided heart failure from a variety of disorders, long-standing mitral disease, or pulmonic stenosis. In this cardiac contour abnormality, an increase occurs in the soft-tissue density within the retrosternal clear space that is best seen on the lateral radiograph (Fig. 3–37). On the PA film, uplifting of the cardiac apex may be seen also. Anterior mediastinal masses may also cause retrosternal fullness and should be included in the differential diagnosis (Fig. 3–38). When the cause is not clear from the conventional radiograph, CT is the next most appropriate test to differentiate between these two considerations.

Cardiac aneurysms, as shown in the patient in Case 3-8 (Fig. 3–34), are almost always the sequelae of myocardial infarction. There are two types of cardiac aneurysms: true and false aneurysms. True aneurysms most frequently occur at the cardiac apex and contain all three layers of myocardium. False aneurysms or pseudoaneurysms occur with disruption of the endocardium, with dissection of blood into the cardiac wall. Pseudoaneurysms, therefore, are not bound by all three layers of the heart wall. Pseudoaneurysms most frequently occur along the free walls of the heart (inferior and lateral walls). Aneurysms are usually diagnosed on the PA chest radiograph as localized soft-tissue outpouchings or irregularities at the apical or anterolateral segments of the left ventricular cardiac contour. A linear rim of dystrophic calcification may develop within the nonviable myocardium after the infarction. With echocardiography, aneurysms show paradoxical enlargement during systole. Because stasis of blood occurs in the aneurysm, blood clots can develop and may be a source of distal emboli. Echocardiography, CT and MR imaging can all be used

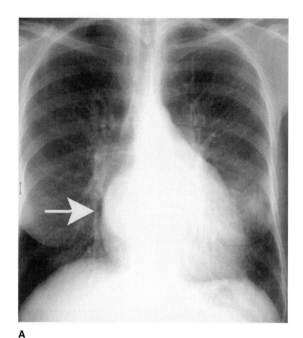

A

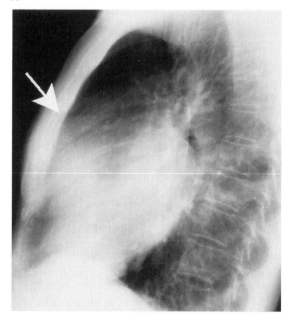

B

Fig. 3–37. PA **A** and lateral **B** views of patient with long-standing mitral stenosis show the double contour (*arrow*) on the PA view and filling in of the retrosternal space (*arrow*) on the lateral view. Right ventricular hypertrophy will be manifested as soft-tissue density in the retrosternal space on the lateral view.

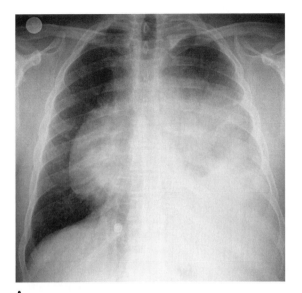

A

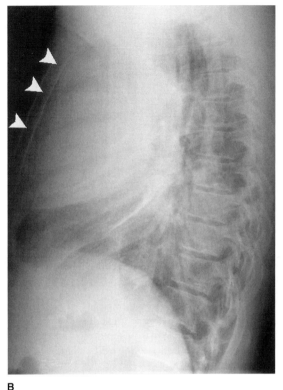

B

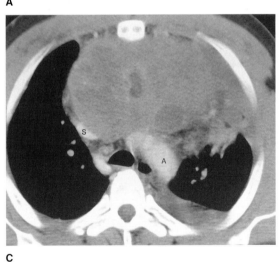

C

Fig. 3–38. PA **A** and lateral **B** views of patient with night sweats show an anterior mediastinal mass, which fills in the retrosternal space on the lateral view (*arrowheads*). A CT scan **C** in the same patient shows the location of the anterior mediastinal mass adjacent to the aortic arch **A**. S = superior vena cava. Biopsy of the mass revealed germ cell neoplasm.

to make the diagnosis of cardiac aneurysm and distinguish between true and false aneurysms. The distinction is important as false aneurysms are at higher risk for rupture and require surgical repair.

Dextrocardia, as shown in Case 3-9 (Fig. 3–35), is usually recognized easily on the PA chest radiograph. However, this finding may be overlooked if the left and right designations on the film are marked incorrectly or are misinterpreted. In most cases of dextrocardia, the aorta descends on the left side and the patient is asymptomatic. If the aorta descends on the right side, a number of other abnormalities should be considered (Table 3–5). The bibliography at the end

Table 3–5. Congenital Cardiac Lesions Associated With Right Aortic Arch

Lesion	Approximate incidence (%)
Corrected great vessel transposition	50
Asplenia syndrome	30–40
Truncus arteriosus	35
Tetralogy of Fallot	
With pulmonary atresia	50
Classic	25
Complete transposition of the great vessels	5–10
Tricuspid valve atresia	5
Large VSD	2

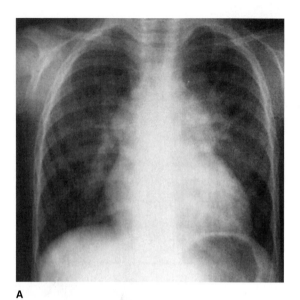

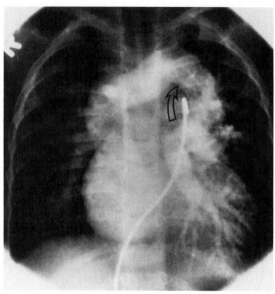

A   B

Fig. 3–39. Frontal radiograph **A** and angiogram **B** of a patient with total anomalous pulmonary venous return shows that the left side of the snowman's head is formed by the left anterior cardinal vein (vertical vein), draining all of the pulmonary veins to the left brachiocephalic vein (*open arrow*). (*Courtesy of Laurence B. Leinbach, M.D., Winston-Salem, NC.*)

of the chapter provides more in-depth discussion of this topic.

The boot shape of the cardiac shadow in Case 3-10 (Fig. 3–36) is secondary to tetralogy of Fallot. The four components of this congenital cardiac anomaly are an overriding aorta, ventricular septal defect, pulmonic stenosis, and right ventricular hypertrophy. It is the right heart enlargement that results in the up-turned cardiac apex. The degree of shunt and pulmonary stenosis dictate the presentation. In cases where the stenosis is severe, infants are cyanotic and a generalized decrease in pulmonary vasculature is seen. If the pulmonary stenosis and degree of left to right shunt are mild, the abnormality may not manifest itself until childhood.

Total anomalous pulmonary venous return has been described as a snowman configuration. The right side of the snowman's head is formed by the dilated SVC, while the left side of the head is formed by the left anterior cardinal vein (vertical vein), draining all of the pulmonary veins to the left brachiocephalic vein. The body of the snowman is represented by the dilated right atrium and ventricle; the atrium bulges to the right and the ventricle expands to the left and superiorly, producing a convex cardiac border comprising the displaced left atrium and ventricle (Fig. 3–39).

EXERCISE 3-3: PULMONARY VASCULARITY

Clinical Histories:

Case 3-11. A 28-year-old man examined in the Emergency Department for chest pain and shortness of breath (Fig. 3–40)

Case 3-12. A 65-year-old woman with a 100-packs-a-year history of smoking (Fig. 3–41)

Case 3-13. An acyanotic 22-year-old man with a systolic murmur (Fig. 3–42)

Case 3-14. A 36-year-old man with asthma (Fig. 3–43)

Case 3-15. A 50-year-old woman with acute shortness of breath (Fig. 3–44)

Questions:

3-11. The most likely cause of the patient's symptoms in Case 3-11 (Fig. 3–40) is

    A. pneumonia.

    B. pulmonary edema.

    C. interstitial lung disease.

    D. anxiety reaction.

    E. pneumothorax.

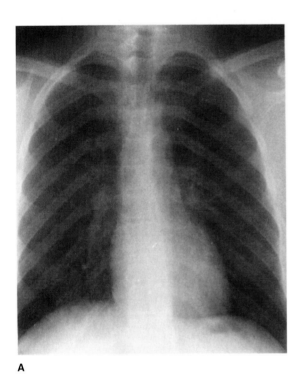

A

B

Fig. 3–40.

3-12. The curved arrow in Case 3-12 (Fig. 3–41*A*) is directed to the
    A. right atrium.
    B. ascending aorta.
    C. right descending pulmonary artery.
    D. main pulmonary artery.
    E. pneumonia.

3-13. The most likely diagnosis in Case 3-13 (Fig. 3–42) is
    A. aortic stenosis.
    B. pulmonic stenosis.
    C. VSD.
    D. pulmonary edema.
    E. normal chest radiograph.

3-14. The appearance of the pulmonary vasculature indicates Case 3-14 (Fig. 3–43) is
    A. enlarged atrial appendage.
    B. partial anomalous pulmonary venous return.
    C. right ventricular hypertrophy.

    D. left atrial enlargement.
    E. pulmonary arteriovenous malformation.

3-15. The most likely etiology of the radiographic findings in Case 3-15 (Fig. 3–44) is
    A. cardiac failure with pulmonary edema.
    B. pulmonic stenosis with pneumonia.
    C. pulmonary embolism.
    D. pneumomediastinum.
    E. pneumothorax.

Radiologic Findings:

3-11. In this case (Fig. 3–40), the chest radiograph was normal in a 28-year-old man seen in the Emergency Department for chest pain. The electrocardiogram was also normal, and there was no obvious cause for the patient's pain. He had just stopped medication for a psychiatric illness and was hysterical. (*D* is the correct answer to Question 3-11.) Note the well-defined pulmonary vessels in the perihilar region and normal branching of

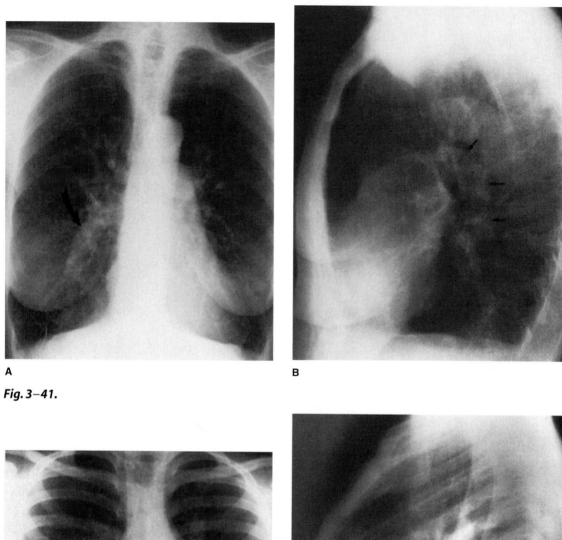

A

B

Fig. 3–41.

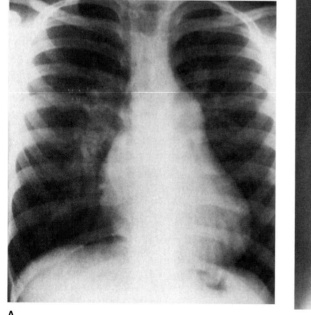

A

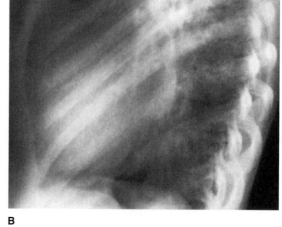

B

Fig. 3–42.

48

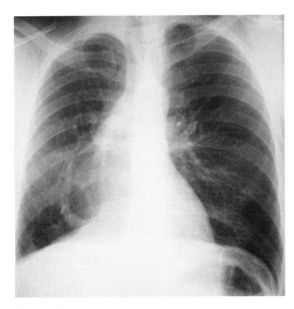

Fig. 3–43.

these vessels into the lungs. There is a gradient of pulmonary vascular markings from the bases to the apices on an upright radiograph due to the increased perfusion to the lower lobes.

3-12. This case (Fig. 3–41) is an example of chronic obstructive pulmonary disease. The large central pulmonary arteries indicate pulmonary arterial hypertension. The curved arrow in Fig. 3–41*A* identifies the enlarged right descending pulmonary artery. (*C* is the correct answer to Question 3-12.) The generalized proximal pulmonary artery enlargement is confirmed on the lateral radiograph by the large left pulmonary artery (Fig. 3–41*B, arrows*). Note the attenuation of vessels in the periphery of the lungs. This constellation of findings is typical of emphysema. There are also large bullae, which result in an absence of pulmonary vessels and hyperlucency of the lungs.

3-13. This case (Fig. 3–42) shows increased pulmonary vascularity in a 22-year-old patient with VSD. (*C* is the correct answer to Question 3-13.) Note the

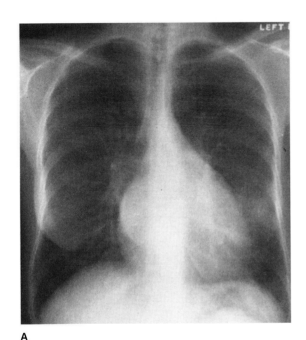

A

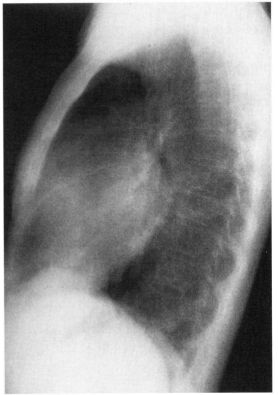

B

Fig. 3–44.

large central pulmonary arteries, the increased linear opacities radiating out into the lungs, and the relatively uniform distribution of the pulmonary vascular shadows. In individuals with long-standing intracardiac shunts and pulmonary hypertension, the pulmonary arterial resistance may exceed systemic pressures resulting in Eisenmenger's physiology, a reversal of an intracardiac shunt from L > R to R < L. In these individuals, the central pulmonary arteries are quite large, but the peripheral pulmonary arteries are markedly attenuated.

3-14. This case (Fig. 3–43) shows the characteristic appearance of venolobar (scimitar) syndrome. (*B* is the correct answer to Question 3-14.) The scimitar vein is the result of partial anomalous pulmonary venous return.

3-15. This case (Fig. 3–44) is an example of a long-standing hypertension in a patient with shortness of breath and pulmonary edema from congestive heart failure. (*A* is the correct answer to Question 3-15.) Note the increased size of the cardiac silhouette, the ill-defined reticular perihilar opacities, and the redistribution of blood flow to the upper lung zones. In this woman, the cause of the pulmonary edema was myocardial infarction.

Discussion:

The main pulmonary arteries are large, the lobar arteries smaller, and each branching segment becomes progressively smaller. On the chest radiograph, this pattern is manifested by linear opacities or shadows that are much more prominent in the central portion of the chest and gradually get less prominent toward the periphery of the lung, as in the normal person in Case 3-11. The right descending pulmonary artery (RDPA) is one important landmark on the PA chest film (see Fig. 3–1). In the normal chest, the lateral border of the RDPA is usually well demarcated, and the artery usually measures less than 15 mm at its widest diameter.

Enlargement of this vessel is caused by a variety of abnormalities (Table 3–6). Chronic obstructive pulmonary disease, with resultant pulmonary hypertension, is the most common cause of pulmonary arterial

Table 3–6. Causes of Pulmonary Arterial Hypertension

Chronic obstructive pulmonary disease
Left-sided obstructive lesions
Mitral stenosis
Intracardiac shunts
Recurrent pulmonary emboli
Vasculitis
Primary pulmonary hypertension (idiopathic)

hypertension and is shown in the patient in Case 3-12 (Fig. 3–41).

Intracardiac shunts that result in increased pulmonary arterial flow can also enlarge the pulmonary vascular system. The most common lesions causing increased vascularity without cyanosis are ASD, VSD, and patent ductus arteriosus. Case 3-13 (Fig. 3–42) is an example of a VSD with increased vascularity. The main cardiac lesions with cyanosis and increased pulmonary vascularity are transposition of the great vessels, truncus arteriosus, and total anomalous pulmonary venous return. The standard texts listed in the bibliography at the end of the chapter provide in-depth discussions of these entities.

One other common cause of pulmonary artery enlargement is mitral disease (either stenosis or regurgitation). In this case, increasing left atrial pressures are transmitted to the pulmonary veins. In time, this raises pulmonary capillary wedge pressures and eventually right heart pressures, similar to cor pulmonale from left heart failure (see Case 3-7).

Venolobar syndrome is a form of partial anomalous pulmonary venous return. Note the right inferior pulmonary vein descending in a curvilinear fashion to empty into the inferior vena cava (Figs. 3–43 and 3–45). Right lung hypoplasia causes the small size of the right hemithorax and results in shift of the heart and mediastinum to the right. Other congenital anomalies may be present.

Pulmonary edema, as exhibited in Case 3-15 (Fig. 3–44), regardless of the cause, is another process that causes the increase in the pulmonary vascularity seen on

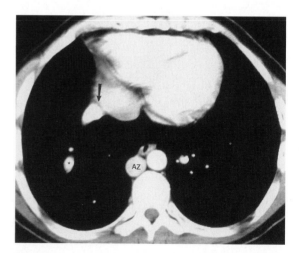

Fig. 3–45. Axial CT with contrast shows anomalous right pulmonary vein descending (*) and entering (*arrow*) inferior vena cava. AZ = azygous vein.

chest radiograph (discussed further in the next chapter). Perihilar indistinctness, caused by interstitial edema, may obliterate the borders of the pulmonary vessels. Associated findings are redistribution of blood flow to the apices, Kerley B lines lines, and pleural effusions (Fig. 3–31).

EXERCISE 3-4: VASCULAR ABNORMALITIES

Clinical Histories:

Case 3-16. A 67-year-old man with a long history of hypertension (Fig. 3–46)

Case 3-17. A 25-year-old man with chest fullness (Fig. 3–47)

Case 3-18. A 76-year-old man with substernal chest pain (Fig. 3–48)

Case 3-19. A 22-year-old man with differential pulses in the legs and arms (Fig. 3–49)

Case 3-20. A 38-year-old man with a systolic murmur (Fig. 3–50) (Courtesy of Laurence B. Leinbach, M.D., Winston-Salem, NC.)

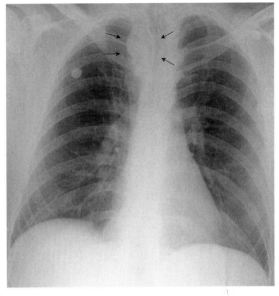

Fig. 3–47.

Questions:

3-16. The abnormal contour of the right heart border in Case 3-16 (Fig. 3–46) is due to
   A. pericardial cyst.
   B. adenopathy.
   C. aortic stenosis.
   D. pulmonary artery aneurysm.
   E. azygous vein.

3-17. The abnormality outlined by arrows in Case 3-17 (Fig. 3–47) is
   A. substernal goiter.
   B. innominate artery aneurysm.
   C. lung cancer.
   D. right aortic arch.
   E. mediastinal adenopathy.

3-18. Causes for the appearance of the chest in Case 3-18 (Fig. 3–48) includes all of the following except
   A. ascending aortic aneurysm.
   B. anterior mediastinal mass.
   C. pleural mass.
   D. lung cancer.
   E. Ewing's sarcoma of rib.

3-19. The arrow in Case 3-19 (Fig. 3–49) is showing
   A. aortic ectasia.
   B. aortic constriction.
   C. pulmonary artery dilatation.
   D. adenopathy.
   E. embolic changes.

3-20. The abnormality shown by the arrow in Case 3-20 (Fig. 3–50) is most likely
   A. enlarged main pulmonary artery.
   B. descending thoracic aorta.
   C. ductus arteriosus.
   D. pulmonary vein.
   E. left superior vena cava.

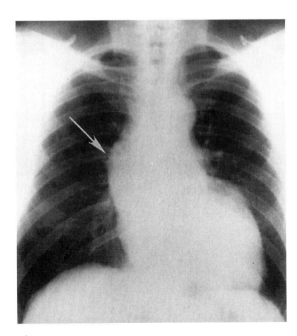

Fig. 3–46.

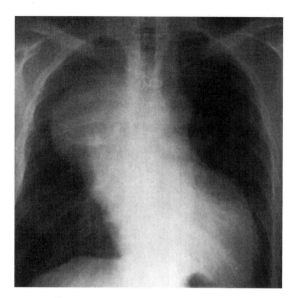

Fig. 3–48.

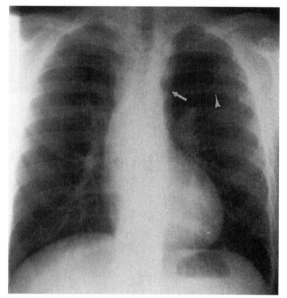

Fig. 3–49.

Radiographic Findings:

3-16. In this case (Fig. 3–46), aortic ectasia (*arrow*) is seen in a patient who has had coronary artery bypass surgery and has a history of long-standing hypertension and aortic stenosis. (*C* is correct answer to Question 3-16.)

3-17. This case (Fig. 3–47) is an example of a right-sided aortic arch in an asymptomatic individual. (*D* is the correct answer to Question 3-17.)

3-18. This case (Fig. 3–48) is a radiograph of the patient in Case 3-16 (Fig. 3–46), 9 years later, and it shows a localized mass in the region of the ascending aorta. The CT image (Fig. 3–51) confirmed the large ascending aorta aneurysm. (*E* is the correct answer to Question 3-18.)

3-19. This case (Fig. 3–49) shows rib notching (*arrowhead*) and a localized constriction of the proximal descending aorta (*arrow*). (*B* is the correct answer to Question 3-19.) These findings are diagnostic of coarctation of the aorta.

3-20. This case (Fig. 3–50) is an example of main pulmonary artery dilation (*arrow*) in a patient with pulmonic stenosis. (*A* is the correct answer to Question 3-20.)

Discussion:

Anomalies of the major vessels are commonly encountered on the chest radiograph. The aortic arch is an easily recognized shadow. On the PA projection, the aorta originates in the middle of the chest and then arches superiorly and slightly to the left (hence, the term *aortic arch*), then curves, crosses the mediastinum at an oblique angle, and continues as the descending thoracic aorta (see Fig. 3–1). The configuration of the

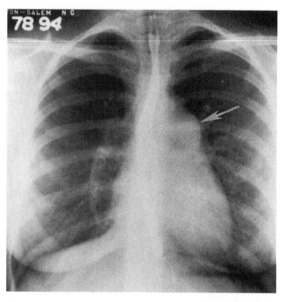

Fig. 3–50.

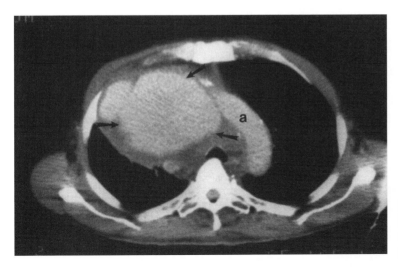

Fig. 3–51. Axial CT image shows large aortic aneurysm (*arrows*) originating from the proximal ascending portion of the aortic arch (a).

aorta changes during life. In the young person, the aortic arch is narrow and smooth and the descending thoracic segment very straight. In the older individual with atherosclerotic disease or aortic stenosis, as shown in Case 3-16 (Fig. 3–46), the ascending aorta becomes more prominent along the right heart border and may have an undulating pattern in the descending thoracic portion.

Other abnormalities of the aortic arch are uncommon. Congenital aortic anomalies include left aortic arch with aberrant branching, right aortic arch, and double aortic arch. The most prominent of these aberrations is the right aortic arch, which occurs in 1 in 2500 people. It can be diagnosed on the conventional radiograph by noting an indentation to and slight deviation of the right side of the trachea and displacement of the SVC shadow, as shown in Case 3-17 (Fig. 3–47, *arrows*). In many individuals, the right arch is discovered incidentally and, in these cases, is usually associated with an aberrant left subclavian artery (Fig. 3–52). The barium swallow can also demonstrate mass effect on the esophagus by the aberrant subclavian and aorta as it crosses from right to left in the chest. When associated with congenital anomalies (tetralogy of Fallot, truncus arteriosus, etc.), the great vessel branching pattern is a mirror image of that seen in a normal left aortic arch.

Aneurysms of the aorta, shown in Case 3-18 (Fig. 3–48), are most often caused by atherosclerosis. Trauma, infection, and connective tissue disorders such as Marfan's and Ehlers-Danlos syndrome are other causes. Aneurysms may be saccular or fusiform in shape, and symptoms include chest pain, hoarseness from compression of the recurrent laryngeal nerve, postobstructive atelectasis from compression of

a bronchus, and dysphagia from esophageal compression. However, aneurysms are most commonly discovered as an incidental finding on an imaging study done for other reasons. An aneurysm of the ascending or transverse aortic segments shows a focal enlargement of the aortic shadow, usually with curvilinear calcification in its wall. A saccular aneurysm of the descending aorta may be misdiagnosed as a lung, mediastinal, or pleural mass, especially if it does not contain linear calcification. In these cases, as mentioned previously, CT is the

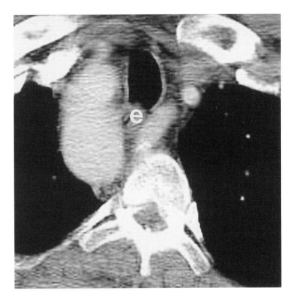

Fig. 3–52. Axial CT shows aberrant left subclavian artery coursing posterior to the esophagus (e).

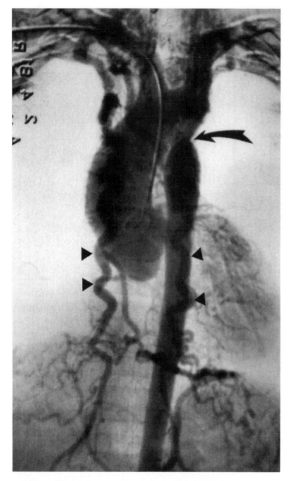

Fig. 3–53. Aortogram of the patient in Case 3-19 shows the characteristic constriction in the descending aorta (*curved arrow*) and the dilated intercostal veins (*arrowheads*).

next best imaging modality to perform (Fig. 3–51). The lack of rib destruction in Case 3-18 strongly argues against a chest wall sarcoma.

A special type of aneurysm is aortic dissection, which is usually caused by atherosclerosis with medial layer necrosis. In this disorder, blood dissects into the aortic wall through a tear of the intima. This process may begin anywhere along the course of the thoracic aorta, but the exact location is very important because it has therapeutic implications. Aortic dissection is most easily classified by the Stanford system. This divides dissections into type A, those involving the ascending aorta, and type B, those that begin distal to the left subclavian. When associated with symptoms, type A dissections are considered surgical emergencies, whereas symptomatic type B dissections often can be managed medically. In the acute setting, the diagnosis is best established by CT because it can rapidly define the entire scope of the dissection as well as show the relationship to other major vessels (Fig. 3–15). Echocardiography can also rapidly detect dissection but provides less anatomic detail. MR imaging is often not used in the acute setting due to time and availability issues. The role of angiography as a diagnostic procedure for dissection has virtually disappeared; however, intravascular therapy including placement of stent-grafts and fenestration of the dissection flap can be performed for treatment in many instances including individuals whose conditions are medically inoperable.

The abnormality in Case 3-19 (Fig. 3–49) is coarctation of the aorta. This congenital anomaly results in partial or complete obstruction of the aorta at the junction of the aortic arch and descending aorta near the ligamentum arteriosum (the *in utero* connection between the aorta and pulmonary arteries). About one-half of these individuals also have a bicuspid aortic valve. The obstruction to flow due to the coarctation results in elevated upper extremity blood pressure and decreased lower extremity blood pressure. A systolic ejection murmur may also be heard. Because of the partial aortic obstruction, collateral flow through the intercostal arteries results in the rib notching seen (Fig. 3–53).

EXERCISE 3-5: HEART AND GREAT VESSEL CALCIFICATIONS

Clinical Histories:

Case 3-21. A 75-year-old woman with "lots of murmurs" when examined by a medical student who was on the first day of clinical rotation (Fig. 3–54)

Case 3-22. A 70-year-old woman who told the medical student she had been very sick as a younger woman and did not know her diagnosis at that time (Fig. 3–55)

Case 3-23. A 65-year-old man with a long history of hypertension hospitalized 6 years ago with an acute illness; lateral chest radiograph (Fig. 3–56)

Case 3-24. A 66-year-old man with long-standing diabetes mellitus; lateral chest radiograph (Fig. 3–57)

Case 3-25. A woman with shortness of breath and decreased exercise tolerance; PA and lateral chest radiographs (Fig. 3–58)

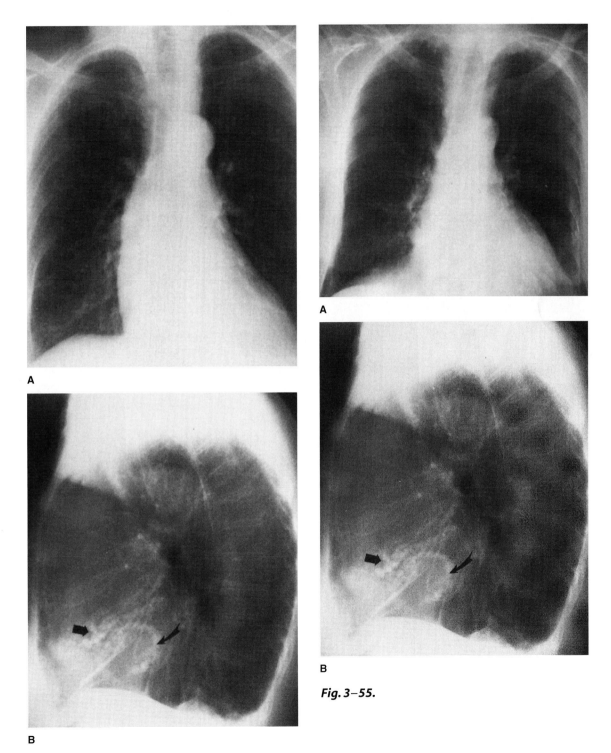

A

B

Fig. 3–54.

A

B

Fig. 3–55.

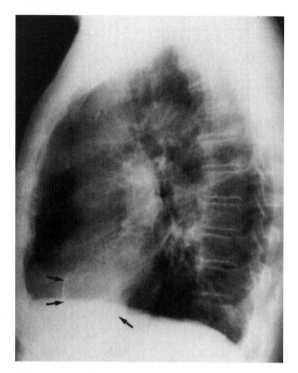

Fig. 3–56.

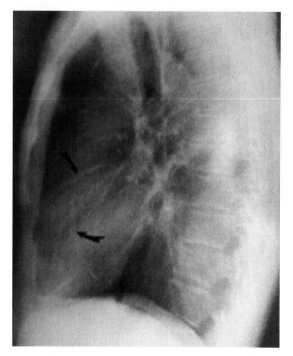

Fig. 3–57.

Questions:

3-21. In Case 3-21 (Fig. 3–54*B*) the straight arrow refers to
A. mitral valve.
B. tricuspid valve.
C. aortic valve.
D. pulmonary embolus.
E. pericardial calcification.

3-22. In Case 3-22 (Fig. 3–55*B*) the arrows are pointing to
A. pulmonary artery calcification.
B. pericardial effusion.
C. pericardial calcification.
D. ascending aortic aneurysm.
E. descending thoracic aortic aneurysm.

3-23. In Case 3-23 (Fig. 3–56) the arrows on the lateral chest radiographs point to calcifications within which cardiac structure?
A. Pericardium
B. Mitral valve
C. Aortic valve
D. Tricuspid valve
E. Left ventricle

3-24. In Case 3-24 (Fig. 3–57) the curved arrows point to calcification within the region of which cardiac structure?
A. Aortic valve
B. Mitral valve
C. Pericardium
D. Coronary artery
E. Aortic aneurysm

3-25. In Case 3-25 (Fig. 3–58) the arrows and arrowheads point to
A. calcified mediastinal mass.
B. calcified left atrial myxoma.
C. pulmonary embolus calcification.
D. aortic valve calcification.
E. mitral valve calcification.

Radiographic Findings:

3-21. The PA and lateral chest radiographs (Fig. 3–54) show irregular linear calcifications in two areas, best seen on the lateral projection. Anteriorly, the curved linear calcifications denoted by the straight arrow reside in the aortic valve. (*C* is the correct answer to Question 3-21.) The curved arrow posteriorly points to calcification within the mitral valve annulus. This woman had rheumatic fever as a young adult, and the calcifications in the aortic valve and mitral annulus resulted from this disease.

3-22. This case (Fig. 3–55) shows pericardial calcification in a woman who had viral pericarditis as a young child. (*C* is the correct answer to Question 3-22.) Note that the calcification is seen much better on the lateral view.

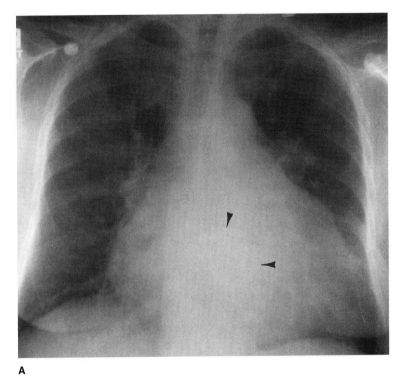

A

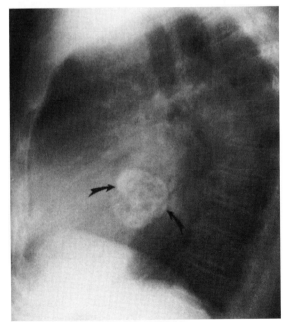

B

Fig. 3–58.

3-23. The lateral chest radiograph in this case (Fig. 3–56) shows linear calcification in a focal area overlying the left ventricle. This calcification resides in a left ventricular aneurysm that this man developed after a myocardial infarction 6 years earlier. (*E* is the correct answer to Question 3-23.)

3-24. The lateral chest radiograph in this case (Fig. 3–57) shows linear tram track calcifications overlying the course of the coronary arteries. These calcifications represent coronary artery atherosclerosis in a patient with long-standing diabetes. (*D* is the correct answer to Question 3-24.)

3-25. In this case (Fig. 3–58), a circular, heavily calcified area overlying the left atrium is seen in both the PA (*arrowheads*) and lateral (*curved arrows*) projections. These calcifications resided within a left atrial myxoma that was causing the patient's symptoms of shortness of breath and decreased exercise tolerance. (*B* is the correct answer to Question 3-25.)

Discussion:

Calcifications, present in almost any area of the cardiovascular system, may be either metastatic or dystrophic in origin. Metastatic calcifications are usually caused by soft-tissue deposition of calcium due to hypercalcemia of any cause. Dystrophic soft-tissue calcifications are responses to tissue injury or degeneration and have no metabolic cause. They can be seen in practically any of the soft-tissue components of the cardiovascular system. We will concentrate on calcifications that can be seen on the conventional radiograph, although CT is a more sensitive test for detecting calcium. Calcium scoring has become a popular way of assessing the degree of atherosclerosis in the coronary arteries, but provides mainly risk stratification rather than site-specific information of stenosis. The utility of this technique over traditional risk factors has yet to be proven. The most common site of calcification seen on the conventional chest radiograph is within the aorta, usually in elderly patients with long-standing atherosclerotic disease or diabetes. In this instance, the calcification is linear and is associated with the aortic wall (Fig. 3–32). These calcifications may also be present in aneurysms (Fig. 3–34).

The aortic valve and mitral valve annulus are the most common intracardiac regions to demonstrate dystrophic calcification, usually secondary to long-standing stenosis or insufficiency from rheumatic fever. Bicuspid valves may also show this type of calcification. The lateral film is best for deciding which valve is calcified. In Fig. 3–59, a line drawn from the hilum (C) obliquely and downward to intersect the anterior cardiophrenic angle (N) will project behind aortic calcifications (A). Calcifications that lie in back of this line are usually mitral annulus calcifications (M).

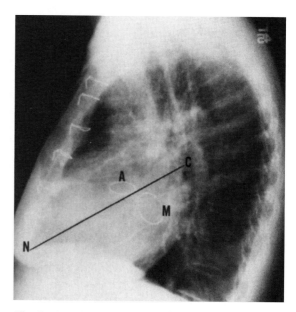

Fig. 3–59. Lateral view of a patient who has undergone replacement of the aortic (A) and mitral (M) valves. The line C–N connects the carina and the anterior cardiophrenic angle. Aortic valves usually lie above this line and mitral valves below it.

Pericardial calcification as in Case 3-22 (Fig. 3–55) is seen in approximately 50% of patients with constrictive pericarditis. It has a characteristic curvilinear appearance outlining the location of the pericardium and is most often seen along the right heart border (Fig. 3–55).

Myocardial calcification, as is seen in left ventricular aneurysms, was discussed in the exercise on altered cardiac contour, and is shown in a slightly different form in Case 3-23 (Fig. 3–56). Thin, focal, linear calcifications overlying the left ventricle should be considered as aneurysms, and echocardiography, CT, and MR imaging are all useful examinations to confirm this diagnosis.

Calcifications within the wall of the coronary arteries, as exhibited in Case 3-24 (Fig. 3–57), are recognized on conventional radiographs as thin, linear, calcific deposits corresponding to the course of the coronary arteries. When discovered by conventional radiographs, it is a late finding of atherosclerosis, and these patients have a high incidence of obstructive coronary artery disease.

Case 3-25 (Fig. 3–58) is an example of the rare primary cardiac neoplasm that may calcify and be detected initially on the plain film. The cardiac tumor that most commonly calcifies is the left atrial myxoma, and calcification occurs in about 10% of these lesions (Fig. 3–58). Rarely, myocardial metastatic disease (such as osteosarcoma) or other primary cardiac tumors may calcify. Finally, primary mediastinal neoplasms such as teratomas may rarely show calcification. In these patients, CT should be performed for diagnosis.

EXERCISE 3-6: MONITORING DEVICES

Clinical Histories:

Case 3-26. Routine supine portable chest radiograph obtained after SG catheter placement (Fig. 3–60)

Case 3-27. Supine chest radiograph obtained after difficult CVP placement (Fig. 3–61) (*Courtesy of Robert H. Choplin, M.D., Indianapolis, IN*)

Case 3-28. Routine supine chest radiograph in ICU patient after placement of several lines and tubes (Fig. 3–62)

Case 3-29. Chest radiograph obtained following pacemaker insertion (Fig. 3–63)

Case 3-30. Chest radiograph obtained following central venous catheter placement (Fig. 3–64); history of prior surgery for congenital heart disease

Questions:

3-26. The complication of Swan-Ganz catheter placement in Case 3-26 (Fig. 3–60) is
A. malposition of the tip.
B. pneumothorax.

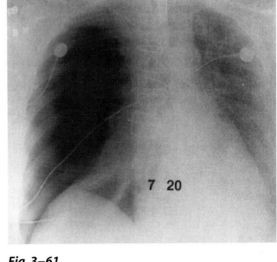

Fig. 3–61.

C. perforation.
D. catheter coiling.
E. catheter thrombosis.

3-27. The complication of CVP catheter placement in Case 3-27 (Fig. 3–61) is
A. malposition of the tip.
B. pneumothorax.
C. perforation.
D. catheter coiling.
E. catheter thrombosis.

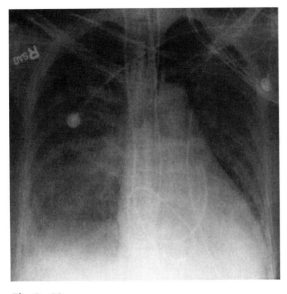

Fig. 3–60.

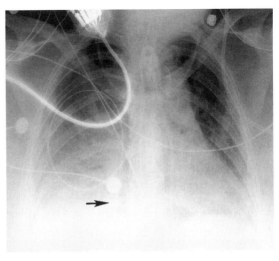

Fig. 3–62.

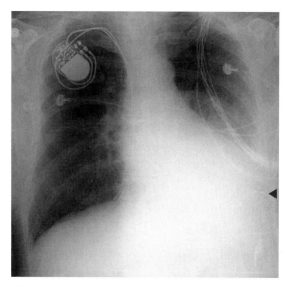

Fig. 3–63.

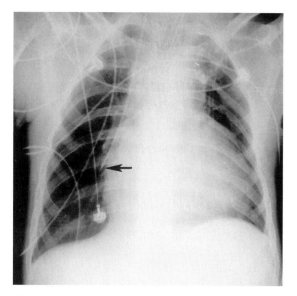

Fig. 3–64.

3-28. The malpositioned catheter in Case 3-28 (Fig. 3–62) is a(n)
    A. tracheostomy tube.
    B. intra-aortic balloon pump.
    C. Swan-Ganz catheter.
    D. nasogastric tube.
    E. none of the above.

3-29. Possible complications from the pacemaker shown in Case 3-29 (Fig. 3–63, *arrowhead*) include all of the following except
    A. pleural effusion.
    B. pneumothorax.
    C. pericardial effusion.
    D. pulmonary infarction.
    E. pacemaker malfunction.

3-30. The catheter in Case 3-30 (Fig. 3–64, *arrow*) is in the
    A. azygous vein.
    B. superior vena cava.
    C. right atrium.
    D. ascending aorta.
    E. right pulmonary artery.

Radiographic Findings:

3-26. The supine portable chest radiograph obtained after SG catheter placement in this case (Fig. 3–60) is coiled within the right ventricle before it terminates in the proximal main pulmonary artery. (*D* is the correct answer to Question 3-26.) This coiling of the catheter in the right ventricle may cause thrombosis or arrhythmia, and it is necessary to reposition this catheter.

3-27. The supine chest radiograph in this case (Fig. 3–61) shows a pneumothorax after a difficult CVP placement. (*B* is the correct answer to Question 3-27.) Pneumothorax is one of the potential complications of subclavian venous catheterization because the apex of the lung is approximately 5 mm below the subclavian vein.

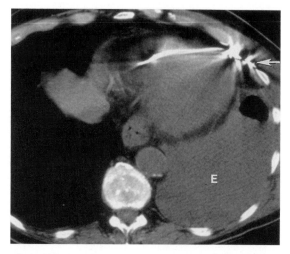

Fig. 3–65. Axial CT shows tip of right ventricular pacing lead outside of myocardium (*arrow*). Note large right pleural effusion (E).

3-28. In this case (Fig. 3–62), the chest radiograph obtained shows a nasogastric tube extending down the right main bronchus into the right lung (Fig. 3–62, *arrow*). (*D* is the correct answer to Question 3-28.)

3-29. In this case (Fig. 3–63), the tip of the right ventricular pacemaker lead extends lateral to the expected border of the myocardium. This positioning may cause the pacemaker to function poorly or cause pleural and/or pericardial effusion. Because the leads are introduced via the subclavian vein, pneumothorax is also a potential complication. (*D* is the correct answer to Question 3-29.) A CT confirmed the pacemaker lead perforation (Fig. 3–65).

3-30. The patient in this case (Fig. 3–64) had hypoplastic left heart syndrome as an infant. To correct this anomaly, numerous surgeries were performed to redirect blood in the setting of a single functional ventricle. As part of this procedure, the superior vena cava is directly anastamosed to the right pulmonary artery (Glenn procedure). (*E* is the correct answer to Question 3-30.) The inferior vena cava is also extended to the right pulmonary artery via a right atrial baffle (Fontan procedure) to complete the flow of deoxygenated blood from the body returning to the lungs. Blood returns from the lungs to the left atrium and finally to the dominant right ventricle via atrial and/or ventricular septal defects.

Discussion:

As mentioned in the subheading of monitoring devices within the chapter, a variety of catheters can be inserted into the heart and great vessels to monitor various hemodynamic parameters, particularly in the ICU setting. Table 3–3 lists the most common monitoring devices, and Table 3–4 shows the most common complications from placement of these devices. It is important to trace and account for each catheter individually. For instance, the nasogastric tube might have initially been mistaken for an EKG lead. The result of instilling fluid through this tube could have been disastrous. Even so, the result of this placement was a pneumothorax.

We have reviewed the normal placement of catheters and some of the more common related complications. The student should be familiar with this aspect of radiography in the ICU setting, and the references cited at the end of the chapter will provide further in-depth learning.

BIBLIOGRAPHY

Chen JT, ed. *Essentials of Cardiac Imaging.* Philadelphia: Lippincott-Raven; 1997.

Elliott LP, ed. *Cardiac Imaging in Infants, Children, and Adults.* Philadelphia: Lippincott; 1991.

Higgins CB. *Essentials of Cardiac Radiology and Imaging.* Philadelphia: Lippincott; 1992.

Manning WJ, Pennell DJ, eds. *Cardiovascular Magnetic Resonance.* Philadelphia: Churchill-Livingstone; 2002.

Miller SW. *Cardiac Radiology: The Requisites.* St. Louis: Mosby; 1996.

Remy-Jardin J, ed. *CT Angiography of the Chest.* Philadelphia: Lippincott Williams & Wilkins; 2001.

Radiology of the Chest

4

Caroline Chiles & Robert H. Choplin

INTRODUCTION

The chest radiograph is the most frequently performed radiographic study in the United States. It should almost always be the first radiologic study ordered for evaluation of diseases of the thorax. The natural contrast of the aerated lungs provides a window into the body to evaluate the patient for diseases involving the heart, lungs, pleurae, tracheobronchial tree, esophagus, thoracic lymph nodes, thoracic skeleton, chest wall, and upper abdomen. In both acute and chronic illnesses, the chest radiograph allows one to detect a disease and monitor its response to therapy. For many disease processes (e.g., pneumonia and congestive heart failure) the diagnosis can be established and the disease followed to resolution with no further imaging studies. There are limitations to the chest radiograph, and diseases may not be sufficiently advanced to be detected or may not result in detectable abnormalities. Other imaging methods are needed to complement the conventional chest radiograph. These imaging methods include computed tomography (CT), magnetic resonance (MR) imaging, ultrasound (US), and radionuclide studies. These techniques, their clinical uses, and case studies are included in this chapter.

TECHNIQUES

Conventional Radiography

THE POSTEROANTERIOR AND LATERAL CHEST RADIOGRAPH

The simplest conventional study of the chest is a posteroanterior and lateral chest radiograph taken in a radiographic unit specially designed for these studies. The x-rays travel through the patient and expose a receptor from which the image is recorded. Most commonly, the receptor is an intensifying screen and radiographic film, but several types of digital radiographic receptors are in use as well. Two of these types receptors are computed radiography and large field-of-view image intensifiers. The digital images may be printed on film by laser printers or viewed on monitors. The two views of a chest radiograph are taken in projections at 90 degrees to each other with the patient's breath held at the end of a maximum inspiration. The first view is obtained as the patient faces the film cassette with the x-ray beam source positioned 6 feet behind the patient. Because the x-ray beam travels in a posterior-to-anterior direction, this view is called a *posteroanterior (PA)* chest radiograph. Another view is then obtained with the patient turned 90 degrees, with the left side against the film cassette and arms overhead. The x-ray beam travels from right to left through the patient and this is called a *left lateral* view. Anatomic features of the chest that are readily identifiable on plain radiographs are shown in Figs. 4–1 and 4–2.

OTHER RADIOGRAPHIC PROJECTIONS

In some clinical situations, patients may not be able to stand or sit upright for the conventional PA and lateral radiographs, and a film must be taken with the patient's back turned to the film cassette and the x-ray beam traversing the patient in an anterior-to-posterior direction. These radiographs are called *anteroposterior* (AP) radiographs. They may be taken in the x-ray department but are more commonly obtained as portable studies at the patient's bedside.

Films may also be obtained with the patient lying on one side in a decubitus position with the x-ray beam traversing the patient either PA or AP along a horizontal plane. These films are designated *lateral decubitus* films. A left lateral decubitus radiograph indicates that the left side of the patient is dependent against the table. A right lateral decubitus radiograph indicates that the right side of the patient is dependent against the table.

THE PORTABLE CHEST RADIOGRAPH

If the clinical situation prevents the patient from coming to the radiology department, a chest radiograph may be obtained at the patient's bedside, and these are almost always AP radiographs. The AP portable radiograph does not provide as much information as PA and lateral chest radiographs for a number of reasons. Because it is a single view, lesions are not as easily or accurately localized along

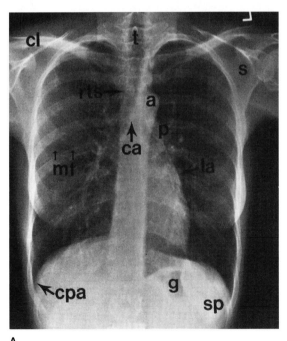

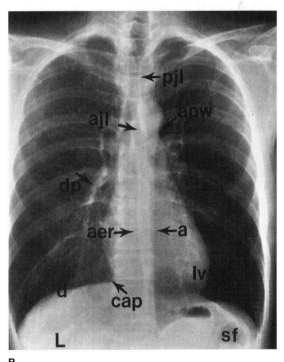

A

B

Fig. 4–1. Normal radiographic anatomy. Posteroanterior chest radiographs. [Key to labels in Figs. 4–1 and 4–2: a = aorta, aer = azygoesophageal recess, ajl = anterior junction line, apw = aortopulmonary window, bi = bronchus intermedius, ca = carina, cap = cardiophrenic angle, cpa = costophrenic angle, cl = clavicle, d = diaphragm, dp = descending (or interlobar) pulmonary artery, g = gastric air bubble, ivc = inferior vena cava, L = liver, la = left atrium, lpa = left pulmonary artery, lul = left upper lobe bronchus, lv = left ventricle, m = manubrium, mf = minor fissure, MF = major fissure, p = main pulmonary artery, pjl = posterior junction line, rpa = right pulmonary artery, rts = right tracheal (or paratracheal) stripe, rul = right upper lobe bronchus, rv = right ventricle, s = scapula, sf = splenic flexure of colon, sp = spleen, svc = superior vena cava, t = trachea, and v = vertebral body.]

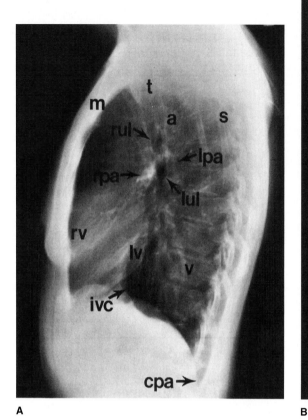

A

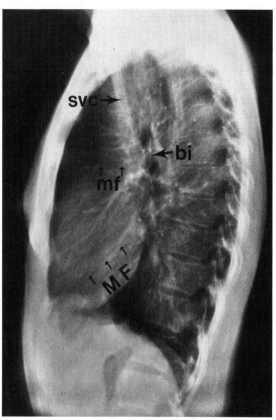

B

Fig. 4–2. Normal radiographic anatomy. Lateral chest radiographs. (See Fig. 4–1 for key.)

the AP axis of the thorax. The patients for whom these films are obtained are usually quite ill and cannot be positioned as well as patients traveling to the x-ray department. They frequently cannot cooperate by holding their breath at total lung capacity. A mobile x-ray generator is typically not as powerful as a fixed x-ray generator, and, therefore, longer exposure times are necessary to obtain sufficient film exposure. The quality of portable chest radiographs, therefore, is often inferior to that of PA and lateral radiographs, as a result of both respiratory and cardiac motion. X-ray grids are used to reduce scatter radiation and improve image quality. Grids are used for most conventional chest films done in radiology departments where fixed equipment is present. Grids are not usually used for portable radiographs, and the result is a high proportion of scattered x-rays that degrade the image. Paradoxically, the portable radiograph may be more expensive than a conventional

PA and lateral chest radiograph, owing to extra labor and equipment costs in obtaining a bedside radiograph.

Computed Tomography of the Chest

Computed tomography is described in detail in Chapter 1. For CT examinations of the chest, intravenous contrast material is frequently administered for opacification of arteries and veins within the mediastinum and hila to facilitate the recognition of abnormal masses or lymph nodes. Anatomic features of the chest that are readily identifiable on CT scans are shown in Figs. 4–3 and 4–4.

Ultrasonography of the Chest

Ultrasound is described in detail in Chapter 1. Ultrasound of the chest is typically performed to evaluate fluid collections within the pleural space. Ultrasound

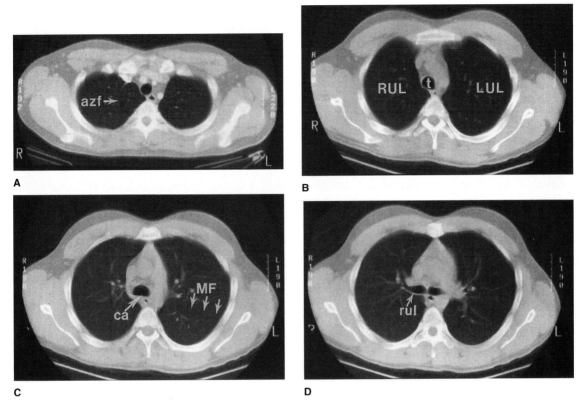

Fig. 4–3. Normal CT anatomy. Axial scans of the chest, contiguous slices at 1 cm of collimation, lung window settings. [Key to labels in Figs. 4–3 and 4–4: a = aorta, aa = ascending aorta, arch = transverse section of the aortic arch, azf = azygos fissure (normal variant), azv = azygos vein, bb = basilar segmental bronchi of lower lobes, bi = bronchus intermedius, ca = carina, cc = common carotid artery, cl = clavicle, da = descending aorta, dp = descending (or interlobar) pulmonary artery, e = esophagus, hazv = hemiazygos vein, h = humerus, im = internal mammary artery and vein, ipv = inferior pulmonary vein, ivc = inferior vena cava, ivs = interventricular septum, l = liver, la = left atrium, lbv = left brachiocephalic vein, lcc = left common carotid artery, Li = lingula segment of the left upper lobe, lij = left internal jugular vein, LLL = left lower lobe, lpa = left pulmonary artery, lsa = left subclavian artery, lul = left upper lobe bronchus, LUL = left upper lobe, lv = left ventricle, m = manubrium, MF = major fissure, r = rib, ra = right atrium, rba = right brachiocephalic artery, rbv = right bronchiocephalic vein, rij = right internal jugular vein, RLL = right lower lobe, RML = right middle lobe, rml = right middle lobe bronchus, rpa = right pulmonary artery, rsa = right subclavian artery, rsv = right subclavian vein, RUL = right upper lobe, rul = right upper lobe bronchus, rv = right ventricle, rvot = right ventricular outflow tract, s = scapula, ss = bronchus to superior segment of lower lobe, st = sternum, svc = superior vena cava, t = trachea, th = thyroid, v = vertebral body.]

may be used to guide thoracentesis, especially when the fluid collection is small or loculated.

Magnetic Resonance Imaging of the Chest

The principles and applications of MR are described in Chapter 1. Anatomic features of the chest that are readily identifiable on MR images are shown in Figs. 4–5 and 4–6.

Nuclear Medicine

Nuclear medicine techniques used in evaluating diseases of the thorax include ventilation-perfusion (V/Q) scanning, scanning for sites of inflammation with gallium-67 or indium-111–labeled white cells, and scanning with tumor-seeking radiopharmaceuticals for tumor staging. The V/Q scan is often the imaging study of choice for a patient with suspected pulmonary thromboembolism. The

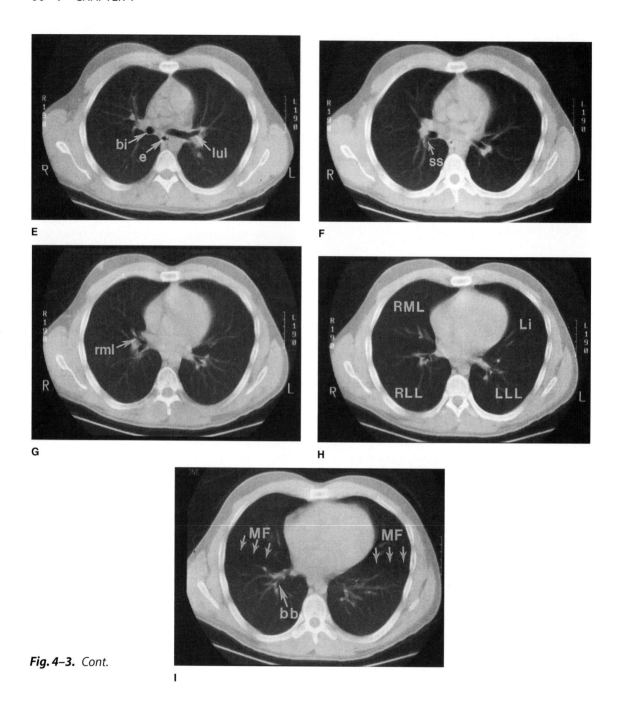

Fig. 4–3. *Cont.*

V/Q scan is noninvasive, and when results are negative, fewer than 10% of patients have pulmonary thromboembolism. The ventilation study is typically performed with the patient inhaling 10 to 30 mCi of xenon-133 while images are obtained with a scintillation camera (Fig. 4–7*A*). Wash-in images are obtained for two con-secutive 120-second periods, an equilibrium image is obtained, and then wash-out images are obtained over 30- to 60-second periods in posterior, and left and right posterior oblique projections. This portion of the study takes about 15 minutes. The perfusion scan is obtained by intra-venously injecting 2 to 4 mCi of technetium-99m-labeled

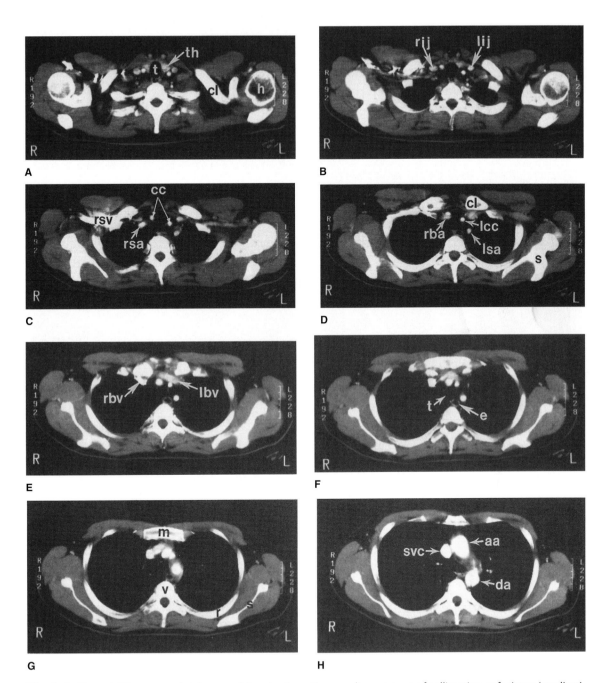

Fig. 4–4. Normal CT anatomy. Axial scans of the chest, contiguous slices at 1 cm of collimation, soft-tissue (mediastinal) window settings. (See Fig. 4–3 for key.)

macroaggregated albumin containing 200,000 to 700,000 particles. The particles range in size from 10 to 100 μm, and they lodge in capillaries and capillary arterioles, accurately reflecting pulmonary blood flow (Fig. 4–7B). The scintillation camera is set so that it obtains

anterior, posterior, both posterior oblique, and both anterior oblique projections for 750,000 counts per image. The perfusion study takes about 30 minutes to perform.

Other radionuclide scans used for the evaluation of suspected pulmonary disease include gallium-67 citrate

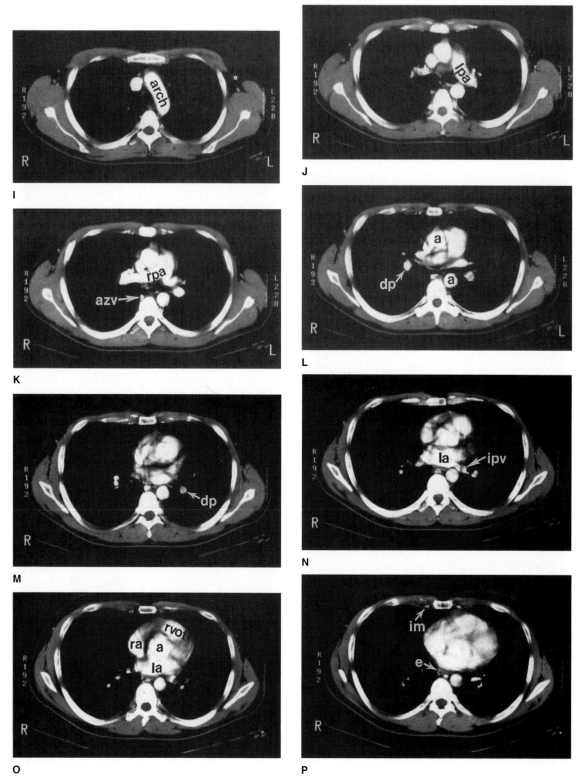

Fig. 4–4. *Cont.*

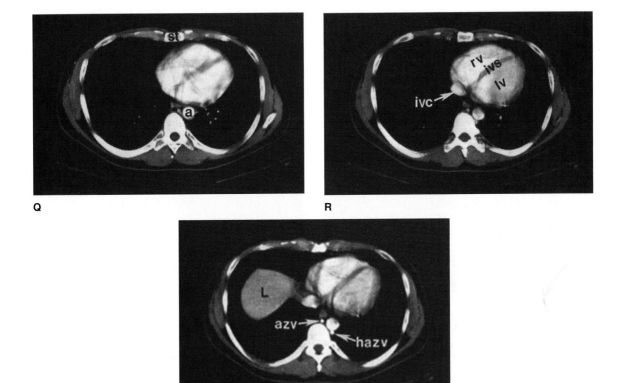

Fig. 4–4. *Cont.*

scans, in which gallium accumulates in leukocytes and in some tumors. After 5 mCi of gallium-67 citrate is injected intravenously, scans are obtained at 24 to 72 hours, allowing time for blood background and colon activity to clear. Abnormal increase in activity in the lungs may be focal or diffuse and may correspond to disease activity in inflammatory diseases, including sarcoidosis, radiation pneumonitis, and idiopathic pulmonary fibrosis, as well as in pneumonia and lung abscess. Gallium activity within the lung is usually reported as a gallium index that is the product of an intensity of 0 to 4 (4 = area of greatest activity, usually the liver) multiplied by the percentage of total lung area involved. The maximum gallium index is 400 (intensity of 4 × 100% involvement). Gallium has affinity for some tumors, including lymphoma, and can be used to detect occult sites of tumor either at presentation or during recurrence.

Another test that can be used to detect occult sites of infection is the indium-111–labeled white blood cell (WBC), or leukocyte, scan. The serous layer of an 80-mL blood sample taken from the patient is centrifuged to produce a white cell button. One to 2 mCi of indium-111 is added to the resuspended white cells. The labeled white blood cells are reinjected into a peripheral vein, and scanning is performed 24 to 48 hours after injection. The activity accumulates in sites of infection, and this test could be used to distinguish between pneumonia or lung abscess and noninfectious lung diseases. In practice, this test is infrequently obtained for pulmonary disease, because CT almost always localizes abnormalities precisely, and fiber-optic bronchoscopy is very effective for diagnosis of pulmonary abnormalities.

Tomography is also available for radionuclide imaging as two other techniques. Single photon emission computed tomography (SPECT) is used for photon emitters (99m Tc, 111 In, ^{123}I). The primary advantage of SPECT is the ability to depict anatomy in three dimensions. SPECT may be used to improve the spatial resolution of radionuclide imaging, including perfusion scans, and gallium- and indium-111–labeled WBC scans. A positron emission tomography (PET) scanner resembles a CT scanner and uses positron emitters (fluorine-18, carbon-11). Today, the most widely used positron emitter is F-18-deoxyglucose (FDG), which is used as a metabolic tracer. The raised metabolic rate can be used to distinguish neoplasm and inflammation from normal tissue. Although PET provides tomographic images, the spatial resolution (0.7–1.0 cm) is somewhat inferior to that of CT.

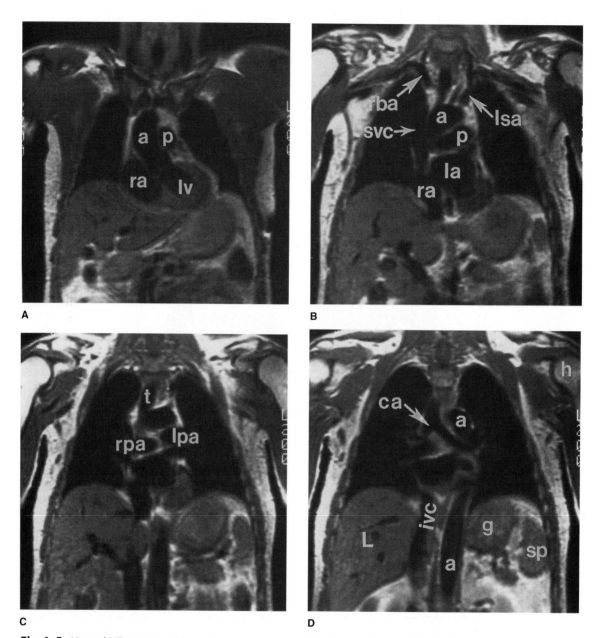

Fig. 4–5. Normal MR anatomy. Coronal spin-echo images of the thorax. [Key to labels for Figs. 4–5 and 4–6: a = aorta, aa = ascending aorta, arch = transverse section of the aortic arch, azv = azygos vein, bi = bronchus intermedius, ca = carina, da = descending aorta, dp = descending (or interlobar) pulmonary artery, e = esophagus, g = gastric fundus, h = humerus, im = internal mammary artery and vein, ipv = inferior pulmonary vein, ivc = inferior vena cava, ivs = interventricular septum, k = kidney, L = Liver, la = left atrium, lcc = left common carotid artery, lpa = left pulmonary artery, lsa = left subclavian artery, lv = left ventricle, m = manubrium, p = pulmonary artery, pc = pericardium, ra = right atrium, rba = right brachiocephalic artery, rca = right coronary artery, rpa = right pulmonary artery, rv = right ventricle, rvot = right ventricular outflow tract, sp = spleen, spv = superior pulmonary vein, st = sternum, svc = superior vena cava, t = trachea, v = vertebral body.]

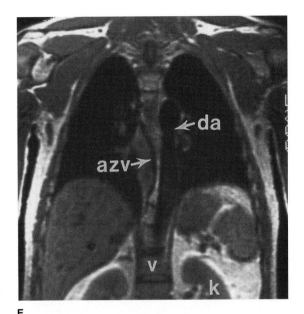

E

Fig. 4–5. *Cont.*

TECHNIQUE SELECTION

The number of diseases and clinical situations for which a chest radiograph may be indicated is so large that an exhaustive listing of individual indications is prohibitive. As a general rule, however, conventional radiographs should be obtained for any patient with symptoms suggesting disease of the heart, lungs, mediastinum, or chest wall. In addition, a chest radiograph is indicated for patients with systemic diseases that have a high likelihood of secondary involvement of those structures. Examples of the former are pneumonia and congestive heart failure and of the latter are a primary extrathoracic neoplasm and connective tissue disease.

In an acutely ill patient, the portable chest radiograph is an invaluable tool for monitoring the patient's cardiopulmonary status. These radiographs are also used for monitoring of life-support hardware, such as central venous access catheters, nasogastric tubes, and endotracheal tubes.

Fluoroscopy provides real-time imaging of the chest. Fluoroscopy may be used to evaluate the motion of the

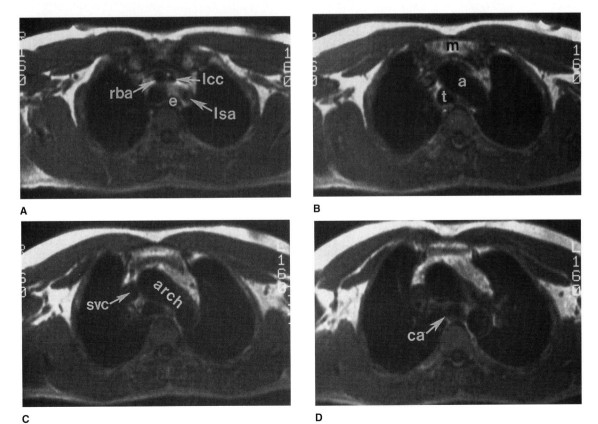

A

B

C

D

Fig. 4–6. Normal MR anatomy. Axial spin-echo images of the thorax. (See Fig. 4–5 for key.)

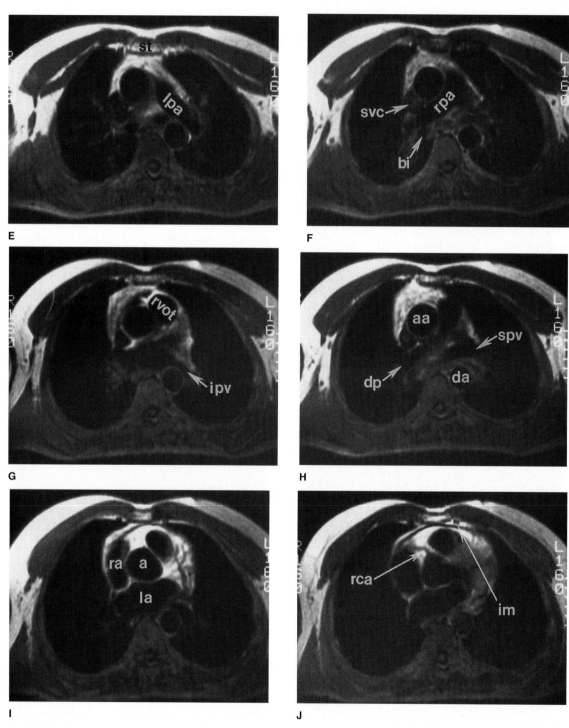

Fig. 4–6. *Cont.*

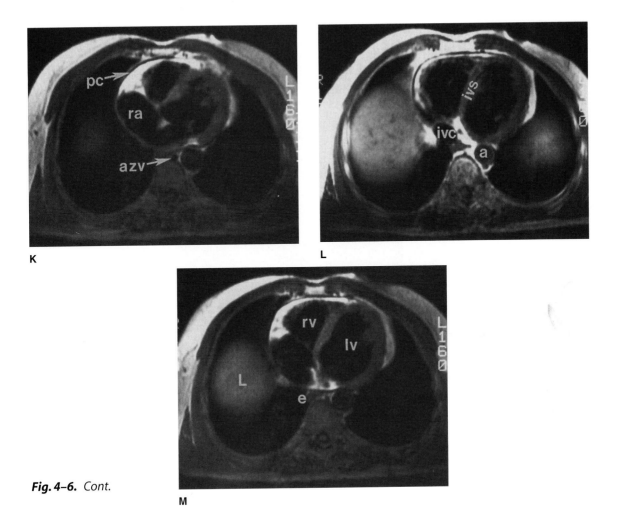

Fig. 4–6. *Cont.*

diaphragm in a patient with suspected diaphragmatic paralysis. A paralyzed hemidiaphragm has sluggish motion as the patient breathes, and as the patient takes in a quick breath of air, the air moves paradoxically upward as the normal hemidiaphragm moves downward ("sniff test"). Fluoroscopy and fluoroscopically positioned spot films are also useful for identification of calcification within a pulmonary nodule, within coronary arteries, or within cardiac valves. Fluoroscopic guidance is commonly used for percutaneous transthoracic needle biopsy of lung masses.

Because the three dimensions of the thorax are captured on a single two-dimensional chest radiograph, superimposition of structures within the thorax may result in confusing shadows. Because CT provides images without this overlap, it is frequently used to clarify confusing shadows identified on conventional radiographs (Table 4–1). These examinations are also used to detect disease that is

occult because of small size or a hidden position. Because of its wider range of density discrimination, CT can

TABLE 4–1. Indications for CT of the Chest

Clarification of abnormal chest radiograph findings
Staging of lung cancer and esophageal cancer
Detecting metastatic disease from extrathoracic malignancy
Evaluation of a solitary pulmonary nodule
Suspected mediastinal or hilar mass
Suspected pulmonary embolism
Evaluation of chronic pulmonary disease (thin-section or high-resolution CT)
Suspected pleural tumor or empyema
Determining source of hemoptysis (e.g., bronchiectasis)
CT-guided percutaneous needle aspiration of lung and mediastinal masses
CT-guided pleural drainage

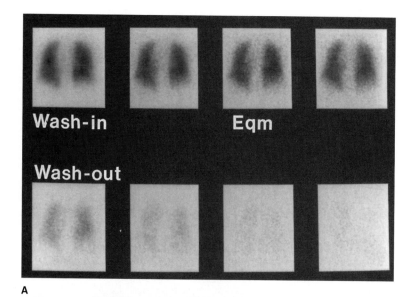

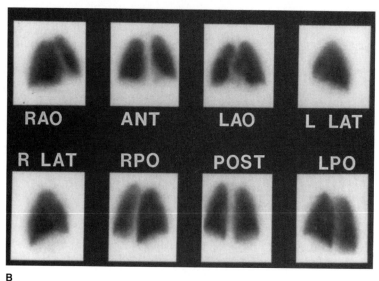

Fig. 4–7. A Ventilation scan performed in the posterior projection shows normal wash of the xenon-133 gas and no retention of gas in any regions on the wash-out views. Eqm = equilibrium. **B** Normal perfusion scans are performed in eight projections of equal profusion of radionuclide throughout all segments of the lungs. RAO = right anterior oblique, ANT = anterior, LAO = left anterior oblique, LLAT = left lateral, RLAT = right lateral, RPO = right posterior oblique, POST = posterior, and LPO = left posterior oblique.

demonstrate mediastinal and chest wall abnormalities earlier than is possible with conventional chest radiography. Abnormalities of hilar structures can be identified on CT scans because of the decreased overlap of the complex structures of the hilum. CT scans of the chest are routinely ordered for oncology patients, both for evaluation of the extent of disease at presentation and for monitoring response to therapy or progression of disease. CT is useful for evaluation of the lung parenchyma, because thin sections (1–2 mm thick) reveal great anatomic detail. Thin-section CT [or high-resolution CT (HRCT)] may enable detection of occult pulmonary parenchymal

disease and may be used for following the course of known pulmonary disease. Because intravenous contrast material may be administered, vascular structures may be evaluated and the technique may be useful in patients with aortic dissection, aortic aneurysm, and superior vena caval obstruction. Because the cost of CT is approximately 10 to 20 times that of a PA and lateral chest radiograph, CT is not practical for monitoring the course of diseases on a daily basis.

Ultrasonography is useful for imaging the soft tissues of the chest wall, heart, and pericardium, as well as fluid collections within the pleural space. Large,

TABLE 4–2. Indications for MR Imaging of the Chest

Evaluation of a mediastinal mass
Suspected Pancoast's (superior sulcus) tumor
Superior vena cava syndrome
Staging of lung cancer, when CT suggests invasion of the heart, great vessel, chest wall, diaphragm
Suspected aortic dissection
Evaluation of the mediastinum and hilum in patients with allergy to iodinated contrast media
Congenital and acquired heart disease

mobile pleural effusions are usually aspirated without sonographic guidance, since these collect predictably within dependent areas of the thorax. On the other hand, loculated pleural fluid collections may be difficult to aspirate without guidance, and the most appropriate entrance site may be marked with sonography for easier access. Ultrasonography has been used for guidance for biopsy of peripheral lung lesions as well.

MR imaging of the thorax is most commonly used for cardiovascular imaging, but there are indications for MR imaging in mediastinal and pulmonary parenchymal imaging as well (Table 4–2). MR is helpful when bronchogenic carcinoma is suspected of invading vascular structures, including the cardiac chambers, pulmonary arteries and veins, and the superior vena cava. In a patient with suspected Pancoast's (superior sulcus) tumor, MR imaging is preferred to CT because of the ability to obtain images in coronal and sagittal planes. The apex of the lung can be difficult to evaluate on axial images alone because of partial-volume effects.

The diseases and situations for which nuclear medicine techniques are helpful are determined for the most part by the radioactive tracer, and these have been outlined in the technique section (Table 4–3).

TABLE 4–3. Indications for Nuclear Medicine Imaging of the Chest

Suspected pulmonary thromboembolism (V/Q scan)
Staging of inflammatory disease (e.g., sarcoidosis) (gallium scan)
Detecting recurrence of lymphoma (gallium scan)
Detecting infection (indium-111–labeled WBC scan)
Differentiation of benign and malignant pulmonary nodule (PET)
Detecting recurrent or metastatic tumor (PET)

EXERCISES

EXERCISE 4-1: THE OPAQUE HEMITHORAX

Clinical Histories:

Case 4-1. A 40-year-old man with fever and dyspnea (Fig. 4–8)

Case 4-2. A 62-year-old man with dyspnea that increased over 2 days (Fig. 4–9)

Questions:

4-1. The most likely diagnosis for Case 4-1 is
   A. massive left pleural effusion.
   B. total atelectasis of the left lung.
   C. right pneumothorax.
   D. aplasia of the left lung.
   E. mediastinal hematoma.

4-2. The most likely diagnosis for Case 4-2 is
   A. left pleural effusion.
   B. collapse of the left lung.
   C. right pneumothorax.
   D. collapse of the right lung.
   E. mediastinal hematoma.

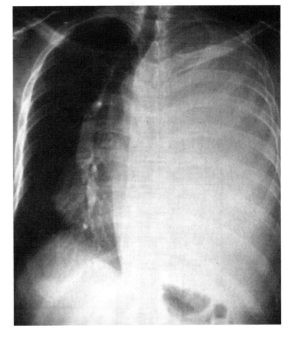

Fig. 4–8.

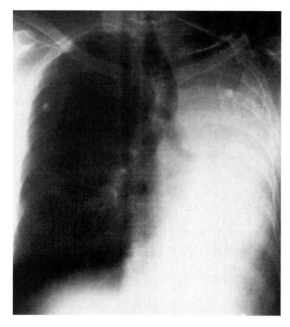

Fig. 4–9.

Radiologic Findings:

4-1. In this case, a frontal chest radiograph (Fig. 4–8) shows that the left hemithorax is opaque. Signs of mass effect are present and suggest a space-occupying lesion in the left hemithorax. There is shift of the mediastinum toward the *contralateral* hemithorax, as evidenced by shift of the trachea and right heart border to the right. If a nasogastric tube were in place, esophageal shift could be inferred from the shift of the nasogastric tube. Space-occupying lesions also cause inferior displacement of the hemidiaphragm. Although the diaphragm itself is not visible, when the process is on the left, one can infer that the diaphragm is depressed by the inferior displacement of the gastric air bubble. Mass effect may also widen the distance between ribs. In this patient, the space-occupying lesion was a large left pleural effusion resulting from tuberculous empyema. A chest CT scan (Fig. 4–10) in this patient shows the large pleural effusion and complete collapse of the underlying left lung against the medial aspect of the left hemithorax. (*A* is the correct answer to Question 4-1.)

4-2. In this case, a frontal chest radiograph (Fig. 4–9) shows that the left hemithorax is also opaque. In contrast to the patient in Fig. 4–8, the patient in Fig. 4–9 has signs of volume loss within the left hemithorax. There is mediastinal shift toward the *ipsilateral* hemithorax, as evidenced by shift of the trachea and the right heart border into the left hemithorax. If more air were visible within the stomach, one would expect that it would be higher in the left upper quadrant of the abdomen than is normally seen, because of elevation of the left hemidiaphragm. The mediastinal window of the chest CT examination (Fig. 4–11*A*) shows the mediastinal shift to the left and total consolidation of the left lung (*arrows*). There is a small left pleural effusion (*arrowheads*). The lung window of the chest CT examination (Fig. 4–11*B*) shows that the right lung is

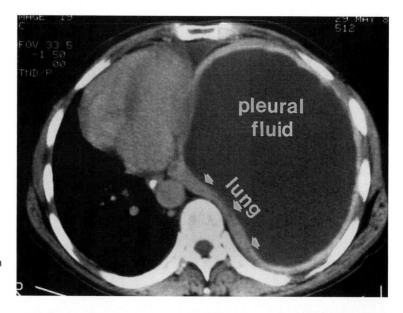

Fig. 4–10. Axial CT scan of the chest of the same patient as in Fig. 4–8 shows filling of the left pleural space by fluid, with compression of the left lung and displacement of the mediastinal contents into the right hemithorax. The pleural fluid in this case represented tuberculous empyema.

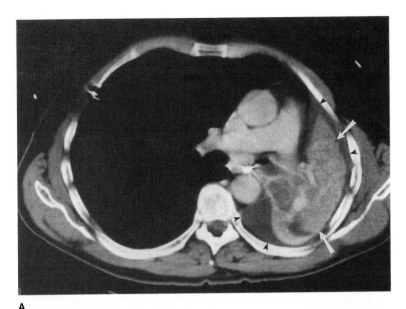

A

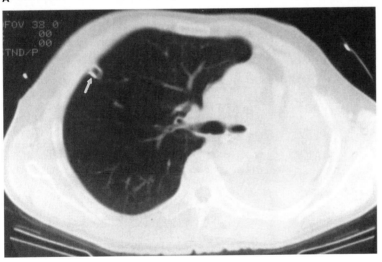

B

***Fig. 4–11.* A** CT scan of the same patient as in Fig. 4–9 shows mediastinal shift to the left, consolidation of the entire left lung (*arrows*), and small pleural effusion surrounding the left lung (*arrowheads*). **B** Lung window shows that the right lung is overexpanded to compensate for the left lung atelectasis. A right-sided chest tube (*arrow*) is noted incidentally.

aerated. In this patient, the left lung collapse is due to a bronchogenic carcinoma in the left main bronchus. This case exhibits the signs of volume loss, as opposed to mass effect. (*B* is the correct answer to Question 4-2.)

Discussion:

This exercise reviews the principal signs that allow one to distinguish mass effect from volume loss. The mass effect caused by a tumor or by a large pleural effusion expands the hemithorax and displaces the trachea, mediastinum, and diaphragm away from the mass. There

may be a subtle increase in the distance between ribs. Volume loss, on the other hand, decreases the size of the hemithorax, and the trachea, mediastinum, and diaphragm move toward the involved hemithorax. The distance between the ribs on the abnormal side will be slightly decreased. In both chest radiographs (Figs. 4–8 and 4–9) the left lung is collapsed. In Fig. 4–8, the opacification of the left hemithorax occurs as a result of massive left pleural effusion, and the left lung is collapsed as a result of both compression by the fluid present within the left pleural space and a loss of the negative intrapleural pressure that keeps the lung in close juxtaposition to the chest wall. In Fig. 4–9, the collapse is due to obstruction of the left main bronchus, resulting in atelectasis (airlessness) of the left lung.

EXERCISE 4-2: LOBAR ATELECTASIS

Clinical Histories:

Case 4-3. A 61-year-old woman with dyspnea (Fig. 4–12*A,B*)

Case 4-4. A 45-year-old woman with chronic cough (Fig. 4–13*A,B*)

Case 4-5. A 62-year-old man with a cough productive of blood-tinged sputum (Fig. 4–14*A,B*)

Case 4-6. A 49-year-old woman with cough (Fig. 4–15*A,B*)

Questions:

4-3. In Fig. 4–12*A,B*, the inferior margin of the opacity in the right upper thorax is due to the

   A. major fissure in RUL collapse without a hilar mass.

   B. minor fissure in RUL collapse with a hilar mass.

   C. minor fissure in RUL collapse without a hilar mass.

   D. major fissure in RUL collapse with a hilar mass.

4-4. In Fig. 4–13*A,B*, all of the following are true with regard to right middle lobe collapse except

   A. a triangular opacity is superimposed on the heart on the lateral radiograph.

   B. the right heart border is obscured.

   C. the minor fissure is inferiorly displaced.

   D. the right heart border is shifted to the left.

4-5. In Fig. 4–14*A,B*, signs of left lower lobe collapse include all of the following except

   A. obscuration of the lateral wall of the descending thoracic aorta.

   B. inferior displacement of the left hilum.

   C. obliteration of the posterior aspect of the left hemidiaphragm on the lateral view.

   D. triangular opacity in the left retrocardiac area on the frontal view.

   E. shift of the major fissure toward the anterior chest wall on the lateral view.

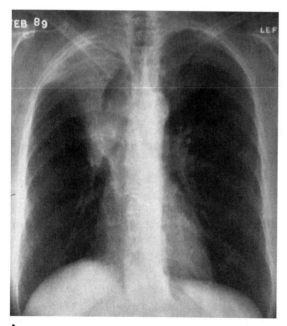

A

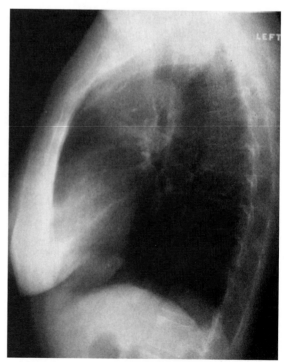

B

Fig. 4–12.

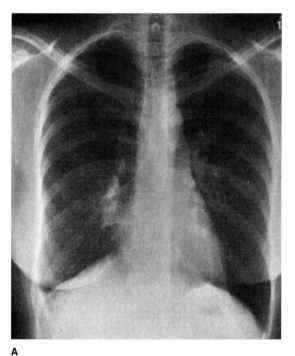

A

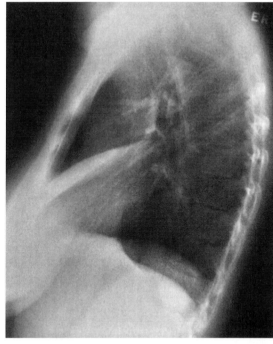

B

Fig. 4–13.

4-6. In Fig. 4–15*A,B,* signs of left upper lobe collapse include all of the following except

  A. crescent of air around the transverse section of the aortic arch resulting from hyperexpansion of the superior segment of the left lower lobe.

  B. anterior displacement of the left major fissure on the lateral view.

  C. obscuration of the left heart border.

  D. tracheal deviation to the left.

  E. inferior displacement of the left hilum.

Radiologic Findings:

4-3. In Fig. 4–12, there is opacity in the right upper lung that is sharply marginated on its inferior border. Volume loss is evidenced by the slight displacement of the trachea into the right hemithorax, the position of the right heart border further to the right of the thoracic spine than normal, and the slight elevation of the right hemidiaphragm, which is normally 1 to 1.5 cm higher than the left hemithorax. The pulmonary vessels of the right hilum are obscured by opacity in the right upper thorax. The configuration of the inferior margin of the opacity is that of a reverse S or an S on its side. The S sign of Golden describes

the appearance of the minor fissure in right upper lobe collapse, which is due to bronchogenic carcinoma. In this case, bulky right hilar lymph node enlargement has caused extrinsic compression of the right upper lobe bronchus and has resulted in right upper lobe collapse. The right hilar mass tethers the medial aspect of the minor fissure to its normal midthoracic position, whereas the lateral aspect of the minor fissure moves freely and collapses superiorly. In patients in whom the minor fissure is incomplete, collateral air drift across the canals of Lambert and the pores of Kohn may allow a lobe to remain aerated despite complete obstruction of its bronchus. In Fig. 4–12*A,* hyperexpansion of the superior segment of the right lower lobe produces the ovoid lucency on the medial aspect of the collapsed right upper lobe. On the lateral radiograph, a V-shaped opacity is seen at the lung apex. A mass-like opacity is superimposed on the suprahilar area, corresponding to a combination of tumor and atelectatic lung. (*B* is the correct answer to Question 4-3.) In patients with right upper lobe collapse without a hilar mass, the fissure is able to rotate in a more straight line and does not result in the reverse S sign. The major fissure is oriented in a coronal plane and is not normally visualized on the frontal chest radiograph. Therefore, the major fissure would not account for the opacity seen on the frontal chest radiograph, either with or without a hilar mass.

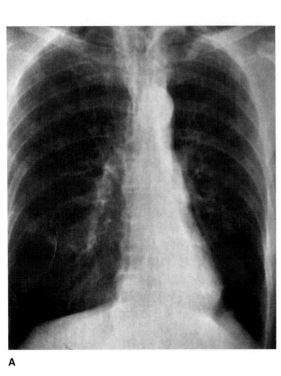

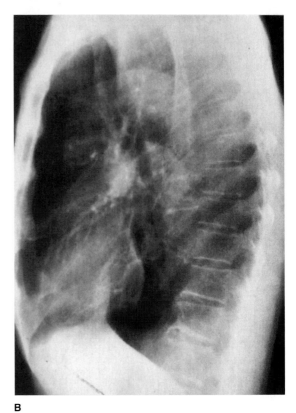

A

B

Fig. 4–14.

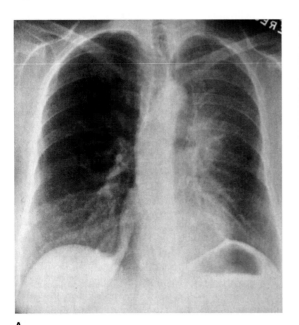

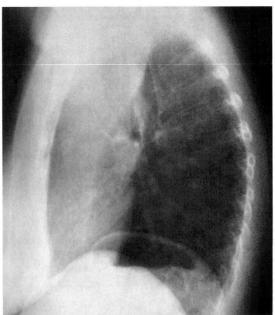

A

B

Fig. 4–15.

4-4. In Fig. 4–13*A,B,* the right heart border is obscured by adjacent opacity on the PA radiograph. The heart is in the midthorax in approximately its normal position. The heart border has not been displaced to the left. On the lateral radiograph, a narrow triangular opacity is superimposed on the heart. The apex of the triangle points toward the hilum, and the base of the triangle is against the anterior chest wall. This is a collapsed right middle lobe. The right hemidiaphragm is slightly elevated, but there are no other signs of volume loss. Right middle lobe collapse may have minimal impact on the overall volume in the right hemithorax because it is the smallest of the pulmonary lobes, and the upper and lower lobes can expand to compensate for its volume loss. Right middle lobe collapse, unlike other lobar collapse, is often due to benign causes and results from extrinsic pressure because of enlarged lymph nodes, which totally surround the bronchus. This enlargement is most frequently due to granulomatous disease of an infectious or noninfectious nature. (*D* is the correct answer to Question 4-4.)

4-5. When the left lower lobe collapses, the result is a triangular opacity, which can be quite subtle, behind the heart. Secondary signs of volume loss, however, should prompt one to look closely for the collapse. These signs include shift of the trachea and heart to the left (note that the right heart border is now superimposed on the thoracic spine), inferior displacement of the left hilum, and elevation of the left hemidiaphragm. On the lateral radiograph, the right hemidiaphragm is visible along its entire contour. However, the left hemidiaphragm is obscured posteriorly because it is "silhouetted" by the collapsed left lower lobe. Because it is tethered medially by the inferior pulmonary ligament, the left lower lobe collapses posteriorly and medially (Fig. 4–16). The major fissure is displaced *posteriorly*, as well as rotated into a more sagittal orientation than the normal coronal orientation. All of the statements in Question 4-5 are correct except shift of the major fissure toward the *anterior* chest wall on the lateral view. (*E* is the correct answer to Question 4-5.) You may have noted the large lung volumes in this patient, which are due to centrilobular emphysema. In this patient, who has a long history of cigarette smoking, a squamous cell carcinoma in the left lower lobe bronchus was responsible for the collapsed left lower lobe.

4-6. The primary sign of volume loss in Fig. 4–15*B* is anterior displacement of the left major fissure on the lateral radiograph. The collapsed left upper lobe is opaque as a result of both airlessness and postobstructive pneumonitis. When there is little pneumonitis within the obstructed lobe, the left upper lobe can collapse completely behind the anterior chest wall, so that only a narrow band of opacity is visible behind the sternum. In this situation, the diagnosis may be suggested by the secondary signs of volume loss. Note the shift of the trachea to the left and the slight elevation of the left hemidiaphragm. The left lower lobe is hyperexpanded. The hyperexpanded superior segment of the left lower lobe produces a crescent of air around the transverse section of the aortic arch on the PA radiograph. A thin opaque line is visible at the apex of the left hemidiaphragm on the PA radiograph. Presence of this line, called a *juxtaphrenic peak,* should prompt one to look for upper lobe collapse. The hilum may be displaced anteriorly in left upper lobe collapse, but it is never displaced inferiorly. Option *E,* inferior displacement of the left hilum, is

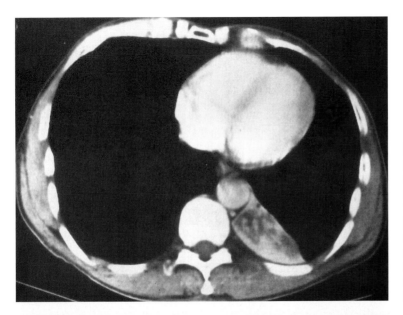

Fig. 4–16. Axial CT scan of the same patient as in Fig. 4–14 shows a triangular mass within the postero-medial aspect of the left hemithorax. This represents the collapsed left lower lobe. The branching areas of decreased attenuation within the mass represent mucoid impaction within the obstructed bronchi. Note the shift of the heart toward the left hemithorax.

therefore false. (*E* is the correct answer to Question 4-6.) Since the lingular bronchus arises from the left upper lobe bronchus, the lingular segment of the left upper lobe is collapsed as well in this patient. The lingula is adjacent to the left heart border and is responsible for the obscuration of the left heart border in left upper lobe collapse.

Discussion:

The term *atelectasis* refers to volume loss, or airlessness, within the lung. The term *collapse* is often used to describe complete atelectasis of an entire lobe or an entire lung. Atelectasis can occur as a result of several pathophysiologic processes. Obstruction of a bronchus by bronchogenic carcinoma should always be considered in an adult with lobar atelectasis. The tumor may be within the bronchus (endobronchial), as occurs with squamous cell carcinoma or small cell undifferentiated carcinoma. The tumor may be outside the bronchus, and enlarged lymph nodes may cause extrinsic compression of the bronchus. In a child, aspiration of a foreign body is a more likely cause of obstruction of a bronchus. Complete obstruction of a lobar bronchus may not always result in lobar collapse because pathways of collateral ventilation are present within the lung. The pores of Kohn and the canals of Lambert allow collateral air drift between adjacent areas of lung but do not extend across pleural surfaces. The visceral pleural surface that covers the lung creates the interlobar fissures (minor fissure, major fissure) that separate lobes of the lungs. These fissures are not always complete, however, and may not extend entirely across the lung. When the right upper lobe bronchus is occluded, for example, the right upper lobe may remain partially aerated as a result of collateral air drift from the right middle lobe, around an incomplete minor fissure. Obstruction of smaller airways can occur as a result of mucous plugs, which are often present in intubated patients and in patients with chronic small airway disease.

Passive atelectasis occurs as a result of a space-occupying process within the pleural space. This is also called *relaxation atelectasis,* since the lung is no longer exposed to the negative intrapleural pressure that normally keeps the lung apposed to the chest wall. Any space-occupying pleural process, including a large pneumothorax (air in the pleural space), pleural effusion, hemothorax (blood in the pleural space), or pleural tumor can cause atelectasis within the underlying lung. *Compressive atelectasis* is the term used to describe atelectasis caused by a space-occupying process within the lung itself. *Cicatrization atelectasis* describes the volume loss that occurs as a result of pulmonary scarring. *Adhesive atelectasis* occurs when there is a loss of the pulmonary surfactant that maintains the surface tension that keeps alveoli open. *Adhesive atelectasis* occurs with pulmonary embolism and with respiratory distress syndrome of the newborn. Atelectasis of small areas of lung is often referred to as *subsegmental atelectasis* and may be recognized as linear bands of opacity, often at the lung bases.

It is helpful to remember the normal positions of the hemidiaphragms, trachea, mediastinum, and hila so that displacement of these structures can be readily noted. In most patients, the left hilum appears slightly higher than the right, since the left hilar opacity is predominantly due to the left pulmonary artery arching over the left main bronchus. The right hemidiaphragm is usually 1.0 to 1.5 cm higher than the left hemidiaphragm. The trachea should be in the midline, and the spinous processes of the upper thoracic vertebrae should be superimposed on the center of the tracheal air column. The right heart border normally lies just to the right of the thoracic spine. Subtle signs of volume loss may be more readily appreciated by comparison of the patient's radiograph with baseline radiographs taken previously.

EXERCISE 4-3: AIRSPACE DISEASES

Clinical Histories:

Case 4-7. A 32-year-old man with fever, cough, and hemoptysis (Fig. 4–17*A,B*)

Case 4-8. A 57-year-old man with fever and a cough productive of purulent sputum (Fig. 4–18*A,B*)

Questions:

4-7. Which of the following is not an accurate descriptor of the opacity in the left upper lobe in Fig. 4–17*A,B*?

    A. Lobar distribution

    B. Ill-defined margins

    C. Reticular pattern

    D. Air bronchograms

    E. Airspace disease

4-8. For Fig. 4–18, which one of the following best explains the opacity in the left hemithorax?

    A. Collapse of the left upper lobe due to bronchial obstruction

    B. Airspace consolidation of the lingula

    C. Empyema loculated within the left major fissure

    D. Carcinoma in the left upper lobe

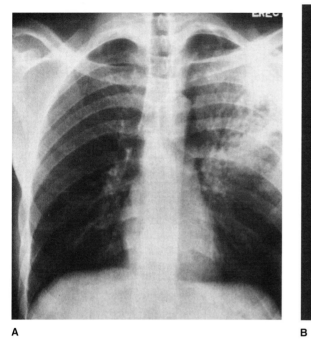

A

Fig. 4–17.

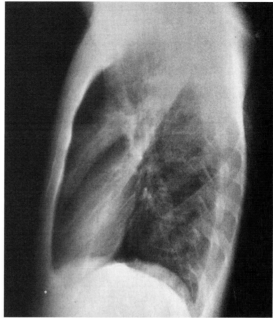

B

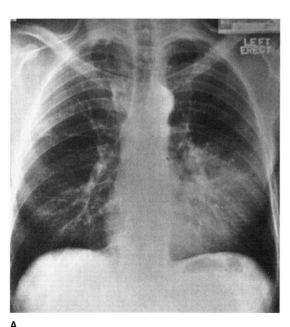

A

Fig. 4–18.

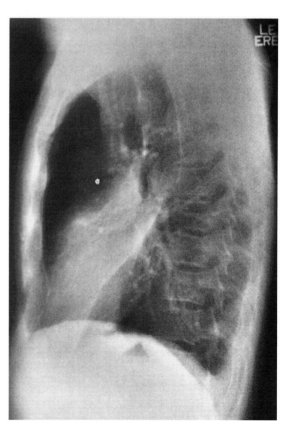

B

Radiologic Findings:

Both of these patients have opacity in the left upper lobe.

4-7. In this case (Fig. 4–17), the opacity is in the upper lung and obscures the margin of the aortic arch. The opacity extends down to the hilum but does not obscure the left heart border. (*C* is the correct answer to Question 4-7; see discussion.)

4-8. In this case (Fig. 4–18), the opacity is lower in the hemithorax and obscures the lateral margin of the heart. On the lateral view of each patient, the posterior margin is sharply demarcated by the major fissure, indicating the lobar nature of the process. Radiolucent structures that exhibit a branching pattern are noted to arborize through both opacities. (*B* is the correct answer to Question 4-8; see discussion.)

Discussion:

The patient in Fig. 4–17 has primary tuberculosis (*Mycobacterium tuberculosis*), manifested as pneumonia in the anterior and apicoposterior segments of the left upper lobe. The patient in Fig. 4–18 has pneumococcal pneumonia (*Streptococcus pneumoniae*) in the superior and inferior lingula segments of the left upper lobe. The opacity seen on both radiographs is best described as airspace disease. The alveoli, or airspaces, that are normally filled with air have become filled with exudate. The exudate-filled alveoli surround the bronchi, so that the air-filled bronchi are visible as radiolucent branching structures within the more radiopaque background (Fig. 4–19). Airspace disease is often either lobar, multilobar, or diffuse in distribution. The process may initially appear as multiple ill-defined nodules that rapidly coalesce. These nodules are the shadows of fluid-filled acini. They are 6 to 10 mm in diameter and always have ill-defined margins. The margins of these coalescing opacities are difficult to outline. Although there can be associated volume loss as the surfactant within the alveoli is lost, the signs of volume loss are often subtle and do not account for the opacity seen within the lung. Once airspace disease is identified, an attempt should be made to determine its cause. Airspace disease that appears suddenly or exhibits change over hours to days is due either to pulmonary hemorrhage or to contusion, pneumonia, or pulmonary edema (blood, pus, or water). The patient's clinical history, physical examination, and laboratory data help to determine the most likely diagnosis. In patients likely to have infectious disorders, the responsible organism is usually not identified at first treatment, and the patient is just given antibiotics. In patients who do not respond to this initial treatment, an attempt should be made to identify the organism.

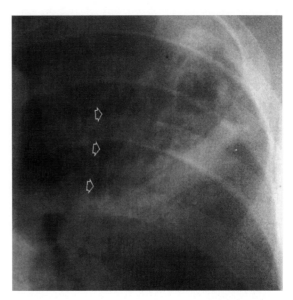

Fig. 4–19. Close-up view of the left upper lobe of the same patient as in Fig. 4–17 shows an ill-defined infiltrate, which is radiopaque. Arborizing through this opacity are radiolucent branching structures representing the air-filled bronchi (air bronchograms) (*arrows*).

In these two patients with fever and productive cough, pneumonia is likely. On the other hand, a patient with rib or sternal fractures as a result of blunt chest trauma is more likely to have pulmonary contusion. Pulmonary edema, which may occur as a result of either cardiogenic or noncardiogenic disease, is discussed later in this chapter.

A reticular pattern is one in which the opacities are linear in nature and the lines range from quite thin to several millimeters thick. The opacities are oriented in multiple directions and appear to overlap so as to create the appearance of a net. This pattern is not present.

EXERCISE 4-4: DIFFUSE LUNG INFILTRATES

Clinical History:

Case 4-9. A 69-year-old man with progressive dyspnea, orthopnea, and pedal edema and a history of hypertension (Fig. 4–20)

Question:

4-9. Which of the following best describes the chest radiograph in Fig. 4–20?

    A. Normal heart size, alveolar pulmonary edema

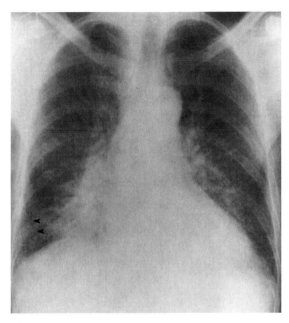

Fig. 4–20.

B. Cardiomegaly, interstitial pulmonary edema, and small bilateral pleural effusions

C. Unilateral interstitial disease

D. Cardiomegaly, oligemia in the right lung

Radiologic Findings:

4-9. Frontal chest radiograph (Fig. 4–20) shows mild enlargement of the heart and indistinct vascularity, particularly at the lower lungs. Interlobular septal lines (*arrowheads*) are visible adjacent to both lower costophrenic angles.

Discussion:

Pulmonary edema can be divided into two major categories: *cardiogenic edema* and *noncardiogenic edema*. Cardiogenic edema occurs as a result of elevation of pulmonary capillary pressure, which is usually due to pulmonary venous hypertension. Noncardiogenic edema occurs as a result of disorders that increase pulmonary capillary permeability. With both types of edema, there is a net movement of fluid out of the microvasculature and into the pulmonary interstitium and alveoli. The most common cause of pulmonary edema is left ventricular failure, which may be due to atherosclerotic coronary artery disease, mitral or aortic valvular disease, myocarditis, or cardiomyopathy. Cardiogenic edema is preceded by pulmonary venous hypertension, which is associated with redistribution of pulmonary blood flow from dependent regions of the lung to nondependent regions. In the erect patient, the radiographic sign of this redistribution is an increase in size of vessels in the upper lungs and a decrease in the caliber of pulmonary vessels in the lung bases. Radiographically, it is often difficult to distinguish pulmonary arteries from pulmonary veins, but for purposes of determination of flow redistribution, the distinction is ignored and multiple vessels are measured at equal distances from the hilum or chest wall.

When seen end-on, normal bronchoarterial bundles may appear as adjacent circles of equal diameter, with the artery opaque and the bronchus lucent. The pulmonary arteries and bronchi are located together in the same interstitial space and arborize adjacent to each other. The pulmonary veins return blood to the heart in a separate interstitial space and have a slightly different arborization pattern. As the pulmonary venous pressure increases, fluid leaks from the pulmonary capillaries into the adjacent interstitium. This interstitial pulmonary edema may be identified by peribronchial cuffing, indistinctness of the perivascular margins, perihilar haziness, and thickening of the interlobular septa and interlobar fissures. As the pulmonary capillary pressure increases further, fluid spills into the alveoli, producing a symmetrical appearance of airspace filling that is predominantly perihilar (central) and basilar in distribution. Cardiogenic edema is greatest in dependent regions of the lungs. In supine patients, the dependent regions are the posterior segments of the upper lobes, and the superior and posterior basilar segments of the lower lobes. The central pattern of pulmonary edema has been called "bat wing" edema. As the pulmonary edema worsens, the pulmonary and pleural lymphatics clear fluid from the lungs, and pleural effusions will develop. In congestive heart failure, the pleural effusions are generally small to moderate in size, and there is typically more fluid within the right pleural space than the left. Isolated left pleural effusion is unlikely to be due to congestive heart failure. In cardiogenic edema, the heart size will be increased. The cardiothoracic ratio is a guide to determining cardiac enlargement. The transverse dimension of the heart is divided by the transverse diameter of the thorax at the same level. When the cardiothoracic ratio is greater than 0.5, cardiomegaly is often (but not always) present. When possible, both the PA and lateral projections should be used to determine cardiac volume. Cardiomegaly may be more readily recognized when comparison is made with prior radiographs. Comparison requires a similar depth of inspiration and similar positioning of the patient (AP versus PA, supine versus erect).

Noncardiogenic edema, or "capillary leak" edema, may be due to a number of conditions, including adult respiratory distress syndrome, fat embolism, amniotic fluid embolism, drug overdose, near drowning, and acute airway obstruction. The cause of pulmonary edema in patients with intracranial injury or tumor (neurogenic pulmonary edema) is uncertain. Similarly, the etiology of high-altitude pulmonary edema is incompletely understood. The common radiographic findings in noncardiogenic edema are symmetric, diffuse areas of airspace filling that is often patchier in appearance and more peripheral in distribution. The heart size is usually normal; pleural effusions and septal lines are typically absent.

Renal failure and volume overload may result in pulmonary edema, which may be chronic. When the amount of edema is small to moderate, patients are often reasonably well compensated and are able to carry out many activities of daily living.

EXERCISE 4-5: AIRWAY DISEASE

Clinical History:

Case 4-10.   A 22-year-old man who has had chronic cough and copious mucous production since childhood (Fig. 4–21A,B)

Question:

4-10.   All of the following are accurate descriptors of his chest radiograph except

  A.   increased lung volume.
  B.   thickened bronchovascular bundles.
  C.   enlargement of the hila.
  D.   right paratracheal lymphadenopathy.
  E.   tram-track lines.

Radiologic Findings:

4-10. In this case, the most prominent radiographic finding in Fig. 4–21A is coarse thickening of the bronchovascular bundles as they radiate from the hila. Thickened bronchial walls may be identified as tram-track lines in the left lower lobe behind the heart and just medial and caudal to the interlobar pulmonary artery on the right. Tram-track lines refer to the appearance of the nearly parallel walls of bronchi oriented longitudinally. Careful inspection shows that these are present throughout both lungs and are located near the hila. Bronchial walls also project as ring-shaped opacities near the hila. (Note that one projects into the middle of

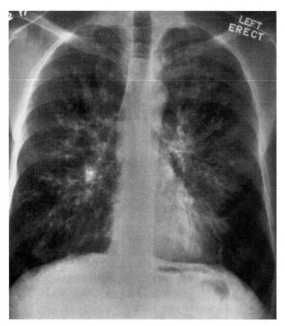

A

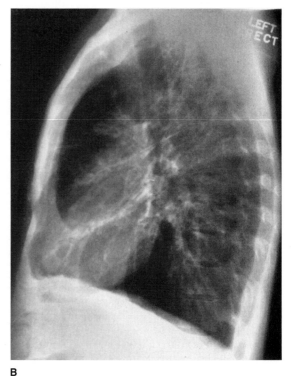

B

Fig. 4–21.

the left interlobar pulmonary artery.) Both of these structures represent the thick walls of dilated bronchi (bronchiectasis). The hila themselves are slightly enlarged as a result of a combination of enlarged hilar lymph nodes and mild pulmonary arterial hypertension. The lung volume is significantly increased. The diaphragms are flatter than normal, especially on the lateral radiograph. The anterior clear space (retrosternal area) is larger and more radiolucent than normal. The right paratracheal stripe, on the other hand, is normal, and there is no evidence of right paratracheal lymphadenopathy. (*D* is the correct answer to Question 4-10.)

Discussion:

The cause of this patient's bronchiectasis is cystic fibrosis. The mucus in patients with cystic fibrosis is thickened, and these patients do not have normal tracheobronchial clearance. This abnormal clearance may cause mucoid impaction, and atelectasis and pneumonia are frequent complications. Bronchiectasis can also occur as a result

of pneumonia in patients without cystic fibrosis. In these patients, the bronchiectasis is more likely to be confined to a single lobe, often a lower lobe. Bronchiectasis is divided into three groups: cylindrical, fusiform (or varicose), and saccular (or cystic). These three groups not only describe the appearance of the abnormal bronchi, but also give an indication as to its severity. *Cylindrical bronchiectasis,* the mildest form, is reversible, and appears as thick-walled bronchi that fail to taper normally. The more severe forms, *fusiform* and *saccular,* are irreversible. *Fusiform bronchiectasis* has a beaded appearance, whereas the bronchi in *saccular bronchiectasis* end with clubbed, cystic areas. If the severe forms are localized, surgical resection may be curative. Medical therapy with bronchodilator and, when necessary, antibiotics is used when surgery is not indicated.

Bronchography was formerly the standard method of diagnosing bronchiectasis (Fig. 4–22*A,B*). Currently, CT is the method of choice for determining the presence and extent of bronchiectasis. It has the advantages of being less invasive and more readily tolerated by the

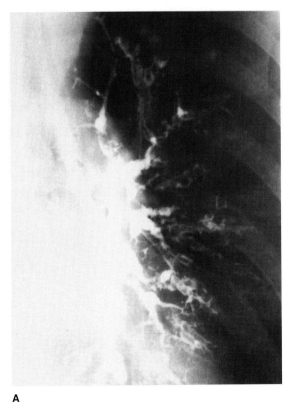

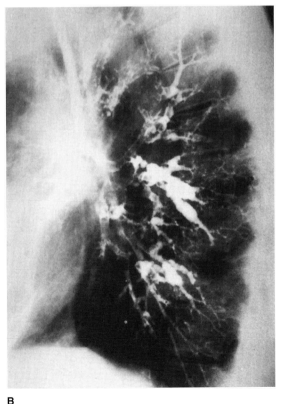

A   **B**

Fig. 4–22. Frontal **A** and lateral **B** views of a bronchogram shows bronchi in the left lung that are beaded and dilated, rather than smoothly tapering.

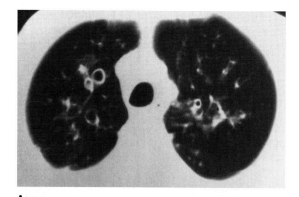

A

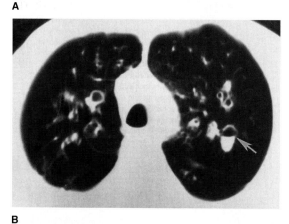

B

C

Fig. 4–23. Axial CT images **A,B** (lung window settings) of the same patient as in Fig. 4–21 show multiple dilated, thick-walled bronchi. Air-fluid levels (*arrow*) are present within areas of cystic bronchiectasis with cystic fibrosis. At the lung bases **C,** thick-walled bronchi are seen longitudinally (*arrowhead*) as they remain within the imaging plane.

patient. When the bronchus is perpendicular to the CT plane of section, bronchiectasis is identified as ring shadows adjacent to an opaque circle. The ring represents the thickened, dilated bronchial walls. The opaque circles represent the pulmonary artery adjacent to the dilated bronchus. Images from the patient show a combination of varicose and cystic bronchiectasis (Fig. 4–23A, B). When the bronchus lies within the plane of section of the CT scan, the dilated bronchial walls project as roughly parallel lines near a vessel (Fig. 4–23C).

EXERCISE 4-6: SOLITARY PULMONARY NODULE

Clinical History:

Case 4-11. A 53-year-old man scheduled for coronary artery bypass grafting; Close-up view of left upper lobe from a preoperative chest radiograph is shown (Fig. 4–24).

Question:

4-11. Characteristics suggesting that a nodule is benign are

    A. size of the nodule does not change over 2 years.

    B. it contains central calcification.

    C. CT attenuation values within the nodule are greater than 200 Hounsfield units (Hu).

    D. all of the above.

Radiologic Findings:

4-11. Close-up view in Fig. 4–24 of the left upper lobe shows a nodule that is smoothly marginated and has a region of central opacity, indicating a calcified central nidus.

Discussion:

Bronchogenic carcinoma, particularly adenocarcinoma, frequently presents as a solitary pulmonary nodule in the periphery of the lung. A new solitary pulmonary nodule or nodule of indeterminate age, therefore, should be considered a possible malignancy. The most common cause of a solitary pulmonary nodule is a granuloma, typically the result of prior granulomatous infection, such as tuberculosis or histoplasmosis. These can frequently be identified as granulomata because of characteristic patterns of calcification.

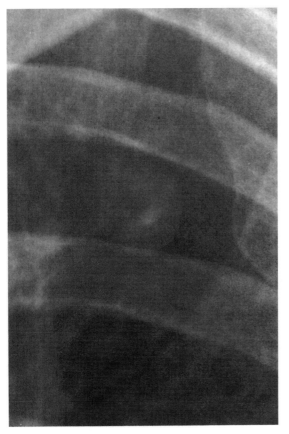

Fig. 4–24.

In attempting to determine whether or not a nodule is benign, the characteristics to consider are the age of the patient, any history of previous malignancy, and the nodule's growth rate, density, shape, and edge characteristics. The most important of these are the growth rate and density. If a nodule has had no growth over a 2-year period and has calcification of the types associated with benign causes, then the nodule is almost certainly benign. Because of the importance of time in assessing growth, comparison with old films is the most important test and the least expensive method of determining whether a nodule is benign. A 2-year interval is approximately four doubling times for an average lung carcinoma; therefore, an increase in diameter of one-third to one-half of the nodule would be expected. The absence of growth over a 2-year period is evidence that the nodule is stable is size and must, therefore, be benign. If radiographs demonstrate growth over this 2-year interval, then the nodule should be assumed to be malignant.

If the nodule is diffusely and completely calcified (Fig. 4–25), if it is calcified centrally (Fig. 4–26), or if it has a laminated pattern (Fig. 4–27), then the nodule may be assumed to be benign. Calcification may not be apparent on the initial radiograph because the most commonly used technique for chest radiography obscures subtle calcification. Demonstration of calcification may require fluoroscopy or repeated chest radiography with low kVp (kiloVoltage* peak) technique to enhance its depiction. When it is not clear from these studies whether calcification is present, CT should be

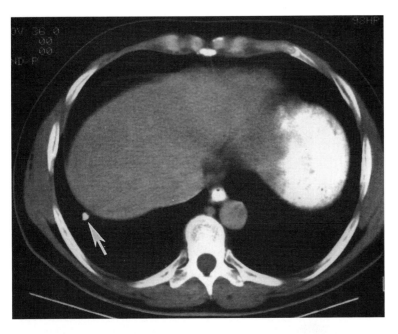

Fig. 4–25. CT scan at a level through the lower lungs shows a nodule (*arrow*) that is completely calcified. Note that the density of the nodule is equal to that of bone.

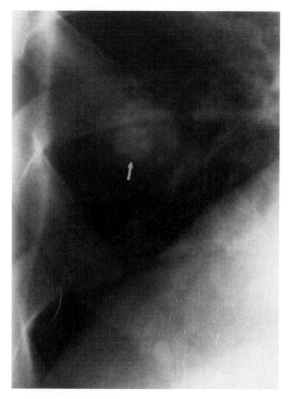

Fig. 4–26. Close-up view of the right lower lung shows a nodule with soft-tissue density and a central nidus of increased density representing a calcified central nidus (*arrow*).

used to identify it. CT has an extended range of tissue discrimination in comparison to plain films. The presence of calcification within a pulmonary nodule can be determined by evaluating the attenuation values within a region of interest (ROI) centered over the nodule (Fig. 4–28A–C). Air within the lung measures −800 Hu, noncalcified nodules measure 30 to 100 HU, and calcified nodules measure greater than 200 HU. Nodules with somewhat dense calcification can be easily identified, but subtle amounts of calcification may require a special phantom for accurate determination. Nodules with attenuation values between 0 and 200 are not necessarily malignant; they just do not have enough calcification to be categorized unequivocally as benign.

If a nodule is not calcified or if it has shown growth over a 2-year period, it should be considered as a possible malignancy and further assessment should be dictated by the clinical circumstances. Most patients will need evaluation for possible surgical resection and tissue biopsy to determine the cause.

Note that the margins of the lesion, whether smooth or spiculated, are of no value in determining the benignity or malignant potential of a lesion. Only uniform or central calcification, absence of growth over a 2-year period, or CT attenuation values greater than 200 HU throughout the nodule are reliable noninvasive indicators of benignity. (*D* is the correct answer to Question 4-11.)

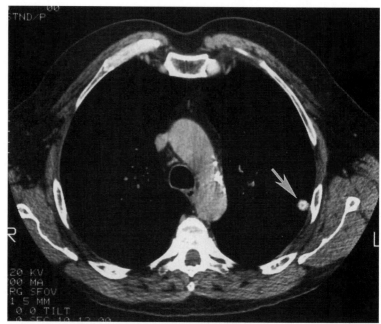

Fig. 4–27. CT scan at the level of the aortic arch shows a nodule in the left lung that has laminar calcification and central and peripheral soft-tissue density (*arrow*).

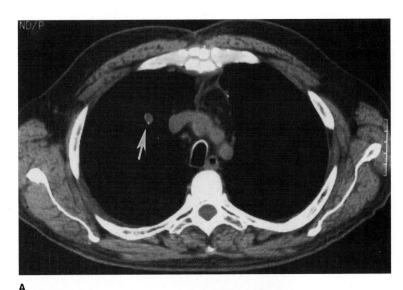

Fig. 4–28. A CT scan just above the aortic arch shows a nodule in the right upper lobe (*arrow*) with at least two eccentric regions of calcification. **B** A region of interest has been drawn on the nodule (*arrow*).

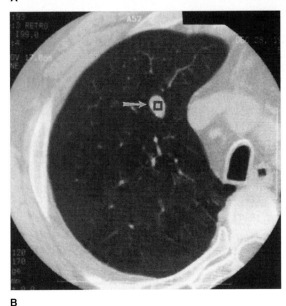

B

EXERCISE 4-7: PULMONARY NEOPLASM

Clinical History:

Case 4-12. A 64-year-old man with cough and weight loss and a 50-pack-per-year history of tobacco use (Fig. 4–29*A,B*)

Question:

4-12. The best description of the chest radiograph in Fig. 4-29*A,B* is
    A.   mass in the left upper lobe.
    B.   left upper lobe collapse.
    C.   mediastinal mass.
    D.   consolidation of the left upper lobe.
    E.   enlargement of the left pulmonary artery.

Radiologic Findings:

4-12. In this case, the chest radiographs show a round opacity projecting just laterally and cephalad to the left hilum. Because the medial margin of the opacity can be seen, a mediastinal mass is excluded. The left pulmonary artery can be seen through the opacity and is normal in size. On the lateral view the opacity maintains a round shape and projects over the anterior portion of the chest. The opacity is smaller than the volume of the left upper lobe, and no air bronchograms are present; this excludes consolidation of the lung as an answer. The posterior margin of the opacity is not a long straight or gently curving line, as is the major fissure, and therefore left upper lobe atelectasis is not the correct answer. The one best description of the radiographic findings is mass in the left upper lobe. (*A* is the correct answer to Question 4-12.) In a patient with cough, weight loss, and a history of tobacco use, bronchogenic carcinoma should be

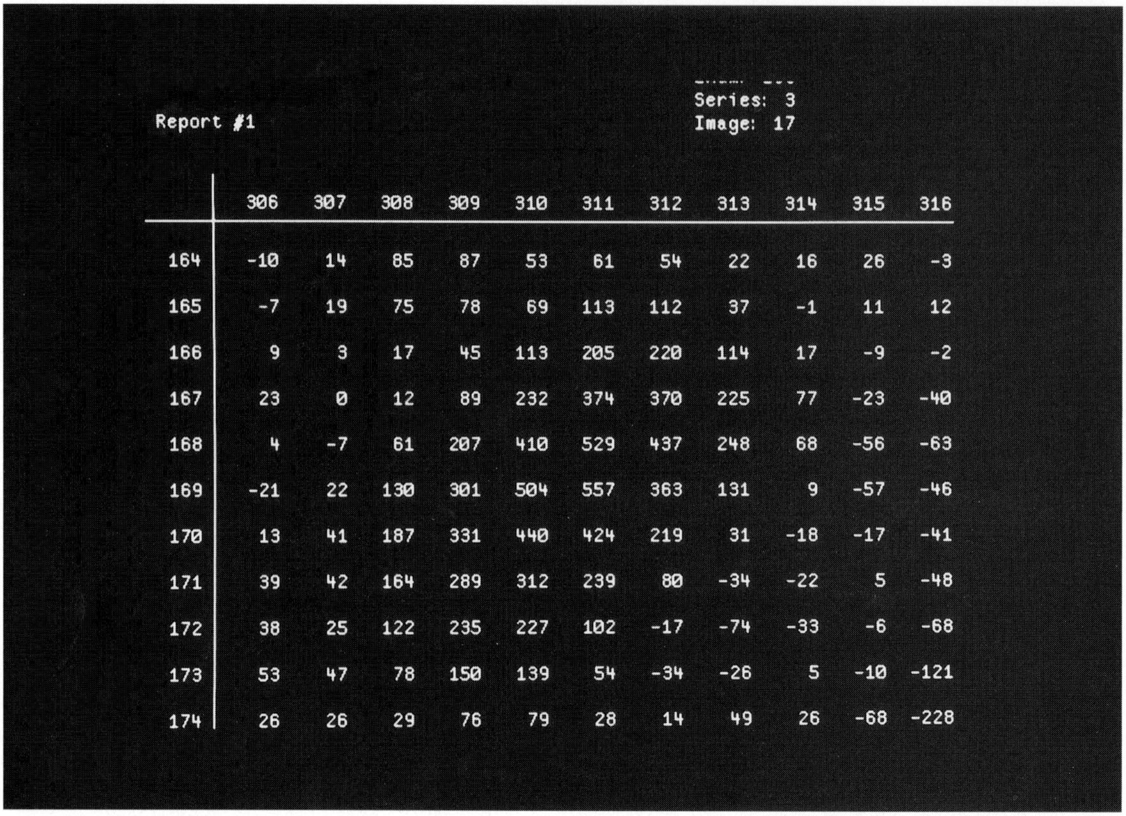

Report #1

Series: 3
Image: 17

	306	307	308	309	310	311	312	313	314	315	316
164	-10	14	85	87	53	61	54	22	16	26	-3
165	-7	19	75	78	69	113	112	37	-1	11	12
166	9	3	17	45	113	205	220	114	17	-9	-2
167	23	0	12	89	232	374	370	225	77	-23	-40
168	4	-7	61	207	410	529	437	248	68	-56	-63
169	-21	22	130	301	504	557	363	131	9	-57	-46
170	13	41	187	331	440	424	219	31	-18	-17	-41
171	39	42	164	289	312	239	80	-34	-22	5	-48
172	38	25	122	235	227	102	-17	-74	-33	-6	-68
173	53	47	78	150	139	54	-34	-26	5	-10	-121
174	26	26	29	76	79	28	14	49	26	-68	-228

C

Fig. 4–28. C The Hounsfield units in each pixel in the ROI are demonstrated. Note the very high numbers in the central portion of the lesion, indicating calcification within those pixels.

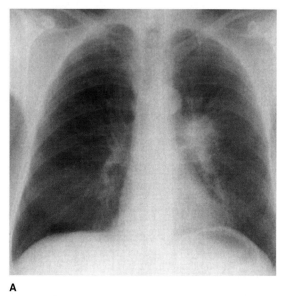

A

Fig. 4–29.

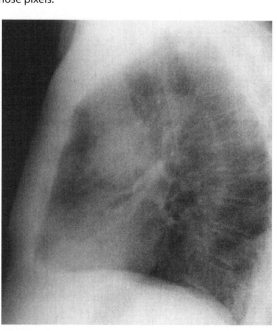

B

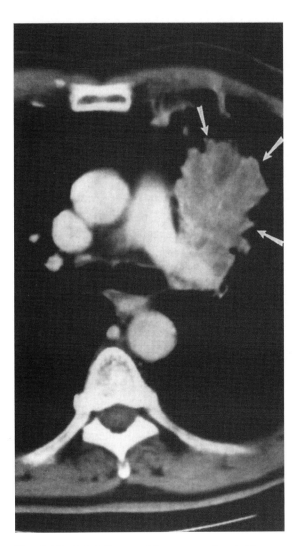

Fig. 4–30. Axial CT scan of the same patient in Fig. 4–29 (mediastinal window setting) shows a lobulated mass (*arrows*) within the left upper lobe. The fact that the mass is adjacent to the left pulmonary artery explains why the left hilum is somewhat obscured on the chest radiograph.

the primary consideration. A CT examination in this patient (Fig. 4–30) shows the mass in the anterior segment of the left upper lobe, which is contiguous with the superior left hilum. A CT-guided percutaneous biopsy of this mass was positive for squamous cell carcinoma.

Discussion:

More than 150,000 new cases of lung cancer, or bronchogenic carcinoma, are diagnosed in the United States each year. *Bronchogenic carcinoma* is the more appropriate term, because most of them arise from the epithelium of the airways and not the lung per se. Because early recognition and surgical resection offer the patient the best chance for cure, it is important to be familiar with the variety of radiographic appearances of lung cancer. Four major cell types account for almost 90% of all lung cancers. The major cell types are squamous cell, adenocarcinoma, large cell, and small cell. For therapeutic purposes, lung cancer is divided into small-cell and non-small-cell carcinoma. This distinction is necessary because small-cell bronchogenic carcinoma is almost always widespread at the time of diagnosis and is best treated by chemotherapy and radiation therapy. Non-small-cell bronchogenic carcinoma, on the other hand, is best treated by surgical resection when the tumor is confined to one lung and regional lymph nodes. The typical radiographic appearance of small-cell carcinoma is bulky hilar or mediastinal lymph nodes or both; and the primary tumor sometimes is visible as a nodule within the lung.

Non-small-cell bronchogenic carcinoma includes adenocarcinoma, squamous cell carcinoma, and large-cell carcinoma. Adenocarcinoma, the most common cell type, typically appears as a solitary pulmonary nodule in the periphery of the lung. Bronchioalveolar cell carcinoma is a subtype of adenocarcinoma that may present as either lobar airspace disease or as diffuse ill-defined pulmonary nodules (Fig. 4–31). Bronchioalveolar cell carcinoma may rarely present as a solitary pulmonary

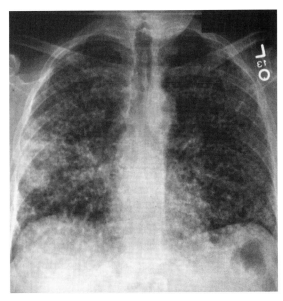

Fig. 4–31. Diffuse pulmonary nodules represent bronchioalveolar cell carcinoma in this patient.

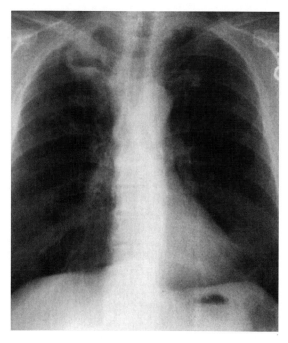

Fig. 4–32. An air-fluid level is present within a thick-walled cavity mass at the right lung apex. This represents squamous cell carcinoma.

nodule. The second most common cell type, squamous cell carcinoma, is associated with cigarette smoking and most often is found as an endobronchial tumor resulting in lobar collapse (Fig. 4–9). The endobronchial tumor is visible bronchoscopically, and sputum cytology is frequently diagnostic in this tumor. Squamous cell carcinoma can also appear radiographically as a solitary

cavitary mass (Fig. 4–32) or noncavitary mass. Large-cell carcinoma is the least frequent cell type. Its appearance is that of a bulky lesion within the lung.

When non-small-cell lung cancer is diagnosed, the patient undergoes a series of clinical and radiologic studies to determine the stage of the tumor. In the TNM staging system (Table 4–4), the categories of disease are stage IA, IB, IIA, IIB, IIIA, IIIB, or IV (Table 4–5). Stages I, II, and IIIA are surgically resectable. Patients with either stage IIIB or stage IV disease are not surgical candidates, but are treated with chemotherapy, radiation therapy, or both. In addition to helping define which treatment the patient should receive, the stage of the tumor helps provide prognosis. Patients with stage I disease have a 60% 5-year survival rate. Patients with stage IV disease have a 10% 5-year survival rate.

EXERCISE 4-8: MULTIPLE PULMONARY NODULES

Clinical History:

Case 4-13. A 70-year-old woman with uterine carcinoma treated with surgical resection 3 years previously. Chest radiograph obtained as part of a routine follow-up examination is shown (Fig. 4–33).

Question:

4-13. The most likely cause of the multiple pulmonary nodules in Case 4-13 is

    A. metastasis.

    B. herpes simplex pneumonia.

    C. histoplasmosis.

    D. Wegener's granulomatosis.

    E. arteriovenous malformations.

TABLE 4–4. TNM Staging System

Tumor	Node	Metastasis
T_1 A tumor 3 cm or less in greatest diameter, limited to the lung, and without invasion proximal to a lobar bronchus	N_0 No lymph node metastases	M_0 No distant metastases
T_2 A tumor larger than 3 cm; a tumor that invades the visceral pleura or produces collapse or consolidation of less than an entire lung; the tumor must be more than 2 cm distal to the carina	N_1 Metastases to ipsilateral hilar lymph nodes	M_1 Distant metastases present
T_3 A tumor invading parietal pleura, chest wall, diaphragm, or mediastinal pleura or pericardium; a tumor less than 2 cm from the carina; or producing collapse or consolidation of an entire lung	N_2 Metastases to ipsilateral mediastinal or subcarinal lymph nodes	
T_4 A tumor of any size with invasion of the mediastinum or involving heart, great vessels, trachea, esophagus, vertebral body, or carina, or producing malignant pleural effusion	N_3 Metastases to contralateral hilar or mediastinal lymph nodes, or scalene or supraclavicular lymph nodes	

TABLE 4–5. Staging Classifications

Stage IA	Stage IB	Stage IIA	Stage IIB	Stage IIIA	Stage IIIB	Stage IV
$T_1 N_0 M_0$	$T_2 N_0 M_0$	$T_1 N_1 M_0$	$T_2 N_1 M_0$	$T_{1-3} N_2 M_0$	T_4 any N M_0	Any T any N M_1
			$T_3 N_0 M_0$	$T_3 N_1 M_0$	Any T $N_3 M_0$	

Radiologic Findings:

4-13. In this case, the chest radiograph shows multiple, smoothly marginated, solid nodules in both lungs. These are water-density nodules that are distributed diffusely and have varying sizes. The heart is normal in size and shape.

Discussion:

The radiographic pattern of multiple pulmonary nodules is frequently encountered. The clinical setting has considerable influence on the differential diagnosis in such cases and should always be taken into account when assessing patients with this pattern. However, the differential diagnosis may be narrowed by assessing the absolute size of the nodules, the uniformity of their size, their marginal characteristics, whether or not they are calcified, and whether or not they are cavitary. In adults the most common causes of multiple nodules are metastatic neoplasm and infectious disease. Metastatic neoplasm may result from carcinoma, sarcoma, or lymphoma. Pulmonary metastases may be of any size and number. In contrast to inflammatory nodules, nodular pulmonary metastases are often of variable diameters. Metastases are usually of soft-tissue density similar to muscle or blood. Metastases may be calcified if the patient has a sarcoma that makes bone or cartilage (e.g., osteosarcoma). Calcified pulmonary nodules are more frequently encountered in patients with healed fungal or mycobacterial disease. Differentiation is most commonly made by the clinical setting or review of old films, but determination of the correct diagnosis may require tissue confirmation.

Multiple pulmonary nodules may also be due to infectious disease, most commonly fungal or mycobacterial infections. In the United States the most common fungus is histoplasmosis (Fig. 4–34), although there are regional variations. Infectious nodules are often not as sharply defined as metastases. This is especially true if the nodules represent acinar shadows. In these instances, the nodule is approximately 5 to 10 mm in diameter and is ill defined or fuzzy on its margin. Acinar nodules develop in patients with viral pneumonias such as herpes pneumonia or chickenpox pneumonia.

Multiple pulmonary nodules may also develop in a wide variety of other disorders, including Wegener's

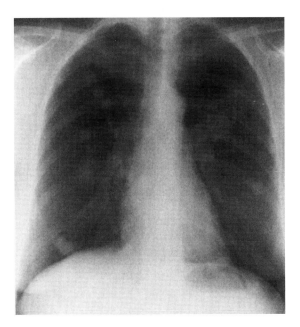

Fig. 4–33.

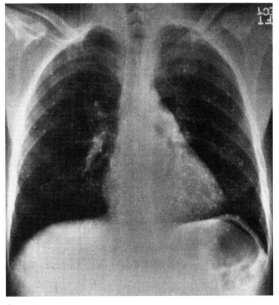

A

Fig. 4–34. Frontal **A** and lateral

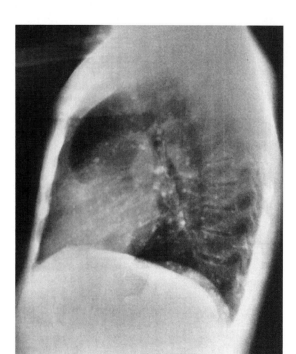

B

Fig. 4–34. **B** chest radiographs show multiple small, rather dense nodules scattered throughout both lungs; these calcified nodules are the residua of a prior histoplasmosls infection. Tuberculosis can also produce calcified granulomata.

granulomatosis and arteriovenous malformations. (*A* is the correct answer to Question 4-13.)

EXERCISE 4-9: CAVITARY DISEASE

Clinical History:

Case 4-14. A 27-year-old man with a history of intravenous drug usage and a 2-week history of fever and malaise (Fig. 4–35*A,B*)

Question:

4-14. The chest radiographic findings in Case 4-14 could be explained by any of the following except

    A. multiple abscesses due to *Staphylococcus aureus*.

    B. pneumatoceles due to *Pneumocystiscarinii*.

    C. Wegener's granulomatosis.

    D. multiple cavities due to *Mycobacterium avium-intracellulare*.

    E. metastases from Kaposi's sarcoma.

Radiologic Findings:

4-14. A close-up view of the chest radiograph (Fig. 4–35*A*) and CT image (Fig. 4–35*B*) of the left upper lobe show multiple thin-walled cavitary lesions. A left

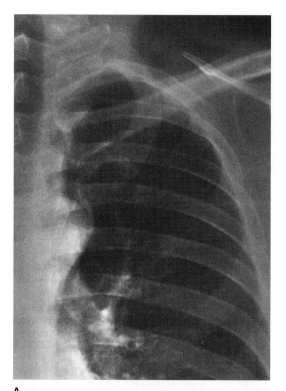

A

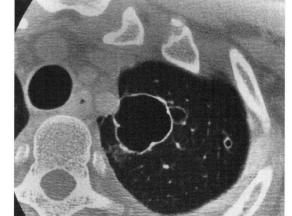

B

Fig. 4–35.

pneumothorax is also present. There is no hilar or mediastinal lymph node enlargement. The heart and skeleton are normal.

Discussion:

Inflammatory lesions are the most common cause of lung cavities. The number of cavities may range from one to many. A wide variety of infecting organisms may result in cavitation, and the radiograph is nonspecific as to etiology. There is considerable overlap in appearances from the various organisms, so that culture or histologic evaluation is the only satisfactory means of identifying the etiology. If the lesion is single, a cavitating pneumonia should be the first consideration, especially if the patient is febrile. If multiple cavities are present, the infection is likely due to hematogenous dissemination, and a source for this dissemination should be sought. The source could be right-sided endocarditis or infected venous thrombi. *Staphylococcus aureus* pneumonias are frequently seen in intravenous drug users and usually appear as multiple cavities. These usually have thin walls (2–4 mm) that are slightly indistinct on their outer borders.

As the AIDS epidemic has progressed, it has been recognized that patients with *Pneumocystis carinii* may develop cavitary lesions in the lungs. These cavities may be reversible and result from pneumatoceles or they may be due to a slowly progressive granulomatous reaction. The cavities are usually in the upper lobes and are thin walled. Pneumothorax can result when a peripheral cavity ruptures through the visceral pleura, into the pleural space.

Cavities may result from pulmonary vasculitis, of which Wegener's granulomatosis is the prototype. Neoplasia, either primary or secondarily involving the lung, may also cavitate (Fig. 4–36A,B). This patient is rather young to have neoplasia. If he did have AIDS and Kaposi's sarcoma, it would be unusual for that to cavitate. (*E* is the correct answer to Question 4-22.)

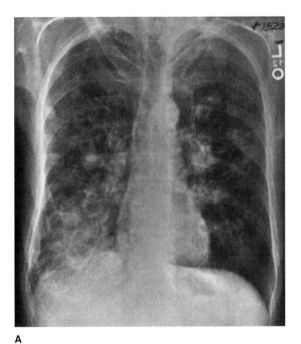

A

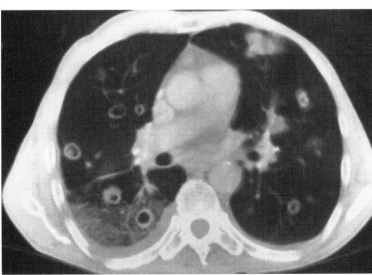

B

Fig. 4–36. Frontal chest radiograph **A** and CT scan **B** of a 60-year-old man with a previous squamous cell carcinoma of the pharynx. Chest radiograph shows multiple pulmonary nodules, many of which have cavitated, in both lungs.

EXERCISE 4-10: OCCUPATIONAL DISORDERS

Clinical Histories:

Case 4-15. A 64-year-old man, who previously worked in a naval shipyard, with a cough productive of blood-tinged sputum (Fig. 4–37*A,B*)

Case 4-16. A 55-year-old man who worked as a coal miner for 30 years (Fig. 4–38*A,B*)

Questions:

4-15. The most likely diagnosis in Fig. 4–37*A,B* is
  A. progressive massive fibrosis, due to silicosis.
  B. pneumonia in a patient with chronic interstitial lung disease.
  C. lung cancer in a patient with asbestosis.
  D. rounded atelectasis in a patient with asbestosis.
  E. berylliosis.

4-16. The most likely diagnosis in Fig. 4–38*A,B* is
  A. progressive massive fibrosis, due to silicosis.
  B. pneumonia in a patient with chronic interstitial lung disease.
  C. lung cancer in a patient with asbestosis.
  D. rounded atelectasis in a patient with asbestosis.
  E. berylliosis.

Radiologic Findings:

4-15. The dense radiopaque lines projecting adjacent to the left diaphragmatic surface on the PA radiograph and over both diaphragmatic surfaces on the lateral radiograph represent calcified pleural plaques. These are better seen on the oblique radiograph (Fig. 4–39*A*) and on the CT (Fig. 4–39*B*). When the pleural plaques are seen en face on the PA radiograph, they produce irregular opacities over the left midlung. These opacities have been described as having a holly leaf appearance. At the lung bases, a network of fine lines is superimposed over the normal vascular shadows. These reticular markings represent interstitial

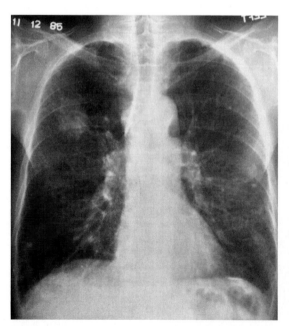

A

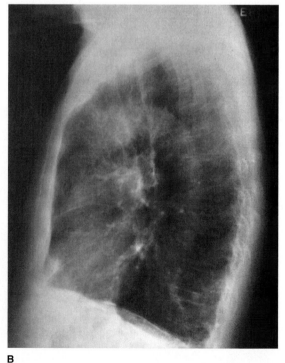

B

Fig. 4–37.

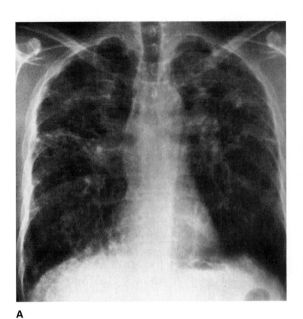

A

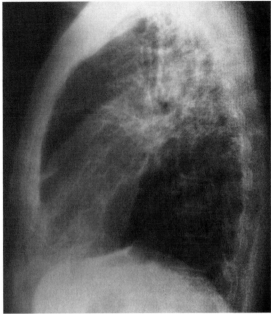

B

Fig. 4–38.

pulmonary fibrosis, which almost certainly represents asbestosis. Also present is a 3.5-cm mass in the anterior segment of the right upper lobe. This is a primary bronchogenic carcinoma. (*C* is the correct answer to Question 4-15.) The oval convexity in the lower right paratracheal region represents regional metastasis to the lower right paratracheal lymph node.

4-16. The patient in Fig. 4–38*A,B* has a myriad of small, rounded pulmonary opacities (nodules) that in some areas have coalesced to form larger pulmonary masses. The nodules are predominantly located in the upper lobes. There is also bilateral hilar lymph node enlargement, which is more evident on the lateral radiograph. Bilateral upper lobe volume loss is indicated by upward displacement of the hila. The superior lateral margin of the large opacity is relatively straight, and there is emphysema lateral to it. Nodular diseases that have an upper lobe preponderance include silicosis, sarcoidosis, and eosinophilic granuloma. In this patient with a history of working in coal mines, the most likely of these is silicosis, or coal worker's pneumoconiosis. (*A* is the correct answer to Question 4-16.)

Discussion:

The two most commonly encountered occupational lung diseases in the United States are asbestosis and silicosis. Development of these diseases is dose dependent,

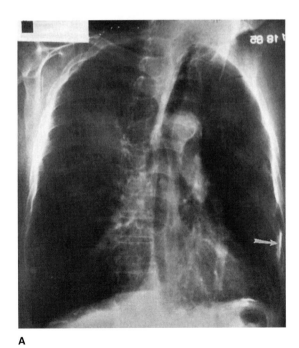

A

Fig. 4–39. **A** Left anterior oblique radiograph shows calcified pleural plaques over the left anterior lung (*arrow*) and over both hemidiaphragms. These are typical of the parietal pleural plaques seen in asbestos exposure.

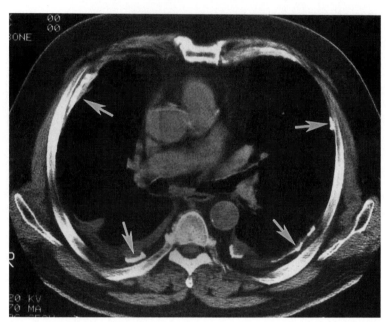

Fig. 4–39. **B** Axial CT image (mediastinal window setting) shows bilateral calcified pleural plaques (*arrows*), as well as pleural thickening posteriorly.

B

and there is a latent period of many years between exposure and disease. Asbestos-related diseases occur after exposure to asbestos particles, which are found in many types of insulation, fireproofing materials, concrete, and brake linings. The patient with asbestos exposure is at an increased risk of developing lung cancer. If the patient also smokes, there is an additive risk, and these patients may be as much as 100 times more likely to develop lung cancer than the nonsmoking individual with no asbestos exposure.

The term *asbestosis* is used to refer to the pulmonary fibrosis that may be incited by the presence of the mineral and is not used in reference to the pleural disease. The pulmonary fibrosis is predominantly distributed in the lung bases. When severe, it is detected with plain chest radiography. When it is more subtle, CT is required for its demonstration (Fig. 4–40). When confined to the pleura, the process is called *asbestos-related pleural disease.* There are five manifestations of asbestos-related pleural disease: asbestos-related pleural effusion, diffuse pleural thickening, pleural plaques, rounded atelectasis, and malignant mesothelioma. Asbestos-related pleural effusion occurs from 7 to 15 years after exposure. It is self-limited and may resolve without sequelae or result in diffuse pleural thickening. Pleural plaques are fibrous plaques that occur predominantly on the parietal pleural surfaces of the lower thoracic wall and diaphragmatic surfaces. Pleural plaques may be up to 8 to 10 mm thick, but are not easily visualized when seen en face. Oblique radiographs (Fig. 4–39*A*) may show plaques

that are projected en face on the PA chest radiograph. The plaques usually occur 10 years or more after exposure. Early in the development of pleural disease, the plaques are not calcified, but with time, the incidence of

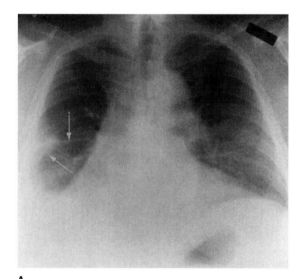

A

Fig. 4–40. **A** Frontal chest radiograph of a 56-year-old man with right-sided chest pain shows pleural opacity on the right with extension into the minor fissure (*arrows*). The patient was exposed to asbestos 20 years earlier.

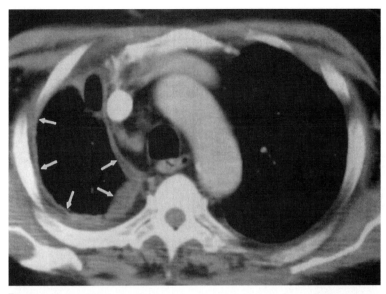

B

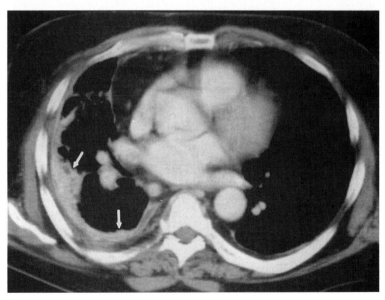

C

Fig. 4–40. **B, C** CT scans through the upper thorax and midthorax show loss of volume in the right hemithorax, with pleural thickening encircling the lung (*arrows*), representing malignant mesothelioma.

calcification increases. CT is the most sensitive method of identifying pleural plaques (Fig. 4–39*B*). Diffuse pleural thickening may result from the scarring of a previous benign asbestos-related pleural effusion or it sometimes is due to confluent pleural plaques. Rounded atelectasis is a piece of folded lung tissue that appears as a mass adjacent to the chest wall. The parietal pleura adheres to an area of lung, usually in the posterior lower lobes, and gradually produces a spiraling folded area of lung, which mimics lung cancer. The comet-tail appearance of bronchi and vessels spiraling into the mass may suggest the correct diagnosis, but because there is such a great increase in the risk of lung cancer in the asbestos-exposed individual, the mass should be closely followed. Surgical resection is often necessary to distinguish the mass of rounded atelectasis from lung cancer. The final asbestos-related disease of the pleura is malignant mesothelioma. This is a malignant tumor of the pleura that usually presents as pleural masses or pleural effusion (Fig. 4–40).

Silicosis is another form of pulmonary fibrosis that occurs after prolonged exposure to silica. Historically, it has most often developed in coal miners. Because of improved ventilation standards and the increased automation of coal mining, silicosis is less commonly encountered today. There is an increased incidence of tuberculosis in coal miners, but no increased risk of lung cancer has been reported. For reasons that are unexplained, silicosis is predominantly an upper lobe process. It appears as small pulmonary nodules, and as the fibrosis progresses, the hila are retracted upward over a period of years. The small granulomatous nodules of simple silicosis coalesce to form larger conglomerate masses. When these reach at least 1 cm in diameter, the disease is called *complicated silicosis,* and as they become larger still, it is designated *progressive massive fibrosis.* Very early disease may be seen only on CT, although in the later stages of the process, the small nodules and conglomerate masses are readily seen on either plain films or CT images (Fig. 4–41*A,B*). Hilar and mediastinal lymph nodes may calcify in the periphery of the lymph node, a type of calcification known as *eggshell calcification* (Fig. 4–42). An acute form of silicosis can occur in sandblasters who inhale a massive amount of sand. This type of silicosis radiographically resembles pulmonary edema. Coal worker's pneumoconiosis is a similar process that results from inhalation of coal of a relatively pure carbon content. This dust is relatively more inert than silica and in-

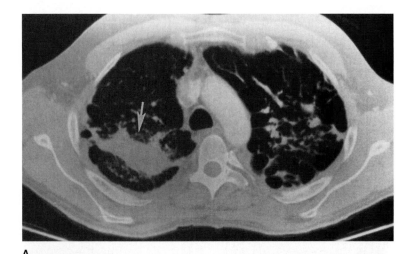

A

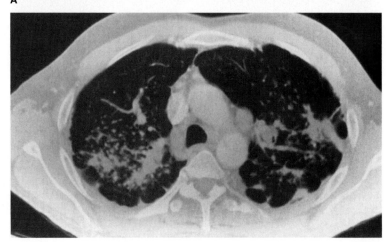

Fig. 4–41. **A,B** Axial CT images (lung window setting) of the same patient in Case 4-16 show multiple small nodules throughout both upper lobes, as well as a platelike area of conglomerate fibrosis in the right upper lobe (*arrow*). These are typical of silicosis, or coal worker's pneumoconiosis with progressive massive fibrosis.

B

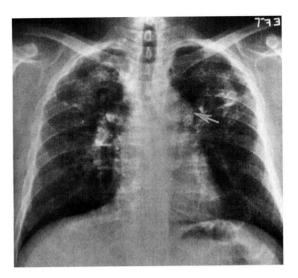

Fig. 4–42. A 49-year-old man who shoveled sand in a glass factory with silica exposure. Eggshell calcification is visible in nodes in both hila and in the aortopulmonary window (*arrow*). Conglomerate masses in the upper lobes are compatible with progressive massive fibrosis.

cites less fibrosis. The nodules are less well defined on their periphery, and there is less tendency to develop progressive massive fibrosis. These distinctions are rather artificial, because rock dust is usually not very pure and contains a mixture of silica, carbon, and other minerals.

EXERCISE 4-11: MEDIASTINAL MASSES AND COMPARTMENTS

Clinical Histories:

Case 4-17. An asymptomatic 37-year-old woman, routine chest radiograph (Fig. 4–43*A,B*)

Case 4-18. A 55-year-old man with multiple subcutaneous nodules (Fig. 4–44*A,B*)

Case 4-19. A 25-year-old woman with a nonproductive cough (Fig. 4–45*A,B*)

Questions:

4-17. The chest radiograph in Fig. 4–43 shows
    A. an anterior mediastinal mass.
    B. a middle mediastinal mass.
    C. a posterior mediastinal mass.
    D. a superior mediastinal mass.

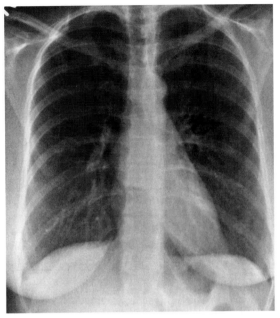

A

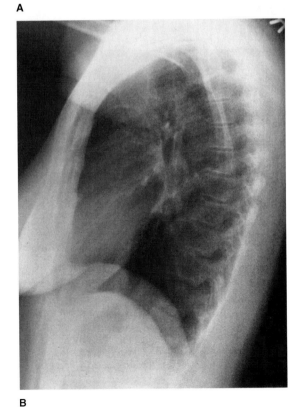

B

Fig. 4–43.

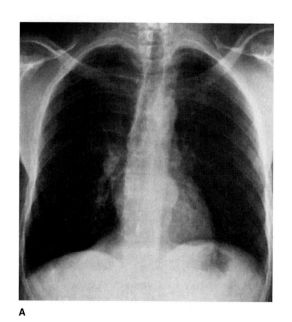

A

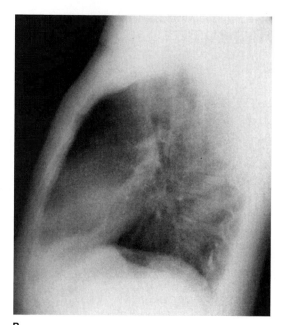

B

Fig. 4–44.

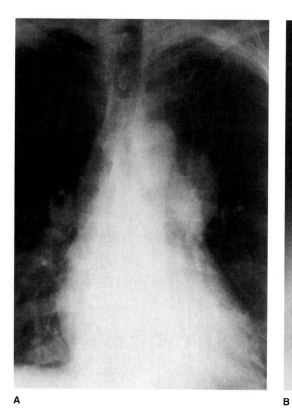

A

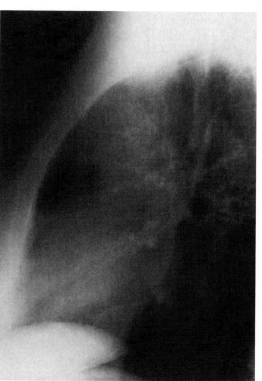

B

Fig. 4–45.

4-18. The chest radiograph in Fig. 4–44 shows

    A.   an anterior mediastinal mass.

    B.   a middle mediastinal mass.

    C.   a posterior mediastinal mass.

    D.   a superior mediastinal mass.

4-19. The chest radiograph in Fig. 4–45 shows

    A.   an anterior mediastinal mass.

    B.   a middle mediastinal mass.

    C.   a posterior mediastinal mass.

    D.   a superior mediastinal mass.

Radiological Findings:

4-17. A spherical mass 4 cm in diameter is present in the subcarinal region on the frontal radiograph (Fig. 4–43*A*) and superimposed on the hilar region on the lateral radiograph (Fig. 4–43*B*). CT (Fig. 4–46) shows that the lesion is of fluid attenuation (greater attenuation than the subcutaneous fat, but less attenuation than muscle). This mass is in the middle mediastinum. (*B* is the correct answer to Question 4-17.) In an asymptomatic individual, this most likely represents a congenital bronchogenic cyst. These masses can grow to sufficient size to cause symptoms such as dyspnea or dysphagia owing to compression of the trachea or esophagus. Bronchogenic cysts may also occur within the lungs and are often surgically resected because of the likelihood of pulmonary infection. The differential diagnosis of a middle mediastinal mass also includes lymphoma, esophageal tumor, hiatal hernia, and aortic arch aneurysm.

4-18. The frontal radiograph (Fig. 4–44*A*) shows a lobulated mass to the left of the lower thoracic vertebrae. Note that the lateral wall of the descending thoracic aorta remains visible, suggesting that this mass is either anterior or posterior to the aorta, but does not displace lung from the wall of the aorta. The mass is not visible on the lateral radiograph. The residual myelographic contrast material visible within the spinal canal hints at the neural nature of these masses. The axial CT images in Fig. 4–47*A,B* show that the masses are bilateral and paraspinal in location. These masses are in the posterior mediastinum. (*C* is the correct answer to Question 4-18.) Neurogenic tumors are the most common cause of posterior mediastinal masses. In this patient with multiple subcutaneous nodules, they most likely are neurofibromas. The differential diagnosis of posterior mediastinal masses also includes paraspinous abscess, descending thoracic aorta aneurysm, Bochdalek hernia, and lymphoma.

4-19. In Fig. 4–45, the frontal chest radiograph (Figs. 4–45*A* and 4–48*A*) shows a mass projecting over the left hilum (*long arrow*, Fig. 4–48*A*) without obscuration of the interlobar pulmonary artery (*short arrow*, Fig. 4–48*A*). Because the mass does not obliterate the margins of the vessel, it must be either anterior or posterior to the hilum. On the lateral view (Fig. 4–48*B*), the anterior clear space is somewhat opaque, and there is a suggestion of margins of the mass (*arrows*). The CT scan (Fig. 4–48*C*) shows the mass, surrounded by fat, in the anterior mediastinum. (*A* is the correct answer to Question 4-19.) The mass is cystic, and the contents have rather low density, suggesting that the mass contains some fat. Notice the thick, irregular wall of the mass. No other abnormalities are present. This is consistent with a teratoma. The differential diagnosis of anterior mediastinal

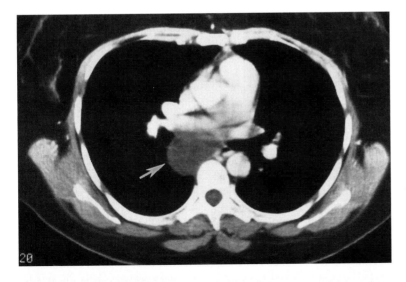

Fig. 4–46. Axial CT image of the same patient in Fig. 4–43 shows a round mass (*arrow*) of fluid attenuation in a subcarinal position. This is a typical appearance of a bronchogenic cyst.

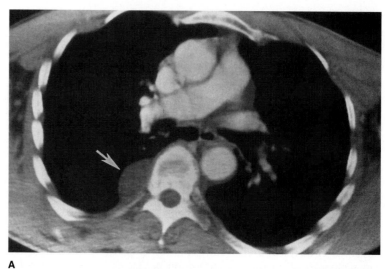

A

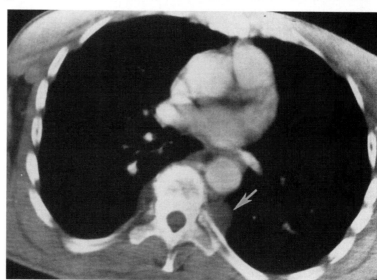

Fig. 4–47. **A,B** Axial CT images of the same patient in Fig. 4–44 show bilateral paraspinal masses (*arrows*).

B

masses also includes lymphoma, thyroid mass, thymoma, and ascending aortic aneurysm.

Discussion:

Two methods of dividing the mediastinum for radiographic purposes are in common use. The radiographic divisions are arbitrary and are intended to provide the most appropriate differential diagnosis for abnormalities that occur in these locations. Neither of the divisions follows the divisions used by anatomists. In the older system, the mediastinum is divided into three compartments. The anterior mediastinum is that portion of the mediastinum

that is anterior to the anterior margin of the trachea and along the posterior margin of the pericardium and inferior vena cava. The posterior mediastinum lies behind a plane that extends the length of the thorax behind a line drawn 1 cm posteriorly to the anterior margin of the vertebral column. The middle mediastinum is the region between these two boundaries. This system has been superseded by a four-compartment model, which designates a superior mediastinal compartment as the space that lies above a plane extending from the sternomanubrial junction to the lower border of the fourth thoracic vertebra. The anterior mediastinum is just caudad to the superior compartment and is anterior to a plane extending along the anterior

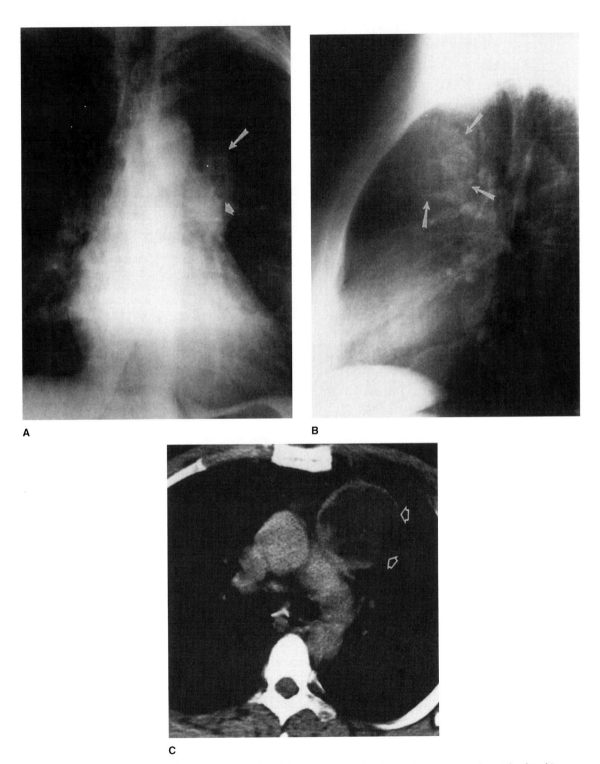

Fig. 4–48. Front **A** and lateral **B** chest radiographs of the same patient in Fig. 4–45. **C** CT scan through a level just below the aortic arch shows a mass in the left anterior mediastinum (*arrows*). The mass has a thick, nodular wall, and the central material is relatively radiolucent. The central portion of this mass is fat, and the mass is a teratoma.

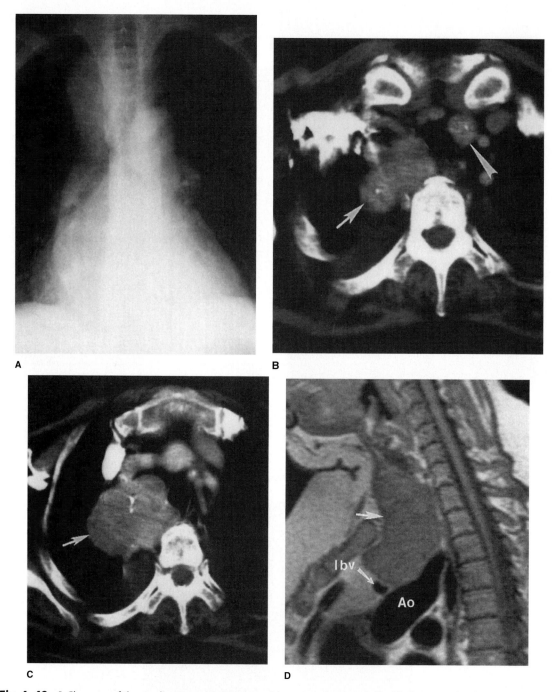

Fig. 4–49. **A** Close-up of the mediastinum in a 75-year-old woman shows a right-sided paratracheal mass with displacement of the trachea to the left. Enlargement of the heart is also seen. **B** CT scan through the lung apices at the thoracic inlet shows the right-sided paratracheal mass (*arrow*), which is of soft-tissue density and has a nidus of calcification within it. A soft-tissue mass is also seen adjacent to the left side of the trachea and has an additional calcification (*arrowhead*). These represent regions of enlargement of the thyroid. **C** CT scan at a level just above the aortic arch shows the mass (*arrow*) extending into the superior mediastinum just lateral to the trachea and displacing the trachea to the left. **D** MR image shows a mass (*arrows*) at the thoracic inlet from thyroid enlargement. Mass displaces the aorta (Ao) and brachiocephalic artery posteriorly and inferiorly. The left brachiocephalic vein (lbv) is also displaced inferiorly.

aspect of the tracheal air column and along the anterior pericardium. Note that the heart shifts from the anterior to the middle mediastinum as the system changes. The middle mediastinum occupies the area from the anterior pericardium backward to a plane 1 cm posterior to the anterior margin of the vertebral column. The addition of the fourth compartment occurred when CT was developed and it became easier to identify structures in each compartment.

The differential diagnosis of lesions occurring in each compartment is in part dependent on the structures that exist there. Note that there are vascular structures and lymph nodes in each of the compartments. Therefore, abnormalities of the blood vessels (e.g., aneurysms) and lymph node diseases (e.g., lymphoma) would have to be included in the differential diagnosis of diseases in all mediastinal compartments. The most common mass to occur in the superior mediastinum is an enlarged substernal thyroid, which may become large enough to extend into the anterior or middle mediastinum (Fig. 4–49A–D).

EXERCISE 4-12: PLEURAL ABNORMALITIES

Clinical History:

Case 4-20. A tall, 21-year-old man who noted the sudden onset of dyspnea, and right-sided pleuritic chest pain (Fig. 4–50A,B)

Question:

4-20. The most likely diagnosis in Case 4-20 is

    A. pulmonary embolism.

    B. overinflation associated with asthma.

    C. pneumothorax.

    D. normal chest, with a skin fold projected over the right hemithorax.

    E. left lower lobe atelectasis.

Radiologic Findings:

4-20. In Fig. 4–50A, there is increased radiolucency in the periphery of the right hemithorax. On the close-up of the right lung (Fig. 4–50B), there is a thin white line (*arrows*) paralleling, but displaced from, the right lateral chest wall. The thin line represents the visceral pleura. There is air-filled lung medial to this thin white line, and there is air within the pleural space lateral to this line. Note the absence of pulmonary vessels lateral to the pleural line. (*C* is the correct answer to Question 4-20.) Note the rounded, thin-walled blebs at the apex of the right lung on the close-up view in Fig. 4–50B.

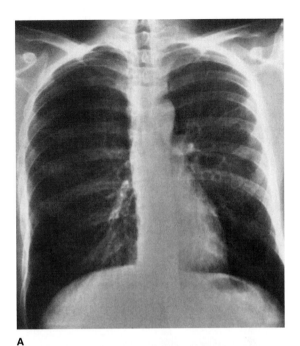

A

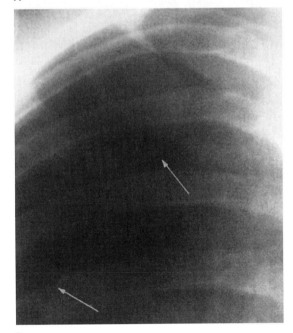

B

Fig. 4–50.

Discussion:

Pneumothorax is the presence of air in the pleural space. The lung collapses away from the chest wall because of its normal elastic recoil. In some instances, a ball valve mechanism is present, and air continues to enter the pleural space and further collapses the lung and displaces the mediastinum away from the side of the pneumothorax. The relationship of the air in the pleural space to the lung and chest wall can be clearly seen on the CT scan of a patient with a left pneumothorax (Fig. 4–51). Note that air rises to the highest point in the thorax, the anterior thorax in a supine patient and the lung apex in an upright patient. The visceral pleura covering the lung is visible as a thin white line on both chest radiographs and CT scans. No pulmonary vessels may be seen extending beyond the pleural line, and the air in the pleural space appears more radiolucent than the adjacent lung.

The most common mimic of a pneumothorax, particularly in a supine patient, is a skin fold. The film cassette for portable AP chest radiographs is placed behind the patient's back. Skin folds may be pressed between the patient's back and the film cassette. Radiographically, a skin fold produces an interface, or an edge of thick tissue outlined by the greater radiolucency of the superimposed lung. If you can distinguish an edge from a line, then you can distinguish a skin fold from a pneumothorax. The absence of pulmonary markings beyond the pleural line is supporting evidence for a pneumothorax. Because the vessels taper as they approach the lung periphery, the vessels in the extreme periphery of the lung may be too tiny to see.

Pneumothorax is spontaneous if it occurs in the absence of trauma (including barotrauma). Spontaneous pneumothorax may be primary and occur in the absence of significant other lung disease, or it may occur secondarily because of lung disease. Apical blebs are present in a high percentage of patients with primary spontaneous pneumothorax, and their rupture is thought to be the most frequent cause of spontaneous pneumothorax. For unknown reasons, it occurs most frequently in tall young men. Secondary spontaneous pneumothorax may occur in association with any cavitary lesion that lies in the periphery of the lung, as well as in emphysema, in bullous disease, and in pulmonary fibrosis of a variety of etiologies.

EXERCISE 4-13: PLEURAL EFFUSION

Clinical History:

Case 4-21. A 45-year-old man with increasing dyspnea and abdominal swelling of 1-week duration (Fig. 4–52A,B)

Question:

4-21. Which of the following radiographic signs suggest the presence of pleural effusion?

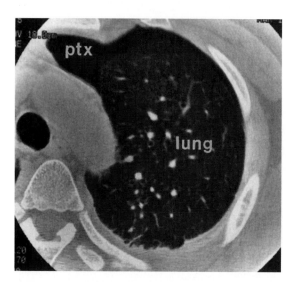

Fig. 4–51. Axial CT image (lung window settings) shows air in the left pleural space (ptx). Note that the pneumothorax in this supine patient rises to the highest part of the thorax. The visceral pleural covering of the left lung is visible as a thin white line.

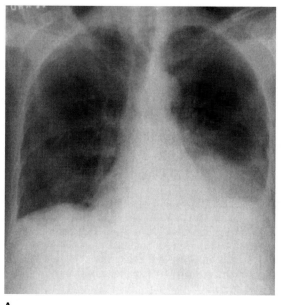

A

Fig. 4–52.

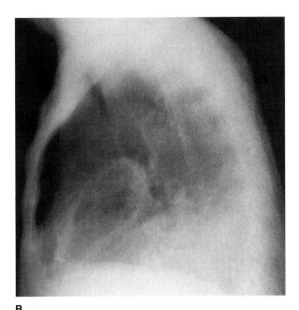

B

Fig. 4–52. *Cont.*

A. Meniscus-shaped opacity in a posterior costophrenic angle on the lateral projection

B. Biconvex lens-shaped opacity projecting in the midthorax on the lateral projection

C. Fluid levels that have different lengths on the PA and lateral views in a hemithorax

D. Homogeneous increased density in a hemithorax with preservation of the vascular shadows in the lungs

E. Separation of the gastric air bubble from the inferior lung margin by more than 2 cm

Radiologic Findings:

4-21. The frontal chest radiograph (Fig. 4–52*A*) shows opacity at the lower left hemithorax, which has a concave border curving upward laterally adjacent to the chest wall. The overall lung volume is low in both the right and left lungs. There is separation of the gastric bubble from the inferior margin of the lung by several centimeters. On the lateral examination (Fig. 4–52*B*), the opacity obscures the posterior heart margin and has a margin curving slightly upward to the posterior chest wall. The findings are those of a pleural effusion on the left. The patient is noted to have slight abdominal pro-

tusion that is seen on the lateral examination. This was due to ascites in this patient with cirrhosis.

Discussion:

The visceral pleura is the outer lining of the lung, and the parietal pleura is the lining of the chest cavity. Normally, these surfaces are smooth and are separated by a minimal amount of pleural fluid. This provides a nearly friction-free environment for movement of the lung within the thorax. The pleural space, therefore, is a potential space that, in the normal individual, contains no more than 3 to 5 cm³ of pleural fluid. Fluid may accumulate within the pleural space as a result of conditions that (1) increase pulmonary capillary pressure, (2) alter thoracic vascular or lymphatic pathways, (3) alter pleural capillary or lymphatic permeability, or (4) affect diaphragmatic peritoneal and pleural surfaces.

Pleural effusions are usually approached clinically according to whether the effusion develops because of alterations of the Starling equation, which controls fluid flow and maintenance in body compartments, or whether the pleura is affected primarily by a disease process. Processes resulting from alterations of the Starling equation include congestive heart failure, hypoproteinemia, fluid overload, liver failure, and nephrosis. These effusions are usually transudates (clear or pale yellow, odorless fluid without elevation of the ratios of pleural fluid: serum protein and LDH). Processes that alter pleural capillary or lymphatic permeability include infections, inflammation, pulmonary embolism, and neoplasms. These effusions are usually exudates (clear, pale yellow or turbid, bloody, brownish fluid; pleural fluid protein: serum protein greater than 0.5; and pleural fluid LDH: serum LDH greater than 0.6). Enlarged lymph nodes or masses within the hila or mediastinum may obstruct lymphatic fluid flow and cause pleural exudates. Abdominal conditions that may produce pleural effusions include pancreatitis, subphrenic abscesses, liver abscesses, ovarian tumors, peritonitis, and ascites.

The most common radiographic sign is pleural meniscus. The volume of fluid necessary to produce a pleural meniscus within a costophrenic angle varies from individual to individual. Approximately 100 cm³ of pleural fluid will cause appreciable blunting of the posterior costophrenic angle on the lateral view; and 200 cm³ will cause blunting of the lateral costophrenic angle on the PA projection in an upright patient (Fig. 4–53*A–C*). A lateral decubitus chest radiograph, with the side containing the pleural effusion placed down (dependent), will demonstrate even smaller amounts of free-flowing pleural effusions (Fig. 4–54). Each millimeter of thickness of pleural fluid in the lateral decubitus projection corresponds to approximately 20 cm³ of pleural fluid. Large pleural effusions may usually be aspirated without guidance

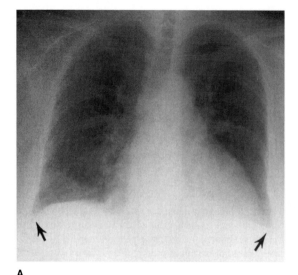

A

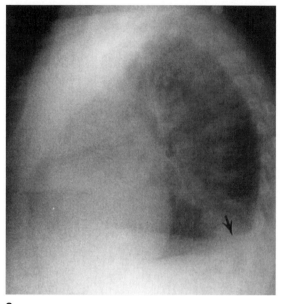

C

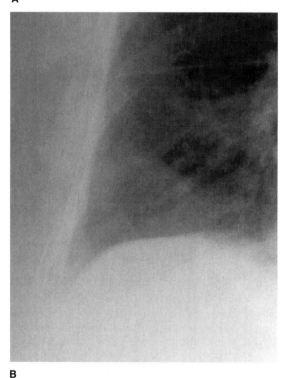

B

Fig. 4–53. Full **A** and close-up **B** frontal views of the chest show blunting of both lateral costophrenic angles (*arrows*) caused by small bilateral pleural effusions. **C** Lateral chest radiograph shows that the posterior costophrenic angles (*arrow*) are also blunted by fluid in both pleural spaces.

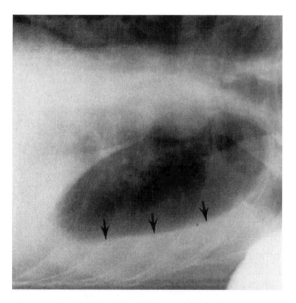

Fig. 4–54. A left lateral decubitus radiograph shows displacement of the lateral margin of the left lung (*arrows*) from the chest wall by free-flowing pleural effusion.

other than the chest radiograph. Small effusions are more difficult to aspirate and, if thoracentesis is planned, additional imaging guidance with ultrasonography or CT may be used. The effusion may simply be marked and aspirated by the clinical physician, or the effusion may be aspirated by a radiologist.

If thoracentesis is attempted and fails for a large pleural effusion, it may be loculated, and further imaging guidance is usually helpful.

When pleural adhesions develop, fluid in the pleural space becomes loculated (Fig. 4–55A,B) and may be trapped in nondependent areas of the thorax. The appearance of pleural fluid may change and, rather than a meniscus shape, may assume the shape of a convex margin away from the chest wall. If fluid is trapped in the fissures, it will assume a biconvex lens shape. If a bronchopleural fistula develops, the patient will have a hydropneumothorax that may be recognized by air-fluid levels of different lengths on the PA and lateral chest radiographs. When cavities develop in the lung, the fluid levels are usually of the same length. (All of the options in Question 4-21 are correct.)

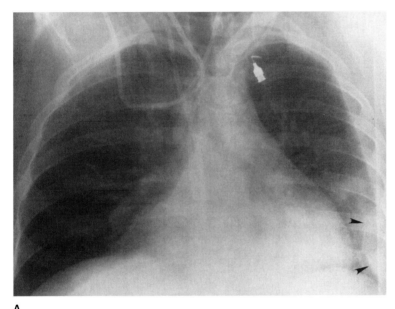

A

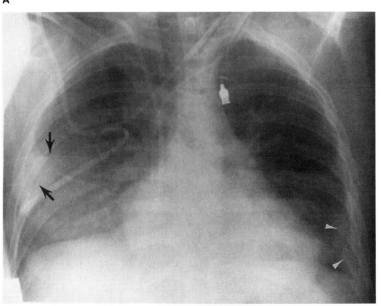

B

Fig. 4–55. **A** Supine radiograph shows displacement of the lung away from the ribs by a homogeneous soft-tissue opacity on the left. This represents a pleural effusion. Note that the contour adjacent to the lower thorax wall is convex, away from the chest wall (*arrowheads*). **B** Right lateral decubitus view of the same patient shows that the homogeneous opacity along the upper chest wall has moved away and allowed the lung to become adjacent to the ribs. Continued presence of the convex contour adjacent to the costophrenic angle indicates a loculation of pleural fluid at the position (*arrowheads*). Note also the displacement of lung away from the right chest wall and tracking of fluid into the minor fissure (*arrows*) on the right.

EXERCISE 4-14: PULMONARY VASCULAR DISEASE

Clinical History:

Case 4-22. A 62-year-old woman with worsening shortness of breath and mild hemoptysis 1 day after receiving intravenous chemotherapy for ovarian cancer. A PA and lateral chest radiograph (Fig. 4–56A,B) and a CT scan with intravenous contrast were obtained (Fig. 4–56C,D).

Question:

4-22. The most likely cause for her dyspnea and hemoptysis is

    A. pulmonary metastases.
    B. malignant pleural effusion.
    C. pulmonary embolism.
    D. septic emboli.
    E. drug-related pneumonitis.

Radiologic Findings:

4-22. The CXR shows small bilateral pleural effusions. These cause blunting of the lateral costophrenic angles on the PA view of the chest (Fig. 4–56A) and of the posterior costophrenic angles on the lateral view of the chest (Fig. 4–56B). The size of the pleural effusions is not sufficient to explain the patient's symptoms. The CT scan (Fig. 4–56C) demonstrates filling defects within the pulmonary arteries bilaterally (*arrows*). At the level shown, thromboemboli are visible within the right interlobar (descending) pulmonary artery and within the basilar segmental arteries on the left. (*C* is the correct answer to Question 4-22.) The lung windows (Fig. 4–56D) show peripheral areas of increased attenuation (*arrows*), consistent with areas of pulmonary infarction.

Discussion:

Pulmonary thromboembolism can occur as a result of deep-venous thrombosis, typically from the veins of the pelvis and lower extremities. These thrombi dislodge (embolize) and travel via the inferior vena cava and right heart chambers to become trapped in the tapering

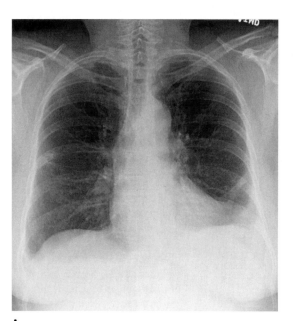

A

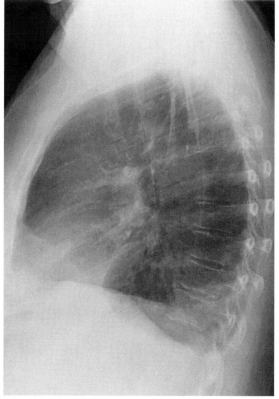

B

Fig. 4–56.

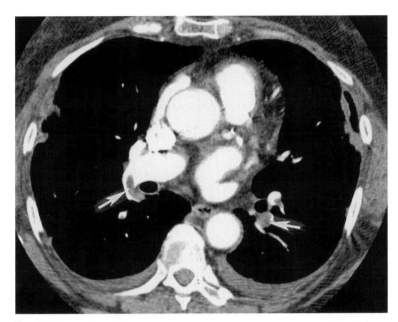

C

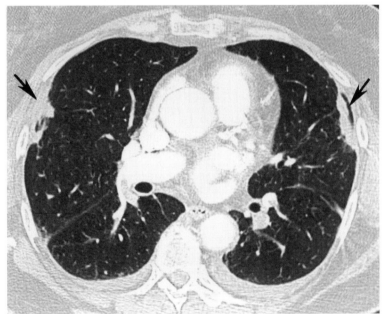

D

Fig. 4–56.

branches of the pulmonary arterial system. Because pulmonary embolism often occurs without pulmonary infarction, the appearance of the chest radiograph is usually normal. The areas of lung deprived of pulmonary arterial flow are perfused by bronchial arterial collateral vessels. The chest radiograph may demonstrate subtle signs of volume loss or a small pleural effusion. Pulmonary opacities develop because of microatelectasis within the region of lung that has had an embolus or from hemorrhage within a pulmonary infarction. Pulmonary infarction may occur if the pulmonary venous pressure is elevated or the bronchial arterial supply to a region is deficient for some reason. The cone-shaped area of pulmonary infarction has been called a Hampton's hump after its original descriptor. An area of radiolucency, corresponding to diminished pulmonary vascularity distal to a pulmonary embolism, is occasionally seen and is called the Westermark sign. There may also be an increase in the size of the pulmonary artery proximal to a large central pulmonary embolus.

Two imaging modalities are widely used in the evaluation of a patient with suspected pulmonary embolism: radionuclide perfusion scan and chest CT. The radionuclide perfusion scan may be the more appropriate examination in the patient with a normal chest radiograph and no preexisting cardiac or pulmonary disease. In the patient with an abnormal chest radiograph, or preexisting cardiopulmonary disease, the V/Q scan is more likely to be interpreted as "indeterminate" and a chest CT becomes the preferred imaging modality. The chest CT also has the advantage of demonstrating unsuspected abnormalities, such as pericardial effusion, emphysema, esophagitis, or aortic dissection, which are responsible for the patient's chest pain or dyspnea.

On chest CT, thromboemboli are visible as filling defects within the contrast-filled pulmonary arteries. These are typically several centimeters long and often are seen draped across the bifurcation of an artery (saddle emboli). In patients with acute pulmonary embolism, the filling defects are seen within the center of the arterial lumen, although they may also completely occlude the artery. In patients with chronic pulmonary embolism, the filling defects are more likely to be found against the wall of the artery. Calcification within the thrombus also confirms the chronic nature of the thrombus.

In some patients, the diagnosis of pulmonary embolism remains uncertain after either a V/Q scan or a chest CT. These examinations can be inadequate for a number of both technical and clinical reasons. The chest CT can be difficult to interpret unless the patient is able to suspend respiration for the duration of the scan. Fortunately, helical CT scans are able to scan the entire thorax in under 30 seconds. Many patients with severe dyspnea, however, are unable to achieve this. Pulmonary angiography can be obtained to further evaluate the pulmonary arterial circulation when either the V/Q scan or chest CT are nondiagnostic.

GLOSSARY OF TERMS IN CHEST ROENTGENOLOGY*

Acinar pattern (synonyms: *alveolar pattern, airspace disease, consolidation*) A collection of round or elliptic, ill-defined, discrete or partly confluent opacities in the lung, each measuring 4 to 8 mm in diameter and together producing an extended, inhomogeneous shadow.

Air bronchogram A branching lucency that represents the roentgenographic shadow of an air-containing bronchus peripheral to the hilum and surrounded by airless lung (whether by virtue of absorption of air, replacement of air, or both), a finding generally regarded as evidence of the patency of the more proximal airway.

Air-fluid level A local collection of gas and liquid that, when traversed by a horizontal x-ray beam, creates a shadow characterized by a sharp horizontal interface between a gas density above and liquid density below.

Airspace The gas-containing portion of lung parenchyma, including the acini and excluding the interstitium and purely conductive portions of the lung.

Anterior junction line A vertically oriented linear opacity approximately 1 to 2 mm wide, produced by the shadows of the right and left pleural surfaces in intimate contact between the aerated lungs anterior to the great vessels. It is usually obliquely oriented, projected over the tracheal air column, below the level of the clavicles.

Aortopulmonary window A zone of relative lucency seen on both the PA and lateral chest radiographs bounded medially by the left side of the trachea, superiorly by the inferior surface of the aortic arch, and inferiorly by the left pulmonary artery. The pleural surface of the aortopulmonary (AP) window is normally concave; convexity of the AP window suggests lymphadenopathy.

Atelectasis Less than normal inflation of all or a portion of lung with corresponding diminution in volume. Qualifiers are often used to indicate extent and distribution (linear or platelike, subsegmental, segmental, lobar), as well as mechanism (resorption, relaxation, compressive, passive, cicatricial, adhesive).

Azygoesophageal recess On the frontal chest radiograph, a vertically oriented interface between air in the right lower lobe, and the adjacent mediastinum containing the azygos vein and esophagus. It projects in the middle of the heart and spine on the frontal view.

Bleb A thin-walled lucency within or contiguous to the visceral pleura.

Bulla A sharply demarcated area of a vascularity (lucency) within the lung measuring 1 cm or more in diameter and possessing a wall less than 1 mm in thickness.

---

*Adapted from "Terms Used in Chest Radiology" in Fraser RS, Muller NL, Colman N, Pare PD. *Fraser and Pare's diagnosis of diseases of the Chest*. 4th ed. Philadelphia: WB. Saunders Co.; 1999: xvii–xxxi.

Carina   The bifurcation of the trachea into right and left main bronchi.

Cavity   A gas-containing space within the lung surrounded by a wall whose thickness is greater than 1 mm and often irregular in contour.

Fissure   The infolding of visceral pleura that separates one lobe, or a portion of a lobe, from another. Radiographically visible as a linear opacity normally 1 mm or less in width. Qualifiers: minor (horizontal), major, accessory, azygos, anomalous.

Ground-glass pattern   A finely granular pattern of pulmonary opacity such that pulmonary vessels remain visible. The degree of opacity is not sufficient to result in air bronchograms.

Hilum   (plural: *hila*): Anatomically, the depression or pit in that part of an organ where the vessels and nerves enter. On chest radiographs, the term *hilum* represents the composite shadow of the bronchi, pulmonary arteries and veins, and lymph nodes on the medial aspect of each lung.

Honeycomb pattern   A number of ring shadows or cystic spaces within the lung representing airspaces 5 to 10 mm in diameter with walls 2 to 3 mm thick that resemble a true honeycomb. The finding implies interstitial fibrosis and end-stage lung disease.

Interface   (synonyms: *edge, border*) The boundary between the shadows of structures of different opacity (e.g., the lung and the heart).

Interstitium   A continuum of loose connective tissue throughout the lung consisting of three subdivisions: (1) bronchoarterial (axial), surrounding the bronchoarterial bundles; (2) parenchymal (acinar), between the alveolar and capillary basement membranes; and (3) subpleural, between the pleura and lung parenchyma and continuous with the interlobular septa and perivenous interstitial space.

Line   A longitudinal opacity no greater than 2 mm in width.

Lobe   One of the principal divisions of the lungs (usually three on the right, two on the left) enveloped by the visceral pleura except at the hilum. The lobes are separated in whole or in part by pleural fissures.

Lucency   (synonym: *radiolucency*) The shadow of tissue that attenuates the x-ray beam less effectively than surrounding tissue. On a radiograph, the area that appears more nearly black, usually applied to areas of air density or fat density.

Lymphadenopathy   (synonym: *adenopathy*) Enlargement or abnormality of lymph nodes.

Mass   Any pulmonary or pleural lesion greater than 3 cm in diameter.

Miliary pattern   A collection of tiny (1–2 mm in diameter) discrete opacities in the lungs, generally uniform in size and widespread in distribution.

Nodular pattern   A collection of innumerable small, discrete opacities (2–10 mm in diameter), generally widespread in distribution.

Nodule   A sharply defined, discrete, circular opacity up to 3 cm in diameter within the lung.

Opacity   The shadow of tissue that attenuates the x-ray beam more than surrounding tissue. On a radiograph, areas that are more white than the surrounding area are said to be more opaque.

Posterior junction line   A vertically oriented, linear opacity approximately 2 mm wide, produced by the shadows of the right and left pleurae in intimate contact between the aerated lungs, representing the plane of contact between the lungs posterior to the trachea and esophagus, and anterior to the spine; the line may project above and below the suprasternal notch.

Posterior tracheal stripe   A vertically oriented linear opacity 2 to 5 mm wide, extending from the thoracic inlet to the bifurcation of the trachea, visible on the lateral radiograph, representing the posterior tracheal wall and contiguous mediastinal tissue (anterior, and often posterior, walls of the esophagus).

Primary complex   The combination of a focus of pneumonia due to a primary infection (e.g., tuberculosis or histoplasmosis), with granulomas in the draining hilar or mediastinal lymph nodes. (Synonym: *Ranke complex*. The term *Ghon focus* describes the pulmonary lesion that has calcified. *Ranke complex* is the term to describe the combination of the Ghon focus and calcified hilar lymph nodes.)

Reticular pattern   A collection of innumerable small, linear opacities that together produce the appearance of a net.

Reticulonodular pattern   A collection of innumerable small, linear, and nodular opacities that together produce the appearance of a net and superimposed small nodules.

Right tracheal stripe   A vertically oriented linear opacity 2 to 3 mm wide, extending from the thoracic inlet to the right tracheobronchial angle. It represents the right tracheal wall and contiguous mediastinal tissue (visceral and parietal pleurae of the right lung).

Septal line   (synonym: *Kerley line*) A linear opacity, usually 1 to 2 mm in width, produced by thickening of the interlobular septa, and often due to either edema or cellular infiltration.

Silhouette sign   The effacement of an anatomic soft-tissue border by either a normal anatomic structure or a pathologic state, such as airlessness of adjacent lung or accumulation of fluid in the contiguous pleural space.

Stripe   A longitudinal opacity 2 to 5 mm in width.

Tramline shadow Parallel or slightly convergent linear opacities that suggest the projection of tubular structures, generally representing thickened bronchial walls.

BIBLIOGRAPHY

Armstrong P. *Imaging of Diseases of the Chest.* 3rd ed. London: Mosby; 2000.

Collins J, Stern EJ. *Chest Radiology: The Essentials.* Philadelphia: Lippincott, Williams & Wilkins; 1999.

Freundlich IM, Bragg DG. *A Radiologic Approach to Diseases of the Chest.* 2nd ed. Baltimore: Williams & Wilkins; 1997.

Groskin SA. *Heitzman's The Lung: Radiologic-Pathologic Correlations.* 3rd ed. St. Louis: Mosby; 1993.

McLoud TC. *Thoracic Radiology: The Requisites.* St Louis: Mosby; 1998.

Reed JC. *Chest Radiology: Plain Film Patterns and Differential Diagnoses.* 4th ed. St. Louis: Mosby; 1997.

Radiology of the Breast

5

Rita I. Freimanis

Imaging of the breast is undertaken as part of a comprehensive evaluation of this organ, integrating the patient's history, clinical signs, and symptoms. Radiography of the breast is known as *mammography* or *radiomammography*. When used periodically in asymptomatic patients, this is called *screening mammography*. When imaging is targeted to patients with signs or symptoms of breast cancer, it is referred to as *diagnostic breast imaging* and usually is a tailored evaluation consisting of some combination of mammography and other techniques described in this chapter. Using the integrated approach, it is often possible to make an accurate diagnosis nonoperatively, and treatment may be individualized according to each patient's needs. The primary purpose of breast imaging is to detect breast carcinoma. A secondary purpose is to evaluate benign disease, such as cyst formation, infection, implant complication, and trauma.

Before the 1980s, when breast imaging was much less widely used, the proportion of surgery for benign breast disease was higher, and treatment for breast carcinoma was initiated at later stages of the disease than at present. Breast imaging has increased the detection of tumors smaller than those found on clinical breast examination and has enabled patients to avoid unnecessary surgery.

The outcome of earlier diagnosis and treatment, however, is yet to be proven. Mortality from breast cancer has remained fairly stable for several decades in spite of the introduction and popularization of screening mammography. Debate continues as to the efficacy of routine breast screening in certain age groups. It is almost universally acknowledged that women older than 50 years of age benefit from periodic screening mammography. Several large population studies have shown a decrease in mortality of around 30% in this group. The greatest current controversy concerns the value of screening mammography for women under the age of 50 years. Because breast cancer has a lower prevalence in this age group, the impediment to mass screening is largely economic; that is, the number of lives saved relative to dollars spent must be justified. Another difference is that in younger women the breast parenchyma is more often dense and nodular. This condition decreases the sensitivity for detection of carcinoma and leads to more false-negative and false-positive results.

Besides a decrease in mortality, a second benefit of earlier diagnosis is that patients with breast carcinoma are afforded more treatment options; lumpectomy with radiation therapy is an option to mastectomy in selected patients.

Mammography has been in common use since about 1980, and breast ultrasonography has been the most often used adjunctive technique during this time. The major contribution of ultrasonography has been its effectiveness in distinguishing cystic lesions from solid masses.

Sonography has, therefore, helped to avoid unnecessary surgery, because asymptomatic simple cysts do not require intervention. Some practitioners also use ultrasonography, together with mammography, to help characterize solid lesions as benign, indeterminate, or suspicious.

Magnetic resonance (MR) imaging of the breast can be used in selected patients. Image-guided needle biopsy of the breast has become the first-line procedure for diagnosis of indeterminate lesions of the breast, with surgical biopsy being reserved for special cases. Nuclear medicine and contrast injection studies (ductography) are occasionally used under special circumstances with specific indications.

TECHNIQUE AND NORMAL ANATOMY

Film-Screen and Digital Radiography (Radiomammography)

The film-screen mammogram is created with x-rays, radiographic film, and intensifying screens adjacent to the film within the cassette, hence the term *film-screen mammography.* The digital mammogram is created using a similar system, but replacing the film and screen with a digital detector.

The routine examination consists of two views of each breast, the craniocaudal (C-C) view and the mediolateral oblique (MLO) view, with a total of four films. The C-C view can be considered the "top down" view, and the MLO an angled view from the side (Figs. 5–1 and 5–2). The patient undresses from the waist up and stands for the examination, leaning slightly against the mammography unit. The technologist must mobilize, elevate, and pull the breast to place as much breast tissue as possible on the surface of the film cassette holder. A flat, plastic compression paddle is then gently but firmly lowered onto the breast surface to compress the breast into as thin a layer as possible. This compression achieves both immobilization during exposure and dispersion of breast tissue shadows over a larger area, thereby permitting better visual separation of imaged structures. Compression may be uncomfortable, and may even be painful in a small proportion of patients. However, most patients accept this level of discomfort for the few seconds required for each exposure, particularly if they understand the need for compression and know what to expect during the examination. Mammography has proved to be more cost effective, while maintaining resolution high enough to demonstrate early malignant lesions, than any other breast imaging

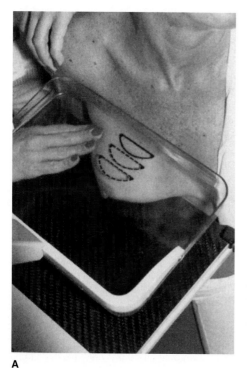

A

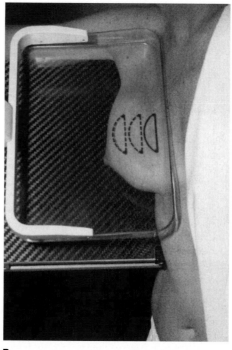

B

Fig. 5–1. Positioning of the patient for **A** the craniocaudal view of the mammogram and **B** mediolateral oblique view of the mammogram.

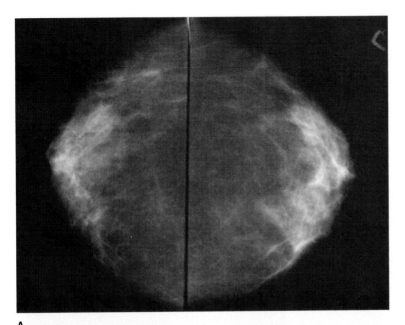

A

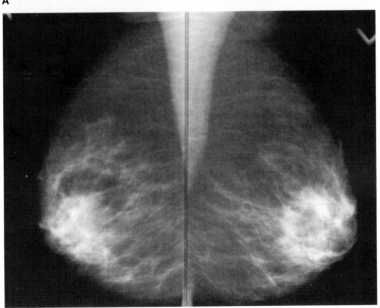

B

Fig. 5–2. **A** Normal bilateral craniocaudal views. **B** Normal bilateral mediolateral oblique views. This patient shows a moderate amount of residual fibroglandular density, having a mixed pattern of dense and fatty areas of the breast.

technique. In its present state of evolution, the sensitivity of radiomammography ranges from 85% to 95%.

LIMITATIONS

Sensitivity is limited by three factors: (1) the nature of breast parenchyma, (2) the difficulty in positioning the organ for imaging, and (3) the nature of breast carcinoma.

The nature of breast parenchyma. Very dense breast tissue may obscure masses lying within adjacent tissue. Masses are more easily detected in a fatty breast.

Positioning. A technologist performing mammography must include as much breast tissue as possible in the field of view for each image. The x-ray beam must pass through the breast tangentially to the thorax, and no other part of the body should intrude into the field of view, so as to not obscure any part of the breast. This requires both a cooperative patient and a skilled technologist. If a breast mass is located in a portion of the breast that is difficult to include in the image, mammography may fail to demonstrate the lesion. Also, because of these practical considerations, routine mammography is not performed in markedly debilitated patients.

The nature of breast carcinoma. Some breast carcinomas are seen as well-defined, rounded masses or as tiny, but bright, calcifications, and are easily detected. Others, however, may be poorly defined and irregular, mimicking normal breast tissue. Rarely, still others may have no radiographic signs at all.

For these reasons, it must be remembered that mammography has significant limitations in detection of carcinoma. It cannot be overemphasized that any suspicious finding on breast physical examination should be evaluated further, even if the mammogram shows no abnormality. Occasionally, additional imaging may reveal an abnormality, but if not, short-term close clinical follow-up or biopsy is warranted.

NORMAL STRUCTURES

Normal breast is composed mainly of parenchyma (lobules and ducts), connective tissue, and fat. Lobules are drained by ducts, which arborize within lobes. There are about 15 to 20 lobes in the breast. The lobar ducts converge on the nipple.

Parenchyma. The lobules are glandular units and are seen as ill-defined, splotchy opacities of medium density. Their size varies from 1 to several millimeters, and larger opacities result from conglomerates of lobules with little interspersed fat. The breast lobes are intertwined and are therefore not discretely identifiable. This parenchymal tissue is contained between the premammary and retromammary fascia.

The amount and distribution of glandular tissue are highly variable. Younger women tend to have more glandular tissue than do older women. Glandular atrophy begins inferomedially, and residual glandular density persists longer in the upper outer breast quadrants. However, any pattern can be seen at any adult age (Fig. 5–3).

Along with glandular elements, the parenchyma consists of ductal tissue. Only major ducts are visualized mammographically, and these are seen in the subareolar region as thickened linear structures of medium density converging on the nipple.

Connective tissue. Trabecular structures, which are condensations of connective tissue, appear as thin (<1-mm) linear opacities of medium to high density. Cooper's ligaments are the supporting trabeculae over the breast that give the organ its characteristic shape, and are thus seen as curved lines around fat lobules along the skin–parenchyma interface within any one breast (Fig. 5–4).

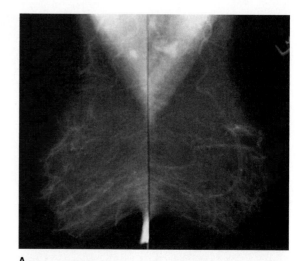

A

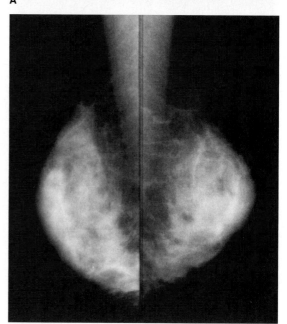

B

Fig. 5–3. Normal mammograms of **A** fatty breasts and **B** dense breasts. Note the extreme variation of the normal breast parenchymal pattern between patients. A small carcinoma would be much more difficult to detect in the patient with dense breasts than in the patient with fatty breasts.

Fat. The breast is composed of a large amount of fat, which is lucent, or almost black, on mammograms. Fat is distributed in the subcutaneous layer, in among the parenchymal elements centrally, and in the retromammary layer anterior to the pectoral muscle (Fig. 5–4).

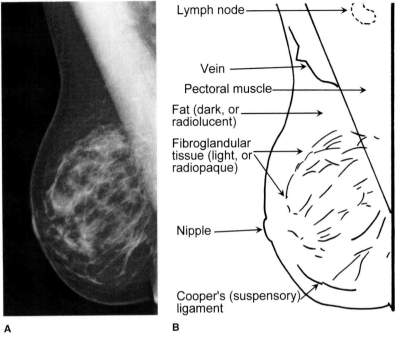

Lymph node

Vein

Pectoral muscle

Fat (dark, or radiolucent)

Fibroglandular tissue (light, or radiopaque)

Nipple

Cooper's (suspensory) ligament

A **B**

Fig. 5–4. **A** Mediolateral oblique view of normal breast. **B** Line drawing with identification of normal structures visible in part A.

Lymph nodes. Lymph nodes are seen in the axillae and occasionally in the breast itself (Fig. 5–4).

Veins. Veins are seen traversing the breast as uniform, linear opacities, about 1 to 5 mm in diameter (Fig. 5–4).

Arteries. Arteries appear as slightly thinner, uniform, linear densities and are best seen when calcified, as in patients with atherosclerosis, diabetes, or renal disease.

Skin. Skin lines are normally thin and are not easily seen without the aid of a bright light for film-screen mammograms. Various processing algorithms with digital mammography may allow better visualization of the skin.

SCREENING MAMMOGRAPHY

The standard mammogram (along with appropriate history-taking) makes up the entire screening mammogram. The indication for this examination is the search for occult carcinoma in an asymptomatic patient. Physical examination by the patient's physician, known as the *clinical breast examination* (CBE), and *breast self-examination* (BSE) are the other two indispensable elements in complete breast screening. Table 5–1 includes guidelines for frequency.

DIAGNOSTIC MAMMOGRAPHY

The diagnostic mammogram begins with the two-view standard mammogram. Additional maneuvers are then used as appropriate in each case, dictated by history, physical examination, and findings on initial mammography. Indications for diagnostic mammography are (1) a palpable mass or other symptom or sign (e.g., skin dimpling, nipple retraction, or nipple discharge that is clear or bloody) and (2) a radiographic abnormality on a screening mammogram. Additionally, patients with a personal history of breast cancer may be considered in the diagnostic category.

Other projections, magnification, and spot compression may be used to further evaluate abnormalities. These techniques provide better detail and disperse overlapping breast tissue so that lesions are less obscured.

TABLE 5–1. American Cancer Society Recommendations for Breast Cancer Detection in Asymptomatic Women

Age group	Examination	Frequency
20–39	Breast self-examination	Monthly
	Clinical breast examination	Every 3 years
40 and older	Breast self-examination	Monthly
	Clinical breast examination	Annually
	Mammography	Annually

Implant views. Patients with breast implants require specialized views to best image residual breast tissue because the implants obscure large areas of the breast tissue with routine mammography. These specialized views, Eklund or "push-back" views, displace the implants posteriorly while the breast tissue is pulled anteriorly as much as possible.

Ultrasonography

The indications for ultrasonography are (1) a mammographically detected mass, the nature of which is indeterminate; (2) a palpable mass that is not seen on mammography; (3) a palpable mass in a patient below the age recommended for routine mammography; and (4) guidance for intervention. Ultrasonography is a highly reliable technique for differentiating cystic from solid masses. If criteria for a simple cyst are met, the diagnosis is more than 99% accurate. Although certain features have been described as indicative of benign or malignant solid masses, this determination is more difficult to make and less accurate than the determination of the cystic nature of a mass.

A limitation of ultrasonography is that it is very operator dependent. Also, it images only a small part of the breast at any one moment. Therefore, an overall inclusive survey is not possible in one image, and lesions may easily be missed.

NORMAL STRUCTURES

The skin, premammary and retromammary fasciae, trabeculae, walls of ducts and vessels, and pectoral fasciae are well seen as linear structures. The glandular and fat lobules are oval, of varying sizes, and hypoechoic relative to the surrounding connective tissue (Fig. 5–5).

Simple cysts are *anechoic* (echo-free) and have thin, smooth walls. Increased echogenicity is seen deep to cysts (enhanced through-transmission). Most solid masses are hypoechoic relative to surrounding breast tissue.

Magnetic Resonance Imaging

Magnetic resonance (MR) imaging is used to evaluate the integrity of breast implants when the specialized mammographic views (Eklund views) are insufficient.

Other current applications include staging of tumor in the breast, search for a primary tumor in patients with cancerous axillary lymph nodes, evaluation of tumor response to neoadjuvant chemotherapy, and differentiation of dense breast tissue or fibrosis from tumor. Because of its present cost, inaccessibility, and lack of standardized interpretation guidelines, however, MR imaging of the breast is not yet widely used routinely.

Selection of pulse sequences and intravenous contrast administration is based on the indication.

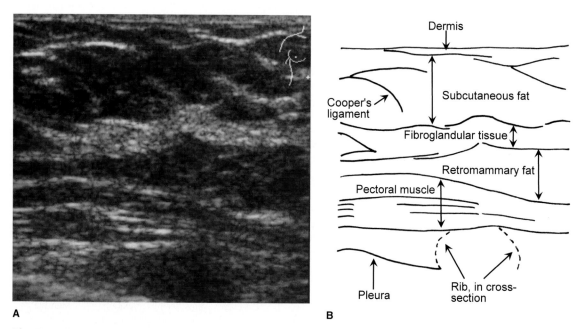

A **B**

Fig. 5–5. **A** Ultrasonographic image of a portion of normal breast. **B** Line drawing identifying normal structures visible on the sonographic image.

The patient lies prone on the scanner table, and a specialized coil surrounds the breast. The patient must remain motionless in the scanner for several minutes at a time. The entire procedure time varies from 20 minutes to 1 hour. Intravenous contrast material is administered if carcinoma is to be ruled out.

NORMAL STRUCTURES

Tissues are differentiated by their pattern of change on different pulse sequences. The skin, nipple and areola, mammary fat, breast parenchyma, and connective tissue are normally seen, in addition to the anterior chest wall, including musculature, ribs, and their cartilaginous portions, and portions of internal organs. Small calcifications are not visible, and small solid nodules may not be detected. Cystic structures are well seen. Normal implants appear as cystic structures with well-defined walls. Their location is deep to the breast parenchyma or subpectoral, depending on the surgical technique that was used to place the implants. The internal signal varies and depends on implant contents, either silicone or saline.

Ductography

Ductography, or galactography, uses mammographic imaging with contrast injection into the breast ducts. The indication for use is a profuse, spontaneous, non-milky nipple discharge from a single duct orifice. If these conditions are not present, the ductogram is likely to be of little help. The purpose is to reveal the location of the ductal system involved. The cause of the discharge is frequently not identified. Occasionally an intraluminal abnormality is seen, but findings have low specificity.

The patient lies in supine position while the discharging duct is cannulated with a blunt-tipped needle or catheter under visual inspection and with the aid of a magnifying glass. A small amount of contrast material (usually not more than 1 cm^3) is injected gently by hand into the duct. Several mammographic images are then made. The procedure requires about 30 minutes and is not normally painful.

NORMAL STRUCTURES

Just deep to the opening of the duct on the nipple, the duct expands into the lactiferous sinus. After a few millimeters, the duct narrows again and then branches as it enters the lobe containing the glands drained by this ductal system. The normal caliber of the duct and its branches is highly variable, but normal duct walls should be smooth, without truncation or abrupt narrowing. With high-pressure injection, the lobules, as well as cystically dilated portions of ducts and lobules, may opacify.

Image-Guided Needle Aspiration and Biopsy

The indications for needle aspiration and biopsy of breast lesions are varied and are variably interpreted by radiologists and referring physicians. Two categories are discussed here.

The first indication is aspiration of cystic lesions to confirm diagnosis, to relieve pain, or both. Nonpalpable cysts require guidance with either ultrasound or mammography. A fine needle (20–25 gauge) usually suffices. The cystic fluid is not routinely sent for cytology unless it is bloody.

The second indication concerns solid lesions. Needle biopsy is used in this case to (1) confirm benignity of a lesion carrying a low suspicion of malignancy mammographically, (2) to confirm malignancy in a highly suspicious lesion prior to initiating further surgical planning and treatment, and (3) to evaluate any other relevant mammographic lesion for which either follow-up imaging or surgical excision is a less desirable option for further evaluation. Guidance for needle biopsy can be accomplished with stereotactic mammography, ultrasound, and MR. The imaging modality for needle guidance is selected on the basis of lesion characteristics, availability of technology, and personal preference of the radiologist. Ultrasound and mammography are most commonly used.

Large core needle biopsy (typically 14 or 11 gauge) has been shown to be more accurate for nonpalpable lesions than fine-needle aspiration (20 gauge or smaller), and is often combined with vacuum assistance to further increase tissue yield.

Mammographic guidance is most easily and accurately performed with a stereotactic table unit. Lesions of only a few millimeters can be successfully biopsied. With stereotactic tables, the patient lies prone with the breast protruding through an opening in the table surface. A needle is mechanically guided to the proper location in the breast with computer assistance (Fig. 5–6). The entire procedure requires 30 minutes to 1 hour.

Image-Guided Needle Localization

When a nonpalpable breast lesion must be excised, imaging is used to guide placement of a needle into the breast, with the needle tip traversing or flanking the lesion. Either ultrasonographic or mammographic guidance can be used, and the choice again depends on lesion characteristics and personal preference. Once the needle is in the appropriate position, a hook wire is inserted through the needle to anchor the device in place. This prevents migration during patient transport and surgery. After needle placement, the patient is taken to the operating area for excision of the lesion by the surgeon.

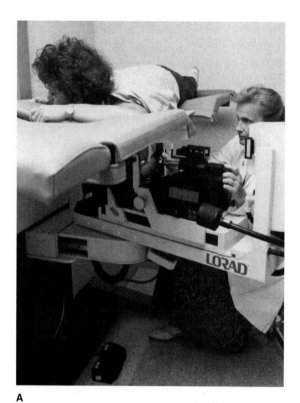

A

Fig. 5–6. **A** Stereotactic biopsy table with patient undergoing core needle biopsy of the breast.

Biopsy Specimen Radiography

When a lesion is excised from the breast, a surgical specimen can be radiographed to document that the mammographic abnormality was removed. This practice is routinely followed with needle-localized lesions, but palpable lesions excised may also be radiographed to confirm that the specimen contains an abnormality that may have been present on the mammogram.

TECHNIQUE SELECTION

As with other organ systems, the task of the referring physician, with regard to breast imaging, is to determine which patients may benefit from these studies and which are the appropriate studies to order. To do this, the physician first categorizes the patient as asymptomatic or symptomatic:

1. *Asymptomatic patients.* As a group, these patients will benefit from routine screening mammography performed according to published national guidelines. A particular patient may require an individualized program for specific reasons. For example, a 30-year-old asymptomatic woman whose mother died of breast cancer at age 35 may justifiably begin yearly screening mammography.

2. *Symptomatic patients.* These are women who have any of the following signs or symptoms: a new or enlarging breast lump, skin changes (primarily dimpling), nipple retraction, eczematoid nipple changes, bloody or serous nipple discharge, and focal pain or tenderness. Diagnostic mammography

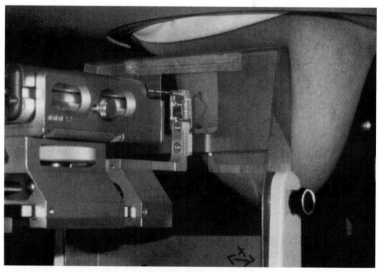

Fig. 5–6. **B** The needle is mechanically guided into the breast with the aid of computer targeting on mammographic images.

B

is indicated in these patients. If the patient is under 35 years of age, the examinations may be differently tailored than for older patients. A telephone call to the radiologist may be helpful in determining a suitable evaluation plan in any patient for whom the usual guidelines are not helpful.

If a diagnostic study is needed, a standard two-view mammogram is obtained first. The need for further studies will be determined by the results of the mammogram. Whether ultrasonography or another modality is needed is best decided by the person interpreting the films, provided that he or she has the necessary clinical information available. For example, it is imperative that the location and description of a suspected mass be made known to the radiologist so that a specific search can be made for a lesion.

Also, knowledge of prior surgery, inflammation, or trauma to the breast is a requirement for accurate image interpretation. The different disease processes may have overlapping appearances on breast images, and refining the differential diagnosis, therefore, depends on accurate breast physical examination and the patient's history.

When it has been determined that an abnormality is present, then the decision as to whether close follow-up, needle biopsy, or excision is warranted is best made by integrating the image-based diagnosis and clinical considerations. Good communication between the radiologist and referring physician is needed to optimize management of breast lesions.

Patient Preparation

For the mammogram, two-piece clothing is most convenient because the patient will need to undress from the waist up. Patients should not apply antiperspirant to the breast or axilla, since it may cause artifacts.

Mammography is generally limited to ambulatory, cooperative patients because of the difficulties in proper positioning and because mammography units are not portable. If a debilitated patient has a palpable mass, then ultrasound would be a reasonable first step, followed by bedside needle aspiration or biopsy if the mass is solid. Screening mammography in markedly debilitated patients rarely has clinical utility.

Patients for whom stereotactic biopsy is being considered should be able to lie in the prone position without moving for about 1 hour.

Conflict with Other Procedures

Coordinating with other techniques is an infrequent problem with breast imaging. One situation that does occasionally cause difficulty occurs in the patient with a palpable mass that is aspirated with a needle prior to imaging. Aspiration of a simple cyst may cause bleeding into the lesion. Subsequent ultrasonography then shows a complex lesion with debris or some apparently solid elements, rather than a simple cyst. A complex lesion requires more aggressive management than does a simple cyst. Therefore, imaging is best performed prior to aspiration.

EXERCISES

The Symptomatic Patient
EXERCISE 5-1: THE PALPABLE MASS

(Please answer questions for this exercise before looking at the images that are presented with the discussion.)

Clinical Histories:

Case 5-1. A 34-year-old woman who noticed a new lump in her breast

Case 5-2. A 60-year-old woman who, on the insistence of her children, went for her first routine physical examination in many years. Her doctor found a mass in her breast.

Case 5-3. A 53-year-old woman who thinks she feels a hard nodule deep in her breast. Her breasts are of dense nodular texture. She had a normal screening mammogram 4 months ago.

Case 5-4. A 78-year-old woman with a soft, rounded mass discovered during physical examination

Questions:

5-1. What test should be ordered first in Case 5-1?
- **A.** Screening mammography
- **B.** Excisional biopsy
- **C.** Ultrasonography
- **D.** Diagnostic mammography
- **E.** Needle aspiration

5-2. What test should be ordered first in Case 5-2?
- **A.** Screening mammography
- **B.** Excisional biopsy
- **C.** Ultrasonography
- **D.** Diagnostic mammography
- **E.** Needle aspiration

5-3. What test should be ordered first in Case 5-3?
- **A.** Screening mammography
- **B.** Excisional biopsy
- **C.** Ultrasonography
- **D.** Diagnostic mammography
- **E.** Needle aspiration

5-4.   With respect to the patient in Case 5-4, which one of the following statements is true?
    A.   A 78-year-old is not likely to benefit from mammography.
    B.   Soft, rounded masses are benign and do not require biopsy.
    C.   This mass should initially be aspirated with a needle.
    D.   If this mass is carcinoma, the patient will probably die of this disease.
    E.   Her physical findings could easily be caused by a lipoma.

Approach to the Palpable Lump

When a breast lump is found, several questions must be answered before proceeding with breast imaging. First, given that lumpy breasts are a normal variant, when is a lump significant? Experts in CBE advise palpation with the flat surface of two to three fingers, and not with the fingertips. With this technique, nonsignificant lumps will disperse into background breast density, but a significant lump will stand out as a dominant mass.

Second, is the lump new or enlarged? A new lump is more suspicious than a lump that has not changed over a few years.

Third, how big is the lump? Tiny pea-sized or smaller lumps, particularly in young women, are often observed closely with repeated CBE, because small breast nodules are extremely common, frequently resolve spontaneously, and are usually benign. Repeating CBE in 6 weeks allows for interval menses, which frequently causes waning or resolution of the lump. If the lump persists, diagnostic mammography is indicated.

Fourth, how old is the patient? If the patient is less than about 35 years of age, then radiation is avoided unless specifically indicated, because the younger breast is more sensitive to radiation. For patients older than 35 years, breast imaging begins with a diagnostic mammogram at the time a lump is deemed to be significant. The mammogram provides a view of the lump, as well as of the remainder of the involved breast and the opposite breast, where associated findings may aid in diagnosis and treatment planning.

If the patient is younger than 35 years of age, a significant lump is usually first examined with ultrasonography to determine whether a simple cyst is present. If there is no cyst, and the patient is younger than 30 years of age, a mammogram may then be obtained. The density of the breast in such a young patient may limit the usefulness of radiomammography, so the mammogram may be limited to one breast or to a single view.

For women between the ages of 30 and 40 years, judgment is needed as to whether other imaging is indicated. Several factors should be weighed, including age, family history of breast carcinoma, reproductive history, and findings at CBE. If the primary care physician is uncertain of the significance of the findings of a CBE, evaluation by a breast specialist may be helpful prior to requesting radiologic tests.

Discussion:

The 34-year-old woman in Case 5-1 indeed has a dominant mass, 2 cm in diameter on CBE. She says it was definitely not present until recently. She has no risk factors for breast cancer. The mass most likely is a fibroadenoma or a cyst, but carcinoma cannot be excluded. The patient now needs breast ultrasonography. (*C* is the correct answer to Question 5-1.)

Ultrasonography is best ordered before attempted needle aspiration because aspiration can alter the appearance of simple cysts, giving a misleading suspicious appearance. Therefore, answer *E*, needle aspiration, is incorrect.

Figure 5–7 shows an image from the ultrasound study, that represents the area precisely in the location of the palpable mass. This area is echo free, with sharply delineated walls and posterior acoustic enhancement (increased echogenicity deep to the anechoic area) consistent with a simple cyst. If these three features are seen, the probability of a simple cyst is greater than 99% and no further treatment is indicated unless the patient has pain and needs cyst drainage for symptomatic relief. Therefore, option *B*, excisional biopsy, is inappropriate because biopsy can be avoided by showing a simple cyst. No further imaging is needed. The patient is under the age of 40 years, not yet of screening age, and radiation should be avoided in young patients. Therefore, answers *A* and *D*, screening and diagnostic mammography, are not viable options until ultrasound is performed. Figure 5–8 illustrates the mammographic features of a cyst. The shape is round or oval, and the margins are smooth and sharply delineated.

Simple cysts are very common in the premenopausal patient and in patients who are being treated with replacement hormone therapy. A complex cyst is one that has internal debris—blood, pus, or tumor. A complex cyst requires further evaluation and a short-term follow-up (6–8 weeks) ultrasound may be sufficient. If the debris is due to attempted aspiration, it may clear on follow-up ultrasonography. Otherwise, excision or needle biopsy is indicated.

The 60-year-old woman in Case 5-2 has a 1.5-cm dominant mass on CBE. It is irregular and not freely mobile. The patient has never had a mammogram. Because she has a palpable mass, however, a screening mammogram is inappropriate, so option *A* is incorrect. Although the mass feels suspicious, she still needs a diagnostic mammogram prior to biopsy (option *B*, excisional biopsy, is incorrect) to exclude other lesions such as multifocal carcinoma. (*D* is the correct answer to Question 5-2.)

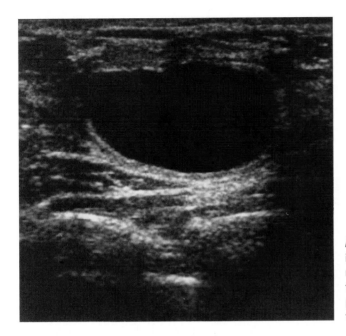

Fig. 5–7. Ultrasonograic image of the patient in Case 5-1. The anechoic, uniformly black area represents a simple cyst. Note that the walls of the cyst are sharp, and there is a brighter echo pattern deep to the cyst (enhanced through-transmission).

The need for ultrasonography in a patient of this age is dictated by the mammographic appearance; therefore, option *C,* ultrasonography, is incorrect.

Her mammogram (Fig. 5–9) shows a very fatty breast, making any abnormal findings readily apparent. There is a mass measuring 1 cm in the upper outer quadrant that corresponds to the area of the palpated mass. The mass is of high density, being white on the mammogram. There is abundant spiculation and stranding around the mass, which is represented by the radiating linear densities around the periphery of the mass. There is also retraction of the linear patterns of the normal breast tissue; this retraction is known as *architectural distortion.* These findings represent the classical features of a malignant lesion on mammography, and this mass must be biopsied. A spiculated mass such as this is the most common appearance of invasive breast carcinoma. Less common signs are a circumscribed mass, asymmetric density, and architectural distortion alone. Intraductal (noninvasive) carcinoma more commonly appears as calcifications.

Spiculation around an invasive carcinoma corresponds to fingers of tumor, as well as to a desmoplastic reaction of adjacent normal breast tissue responding to the presence of tumor. This patient has an invasive ductal carcinoma. About 90% of primary breast carcinomas are ductal carcinomas, and the other 10% are lobular carcinomas.

Besides carcinoma, the primary differential diagnosis for a spiculated mass includes postsurgical change, other trauma with hematoma, fat necrosis, infection, and radial scar (a complex, spontaneous benign lesion involving ductal proliferation, elastosis, and fibrosis).

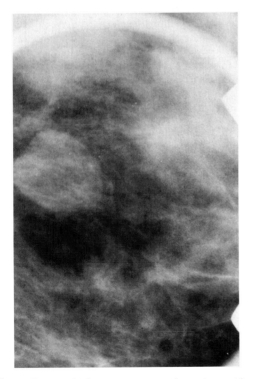

Fig. 5–8. Detail of a mammogram of a patient with a simple cyst. The smoothly circumscribed margin and the round-to-oval opacity, through which normal breast structures are visible, are characteristic of a simple cyst.

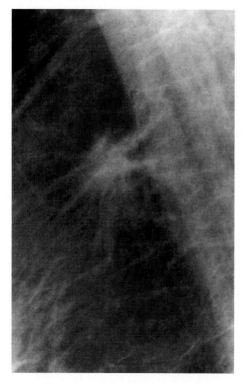

Fig. 5–9. Detail of a mammogram of the patient in Case 5-2. Note the spiculated mass in the upper outer quadrant of this otherwise fatty breast. Diagnosis: invasive ductal carcinoma.

There are no other lesions in this patient's breast, and the other breast appears normal. By mammographic criteria, then, the patient is a good candidate for treatment with lumpectomy and radiation therapy rather than mastectomy. Her tumor is solitary localized to one quadrant and her breast tissue is otherwise easy to evaluate mammographically. Recurrent tumor or additional lesions should, therefore, be readily seen on post-treatment follow-up mammograms.

For a mass that feels malignant and appears suspicious on a mammogram, fine-needle aspiration (FNA) at the bedside may provide a rapid cytological diagnosis of carcinoma. Because FNA best follows mammography, option *E*, needle aspiration, is incorrect. FNA may then be followed by definitive surgical treatment at a later date, after the patient has had time to consider the treatment options available. If FNA fails to disclose carcinoma, then excisional biopsy is required because of the suspicious findings on mammography and CBE. The occasional false-negative FNA occurs with tumors that do not shed cellular material readily.

Cytology of this palpable mass revealed ductal carcinoma and this patient chose to have a lumpectomy.

The 53-year-old patient in Case 5-3 has an ill-defined 1.5-cm hardened nodular area in her breast. Results of screening mammography less than 1 year ago were normal. Her breast tissue is not fatty, as in Case 5-2, but she has quite dense, nodular, fibroglandular tissue, which may obscure small masses. The average doubling time of breast carcinoma makes it unlikely that she has a palpable carcinoma that is entirely new since her last mammogram. It is quite possible, however, that she has had a smaller cancer for a few years and that it has now grown large enough to be palpated. Breast tumors are typically not palpable unless they are at least 1 cm in diameter. Before this stage, in the preclinical phase, the tumor may be visible up to 2 to 3 years earlier on the mammogram if the breast is fatty. In dense breasts, as discussed previously, tumors may not be seen on the mammogram until later stages. For this reason, regular BSE and CBE are important. Mammography will miss some cancers, regardless of the situation, at a rate variably reported to be between 5% and 15%.

With a new area of abnormality on physical examination, being in a high-risk age group (more than 50 years old), and having a dense parenchymal pattern, the patient needs another mammogram, this time a diagnostic mammogram of the involved breast only. (*D* is the correct answer to Question 5-3.) Option *A*, screening mammogram, is incorrect, because it is too soon to repeat screening mammography at this time and the patient does have a palpable finding—as contraindication for a screening study.

Figure 5–10*A* shows a vague, rounded opacity within dense fibroglandular tissue. This is in the area of the palpable mass, as indicated by a small metallic marker (much like a BB pellet) taped on the skin over the abnormality. Detail is not adequate to make a judgment as to the possibility of malignancy here, or even to confirm that a real lesion is present. The appearance may merely be due to superimposed normal breast shadows. Compression spot films are needed to confirm the presence of a mass and to better define its borders.

Figure 5–10*B* shows spot compression of the questioned opacity seen on initial images. This localized compression with a smaller paddle placed directly over the abnormality achieves two things. First, it separates the opacity from adjacent breast tissue, demonstrating this to be a discrete mass with high density and not merely a superimposition of normal shadows. Second, it elicits clear spiculation and architectural distortion around the mass. These features are classic for breast carcinoma, and biopsy is therefore required. Biopsy of this lesion showed invasive ductal carcinoma.

The 78-year-old patient in Case 5-4 has a soft mass in her breast and clearly needs a diagnostic mammogram

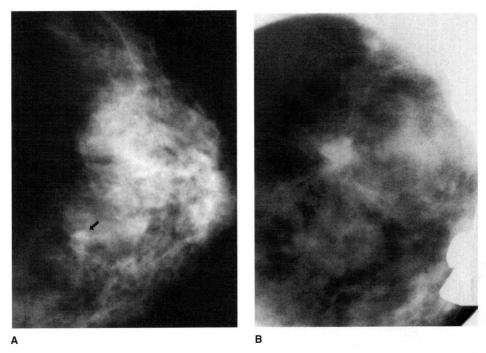

A   **B**

Fig. 5–10. **A** Detail of a mammogram of the patient in Case 5-3. There is a dense nodular breast pattern with a vague, small, rounded opacity (*arrow*). **B** Spot compression view of the region of suspected abnormality in part A. Note how much easier it is to see the lesion and the spiculation (around it) with spot compression. Note also the difficulty in detecting and evaluating this tumor within dense glandular tissue, compared with the fatty breast in Case 5-2.

because of her age and the palpable findings. Soft, rounded masses on physical examination are often benign fibroadenomata or cysts, but carcinoma may also present this way. (Statement *B* is false.)

Other benign causes of these physical findings include hematoma, abscess, and lipoma. (Statement *E* is true and the correct answer to Question 5-4.) Therefore, a mammogram may be beneficial for two reasons: (1) If a benign finding is revealed, biopsy may be avoided; and (2) if findings suggest malignancy, optimal treatment can be planned on the basis of the extent of the lesion and the presence or absence of additional lesions. (Statement A is false.)

Her mammogram (Fig. 5–11) shows two findings. There is a rounded mass with multiple lobulations and circumscribed borders. The fact that the borders are not sharply outlined on all sides raises the suspicion level for this finding. Masses that are sharply delineated may be followed with serial mammograms at 6-month intervals if they are known not to be new, are nonpalpable, and show no other features of malignancy. This is not the case with the patient in Case 5-4. Note the fading margin along portions of the mass. This mass corresponds to the palpable finding. Ultrasonography would be useful to exclude a multiloculated cyst and show the lesion to

be solid. Biopsy is indicated, but needle aspiration without imaging would have been inappropriate. (Statement *C* is false.)

A circumscribed mass representing carcinoma is seen less often than a spiculated mass. About 10% of invasive ductal carcinomas represent the better differentiated subtypes, including medullary carcinoma, mucinous (colloid) carcinoma, and papillary carcinoma, all of which are frequently seen as circumscribed masses. They tend to have a better prognosis than the less well-differentiated garden-variety ductal carcinomas.

The differential diagnosis for the circumscribed mass on mammography includes carcinoma (primary as well as metastatic), fibroadenoma, and cysts; hematoma, abscess, and miscellaneous benign lesions are seen much less often. Correlation with clinical history and physical examination can help to narrow the differential diagnosis. When carcinoma cannot be excluded, either needle aspiration or excisional biopsy is required.

This patient had a needle biopsy. Because palpation alone could not reliably localize this lesion for needle biopsy because of its soft nature and the difficulty in fixing its position, stereotactic mammographic guidance was used in localizing the lesion for this procedure. The

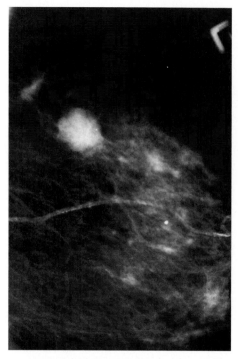

Fig. 5–11. Detail of a mammogram of the patient in Case 5-4.

diagnosis of mucinous carcinoma was made by microscopic inspection of the specimen.

Now, were you astute enough to perceive the second lesion? Above and to the left of large mass is a smaller, dense spiculated mass. This was also biopsied and proved to be a carcinoma of the very well-differentiated tubular type. Even though the patient has two lesions now, both carry an excellent prognosis and she will be unlikely to die from breast carcinoma. (Statement *D* is false.) In fact, although mastectomy is certainly a reasonable treatment for her, local excision would also be an option with these nonaggressive lesions.

EXERCISE 5-2: LUMPINESS, NIPPLE DISCHARGE, AND PAIN

Clinical Histories:

Case 5-5. An 82-year-old woman who complains of newly lumpy, painful breasts. Figure 5-12 is the same breast; part *A* was taken 1 year before *B*.

Case 5-6. A 45-year-old woman with a serous nipple discharge. Ductography was performed (Fig. 5–13).

Case 5-7. A 37-year-old woman who comes to the emergency department with a reddened, swollen, painful left breast. The right (*A*) and left (*B*) breast are shown in Fig. 5–14.

Case 5-8. A 52-year-old woman with soreness in the right breast, the mammogram of which is seen in Fig. 5–15.

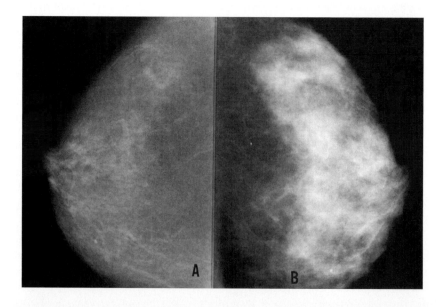

Fig. 5–12.

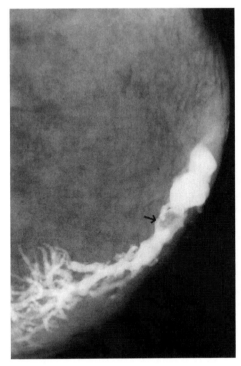

Fig. 5–13.

Questions:

5-5. The most likely explanation for the patient's symptoms and mammographic change in Case 5-5 is
   A. hormone effect.
   B. infectious mastitis.
   C. carcinoma.
   D. congestive heart failure.
   E. cystic disease.

5-6. For Case 5-6, with respect to ductography and this patient's condition, which of the following statements is true?
   A. Ductography should be performed in all patients with nipple discharge.
   B. The cause for this patient's discharge is more likely to be malignant than benign.
   C. This ductogram shows an extraluminal filling defect.
   D. Ductography has a high specificity for malignant lesions.
   E. Ductography is helpful in guiding the surgeon's approach.

5-7. With respect to Case 5-7, which of the following statements is false?
   A. There is diffuse abnormality on the left.
   B. Inflammatory carcinoma is high on the differential diagnostic list.
   C. Infectious mastitis is unlikely to be the cause in this nonlactating patient.

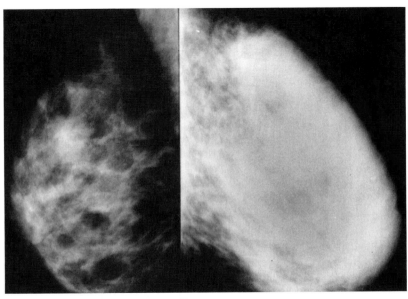

Fig. 5–14.

A   B

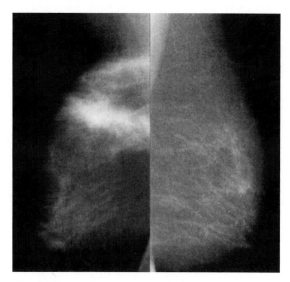

Fig. 5–15.

D. The mammographic appearance is non-specific.

E. Follow-up imaging after a course of antibiotics would be appropriate.

5-8. With respect to Case 5-8, which one of the following statements is true?

A. The soreness indicates a benign process.

B. The appearance is malignant, and biopsy is necessary.

C. Findings on physical examination and history may radically alter our management decision.

D. Bleeding, such as that due to anticoagulation therapy, would not have this appearance.

E. The most likely diagnosis is fibrocystic change.

Radiologic Findings:

5-5. The mammograms of Fig. 5–12 show a diffuse marked increase in mammographic density with a nodular character.

5-6. In the ductogram of Fig. 5–13, contrast has been injected into a portion of a single ductal system with opacification of the lactiferous sinus and larger branching ducts. Most of the walls are smooth, as they should be. However, there is a filling defect in one of the major branches, as exhibited by the lucency outlined by contrast on all sides and indicated by the arrow. (Statement *C* is false.)

5-7. Mammograms of the right and left breast (Fig. 5–14) show that the entire left breast (*B*) is abnormally dense.

5-8. Mammogram (Fig. 5–15) shows a large band of high density with markedly spiculated margins in the upper part of the breast.

Discussion:

Lumpy breasts are a variant of normal and, as such, require careful physical examination and mammography to detect any carcinoma and to avoid unnecessary surgery. Diffuse lumpiness is not a contraindication to screening mammography, but when a particular lump becomes dominant, a diagnostic study is indicated.

The two mammograms of the patient in Fig. 5–12 were obtained 1 year apart. Between these two exams, the patient began to exhibit menopause symptoms and was started on hormonal replacement therapy. (*A* is the correct answer to Question 5-5.) The breasts, which were previously largely fatty (*A*), have become moderately dense and very lumpy on palpation 1 year later (*B*). This change can also be seen, although not usually as dramatically, in the perimenopausal time of estrogen flare.

Such changes can be seen asymmetrically or unilaterally, and it is useful to remember the estrogen effect when evaluating mammograms with interval changes. Correlation with clinical history is then needed.

Answer *B,* infectious mastitis, and answer *C,* carcinoma, are incorrect because both of these entities are usually unilateral and focal. Option *D,* congestive heart failure (CHF), is incorrect because CHF causes bilateral changes that have a more linear pattern of trabecular thickening on mammography, rather than the patchy, ill-defined nodular pattern characteristic of glandular and cystic densities seen here. Answer *E,* cystic disease, is incorrect. Cysts are seen as a component of hormone-related breast changes, but spontaneous cystic disease alone is rare at this age.

In the patient in Case 5-6, a single intraluminal filling defect is seen on ductography (Fig. 5–13). However, we cannot determine from these findings alone whether the defect is due to a benign or a malignant nodule (statement *D* is false), although approximately 90% of nipple discharges are due to benign causes (statement *B* is false). The filling defect in this woman was a benign papilloma, the most common cause of bloody or serous discharge. Mammograms usually do not show these small, intraductal nodules.

Whether or not a filling defect is seen on a ductogram, biopsy is needed to rule out carcinoma, and the ductogram may be helpful in showing the surgeon which area of the breast harbors the cause of discharge. (Statement *E* is true.) However, many surgeons are able to identify the lobe(s) involved by the pathology by inspecting the nipple, noting the location of the discharging duct, and by palpation, observing which portion of the breast produces discharge when compressed. In normal patients, ductography is not easily performed and is of limited usefulness when discharge is not spontaneous, profuse, and confined to a single duct. Therefore, statement A is false; ductograms should not be performed on all patients with nipple discharge. Furthermore, only bloody or serous discharges are of concern. A large portion of patients with discharge have secretions typical of fibrocystic change (i.e., a dark brownish or greenish fluid rather than a truly bloody or serous discharge). Milky discharge is normal.

In Case 5-7 (Fig. 5–14), the patient's entire left breast is abnormally dense. (Statement A is true.) There is skin thickening as well. This is a nonspecific appearance (statement D is true); infection and inflammatory carcinoma are both high on the differential diagnosis list. (Statement B is true; C is false and therefore the correct answer.) Breast carcinoma may incite an inflammatory response in the breast, mimicking a benign infectious process both clinically and radiographically. The patient turns out to have an elevated white blood cell count and fever with marked pain. This information now makes infection more likely than tumor, and a course of antibiotics with follow-up imaging to monitor resolution is appropriate. (Statement E is true.)

Figure 5–16 shows the follow-up mammogram after significant clinical resolution. The mammographic findings have resolved, and the left breast now appears very similar to the right one.

Infectious mastitis occurs more frequently in lactating women but is not uncommon in nonlactating women, particularly in diabetic patients. Imaging (mammography or ultrasound) is useful to exclude a drainable abscess collection and to provide a baseline for monitoring resolution to exclude carcinoma.

Case 5-8 illustrates the importance of correlation with history and physical examination. This patient has pain, as in the last case, but her mammographic abnormality (Fig. 5–15) is much more localized and appears more like a malignant mass, being a high-density opacity with excessive spiculation. However, this, too, is a benign process. The patient was in a motor vehicle accident 2 months earlier and sustained a severe injury to the right side of her chest. Physical examination shows a resolving laceration and contusion that extends in a linear fashion over the right breast. (No wonder she is sore!) A CT scan performed at the time of trauma showed the acute injury precisely in the area shown on the mammogram. These mammographic features are consistent with resolving (or acute) trauma. Therefore, no further action is warranted at this time, other than follow-up. (Statement C is true and is the correct answer to Question 5-8.) Although pain is not a prominent feature of carcinoma, patients with cancer may be symptomatic. Therefore, pain does not always mean benignancy. (Statement A is false.)

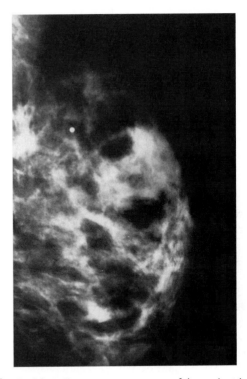

Fig. 5–16. Follow-up mammogram of the patient in Case 5-7 after a short course of antibiotics. Note the resolution of abnormal findings and the resultant symmetrical appearance compared with that of the opposite breast.

The mammographic appearance would certainly be highly suspicious for invasive carcinoma in the absence of clinical information, but with careful correlation we are able to avoid biopsy in this case. (Statement B is false.)

Anticoagulation therapy with resultant bleeding could also have this appearance. (Statement D is false.)

Fibrocystic change, although very common, is an unlikely diagnosis. Fibrocystic change appears as increased cloudy densities, nodular densities, and occasionally some thickened linear densities, but rarely as a spiculated mass. (Statement E is false.)

THE ASYMPTOMATIC PATIENT

EXERCISE 5-3: THE FIRST MAMMOGRAM

Clinical Histories:

Case 5-9.   A 40-year-old woman whose mother died of breast carcinoma (Fig. 5–17)

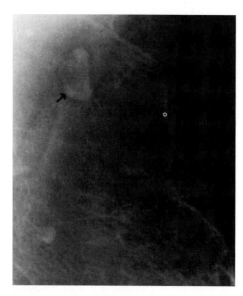

Fig. 5–17.

Case 5-10. A 42-year-old woman with no risk factors for breast carcinoma. She has no symptoms (Fig. 5–18)

Case 5-11. A 45-year-old woman, asymptomatic, with no risk factors (Fig. 5–19)

Questions:

5-9. According to the American Cancer Society, the best program of breast screening for the woman in Case 5-9 includes all of the following except
    A. monthly breast self-examination.
    B. yearly mammograms from age 40.
    C. cessation of routine mammograms at age 65.
    D. annual clinical breast examination.

5-10. The most likely diagnosis in Case 5-10 is
    A. complex cyst.
    B. fibroadenolipoma.
    C. galactocele.
    D. ductal carcinoma.
    E. oil cyst.

5-11. The differential diagnosis in Case 5-11 includes all of the following except
    A. invasive ductal carcinoma.
    B. cyst.
    C. intraductal comedocarcinoma.
    D. fibroadenoma.
    E. mucinous carcinoma.

Radiologic Findings:

5-9. Detail of mammogram (Fig. 5–17) of the patient in this case shows a smoothly marginated small mass with a lucent center (*arrow*).

5-10. The mammogram in this case (Fig. 5–18) shows a circumscribed mass (*arrows*) with internal lucency as well as opacity.

5-11. The mammogram of the patient in Case 5-11 (Fig. 5–19) shows a nodular density (*arrow*), with indistinct margins.

Discussion:

In Case 5-9 (Fig. 5–17), the 40-year-old woman has a strong family history of breast cancer, which puts her at high risk for developing the disease. As stated in the introduction to this chapter, great controversy exists concerning when mammographic screening should be initiated and the appropriate frequency of examinations in different groups. Most experts agree, however, that patients with a strong family history will benefit from screening beginning

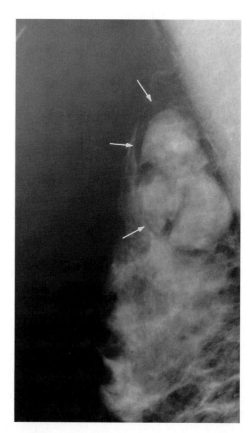

Fig. 5–18.

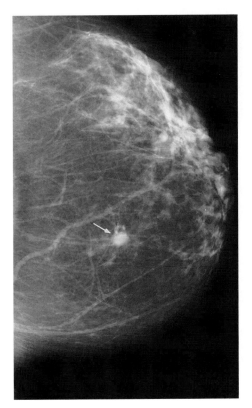

Fig. 5–19.

at age 40. The American Cancer Society (ACS) recommends annual screening above age 40 in all female patients; therefore, *B* is not the correct answer.

Although the upper age limit for mammographic screening has not been defined, we certainly cannot recommend cessation over age 65, since the prevalence of breast cancer is greatest in women in their fifties and sixties. (*C* is the correct answer to Question 5-9.) Current ACS guidelines recommend yearly mammograms for all women older than 40 years. Appropriate age for termination of screening is best judged by the patient's physician, weighing life expectancy against potential benefits from screening.

ACS also recommends yearly physical examination by the physician and monthly BSE by the patient to detect tumors missed by mammography, as well as those that become detectable between routine mammograms (interval cancers). Therefore, *A* and *D* are not correct answers to Question 5-9.

The mammogram for the patient in Case 5-9 (Fig. 5–17) is normal and demonstrates a typical normal lymph node. The node is smoothly marginated and has a fatty hilum, indicated by the darker center.

In Case 5-10, there is a circumscribed mass in the axillary tail of this breast (Fig. 5–18). The key to diagnosis is the mixture of densities within the lesion. Medium-density opacities are interspersed with lucencies within a smoothly marginated mass. This appearance is pathognomonic for a fibroadenolipoma, sometimes called by the misnomer *hamartoma*. (*B* is the correct answer to Question 5-10.) Being composed of elements of normal breast (fatty, glandular, and fibrous tissues) organized within a thin capsule, a fibroadenolipoma forms a "breast within a breast." As such, it is benign and needs no further evaluation. It may be palpable as a soft mass.

The point to remember here is that fat-containing masses are always benign. Answer *D*, ductal carcinoma, is incorrect. The differential diagnosis of a fatty mass, besides fibroadenolipoma, includes lymph node, as in Case 5-9, galactocele, lipoma, and oil cyst. Galactoceles are usually smaller and are seen in lactating women. (Answer *C* is incorrect.)

Oil cysts result from fat necrosis and are usually smaller. Typically, they are entirely lucent, because they are filled with oil, except for a thin wall. (Answer *E* is incorrect.)

Option A, complex cyst, is incorrect because this entity would not contain fat. A cyst, whether it contains serous fluid, blood, or pus, is always opaque and of low to high density, not lucent.

In Case 5-11, an asymptomatic 45-year-old woman's first mammogram (Fig. 5–19) shows a 1-cm nodule centrally located in this breast. The differential diagnosis remains broad without further studies to help characterize this nodule. All choices except option *C*, intraductal comedocarcinoma, may have this appearance. Intraductal carcinoma, when not mammographically occult, usually appears as microcalcifications. Because the margins are indistinct, however, the patient must be recalled for additional imaging to rule out carcinoma.

The sonographic image shows a solid lesion, ruling out a simple cyst. Spot compression is then used to evaluate the borders. If all margins were to appear smooth, one acceptable course of action would be serial 6-month follow-up mammograms for a period of 2 years to demonstrate stability. If any change occurs during this time, biopsy is indicated.

Spot compression (Fig. 5–20*A*) reveals that portions of the border are not smooth, raising the level of suspicion for malignancy. To exclude carcinoma, biopsy is needed.

Biopsy may be accomplished with excision or with needle biopsy. Excision would require needle localization of the nodule for the surgeon, since this is a nonpalpable lesion. Core needle biopsy, either stereotactic or ultrasound guided, is preferable because it is minimally invasive, causes less morbidity to the patient, leaves no distortion in the breast or on the skin, and is often less expensive than surgical excision. Accurate needle biopsy devices, however, are expensive and are not universally available.

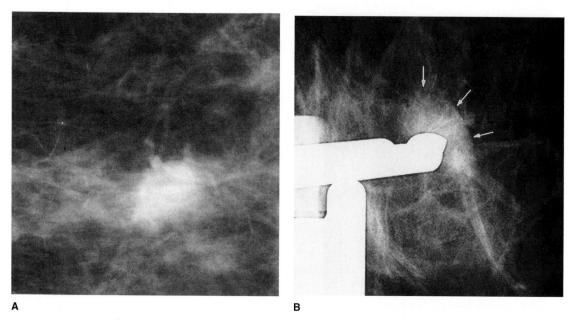

A

B

Fig. 5–20. **A** Spot compression of nodule seen in Fig. 5-19. The margins are indistinct and the shape is somewhat irregular. Biopsy is recommended. **B** Mammographic image obtained during stereotactic needle biopsy of the nodule in Case 5-11. The needle tip is about to pierce the nodule (*arrows*).

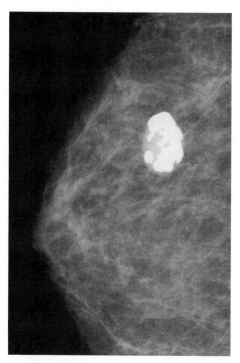

Fig. 5–21. Characteristic appearance of heavily calcified involuting fibroadenoma.

This nodule was diagnosed as a fibroadenoma with stereotactic core needle biopsy (Fig. 5–20*B*). Fibroadenomas are very common and are frequently the cause of benign breast biopsy. They occur in very young women (teenagers and women under 30 years of age) and persist undiscovered, through the age at which the first mammogram is obtained, then on discovery, become a concern of both physician and patient. They may also become palpable or mammographically visible in older women after previously normal mammograms. They continue to be a management problem, because fibroadenoma and carcinoma have overlapping mammographic features and both are common lesions in middle-aged women. With age, fibroadenomas become involuted and heavily calcified, thereby revealing their true identity (Fig. 5–21). Without this appearance, however, biopsy is often necessary.

A high index of suspicion and careful evaluation, together with either close follow-up or liberal use of needle biopsy, are needed to minimize both false-negative impressions and excessive breast surgery.

EXERCISE 5-4: ARCHITECTURAL DISTORTION AND ASYMMETRIC DENSITY

Clinical Histories:

Case 5-12. A 51-year-old woman evaluated with screening mammography (Fig. 5–22)

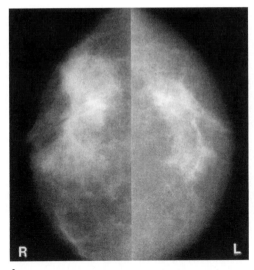

A

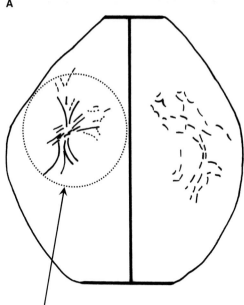

Area of architecture distortion, seen as retraction of parenchymal lines to a central point

B

Fig. 5–22.

Case 5-13. A 61-year-old woman evaluated with screening mammography (Fig. 5–23)

Questions:

5-12. Concerning the architectural distortion in the right breast (Fig. 5–22*A*), which statement is false?

A. Without history of biopsy, scarring is unlikely.

B. Previous mammograms could be very helpful.

C. It is probably nonmalignant because the patient does not complain of a mass.

D. Invasive lobular carcinoma commonly has this appearance.

E. This is probably not an asymmetric response to hormone therapy.

5-13. The mammographic appearance in (Fig. 5–23) is least likely to be caused by

A. normal breasts.

B. postsurgical change.

C. trauma.

D. cystic disease.

E. tumor.

Radiologic Findings:

5-12. Bilateral craniocaudal views (Fig. 5–22*A*) show architecture distortion in the right breast without a discrete dominant mass.

5-13. Bilateral mediolateral oblique views of the patient in this case (Fig. 5–23) show areas of asymmetric density in the left upper and right lower breast. The densities are interspersed with fat. Margins are generally concave and there is no architectural distortion.

Discussion:

Although normal breast tissue is remarkably symmetric, it is never exactly the same on both sides. The challenge in mammography is to recognize normal variation and to be able to distinguish nonpathologic asymmetry from disease. This is not always possible, particularly in the asymptomatic group. A high index of suspicion is needed when evaluating the screening mammogram, just as in the baseline CBE. Once asymmetry is noted mammographically, a careful, focused breast examination is needed. If no suspicious areas are detected and if the radiographic features suggest fibroglandular tissue, then follow-up alone is adequate. Radiographically, we look for a homogeneous, nondistorted pattern of fat interspersed with lobular densities. Any dominant mass or architectural distortion should cause concern.

In Case 5-12 (Fig. 5–22*A*), one area shows a different architectural pattern. The lines of tension appear to pull to a central focus. This is a classic appearance of invasive lobular carcinoma. Remember that 90% of the breast cancers are ductal in origin, and the other 10% are lobular, as in this case. This type of carcinoma shows a subtle infiltrating pattern much more often than does ductal carcinoma. (Statement *D* is true.)

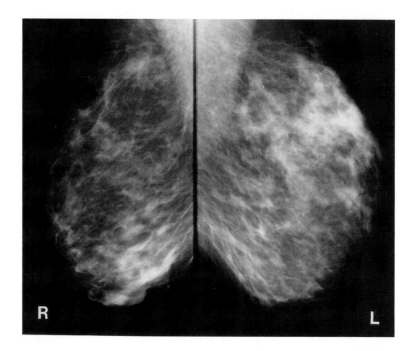

Fig. 5–23.

One of the problems with this disease is that it is difficult to describe the extent of tumor mammographically. There is a large area of asymmetric architecture in this patient, but where tumor ends is unclear. This patient had a carcinoma that measured 4 cm.

A correlated clinical examination often reveals abnormalities not detected without the guidance of mammographic findings. (Statement *C* is false and is the correct answer to Question 5-12.) Biopsy of any suspicious-feeling area is strongly recommended. Studies have shown that a high percentage of carcinomas "missed" at mammography appear as architecture distortion or asymmetric density. This patient did have a large area of thickening in the upper aspect of this breast, confirming the suspicious nature of the mammographic findings.

Previous mammograms are definitely useful in evaluating architecture distortion and asymmetric density. If the finding is unchanged over time, no further action may be needed. If the finding is new or is increasing, it is more easy to recognize. (Statement *B* is true.) Hormonal therapy may indeed have an asymmetric effect (statement *E* is true), but it does not take the form of architecture distortion.

Surgical biopsy may result in such distortion of the architecture, but precise correlation with location and timing of the surgery is needed. (Statement *A* is true.)

Unlike the previous patient, the woman in Case 5-13 has multiple areas of breast asymmetric density (Fig. 5–23). There is a large area in the upper part of the left breast and a smaller area in the lower part of the right breast. Both areas show fat interspersed with fibroglandular densities. There is no architectural distortion. Margins of the larger opacities are generally concave—a sign of benignity. There are no dominant or circumscribed masses, and cystic disease therefore would not be part of the differential diagnosis, because cysts are rounded masses. (*D* is the correct answer to Question 5-13.) Having learned from the previous case that missed carcinoma often presents as asymmetric density, tumor must remain in the differential diagnosis, and answer *E* is incorrect.

Both trauma and postoperative change can lead to ill-defined asymmetric density. With trauma there may be bleeding, contusion, or actual deformity, if severe. With surgery, asymmetry results both from removal of normal tissues, leaving less density on the operated side, and from surgical trauma (hematoma and distortion) that causes increased localized densities. Therefore, options *B* and *C* are both incorrect. The most likely cause of this woman's mammographic appearance is normal breast tissue, and answer *A* is incorrect. The multiplicity and bilaterality of areas of asymmetry, the lack of signs or symptoms of breast cancer, and the fibroglandular characteristics of the densities all support this diagnosis.

EXERCISE 5-5: THE FOLLOW-UP MAMMOGRAM

Clinical Histories:

Case 5-14. A 70-year-old woman who had two screening mammograms 1 year apart Figure 5–24*A* is the first mammogram and Part *B* is the one obtained a year later.

Case 5-15. A 66-year-old woman with this screening mammogram after a previously normal mammogram (Fig. 5–25)

Case 5-16. A 55-year-old woman who had a normal mammogram the previous year (Fig. 5–26)

Questions:

5-14. Which of the following statements is false?
  A. The abnormal finding is a spiculated mass.
  B. The rate of change is too slow for a breast cancer.

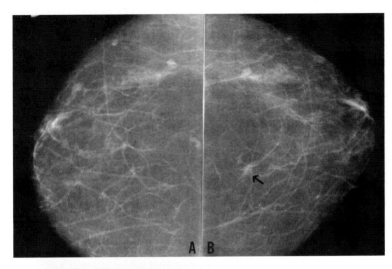

Fig. 5–24.

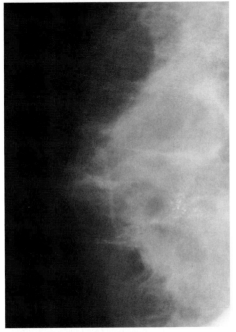

Fig. 5–25.

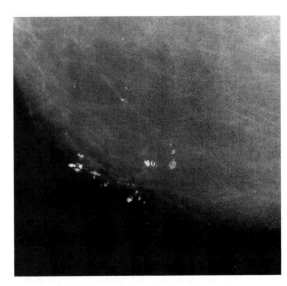

Fig. 5–26.

C. A malpractice claim should not be encouraged.
D. The lesion is probably not palpable.
E. This change warrants biopsy.

5-15. With respect to the calcifications, which statement is false?
A. They may be described as pleomorphic.
B. The coarse nature of some of the calcifications suggests this is a benign process.
C. They signal an aggressive malignancy.
D. They are most likely due to necrosis in duct walls.
E. Magnification should be performed to assess the extent of disease.

5-16. With respect to the calcifications, which statement is true?
A. They may be described as granular.
B. The regional distribution makes them highly suspicious.
C. Follow-up alone would be inadequate.
D. The new onset indicates a high probability of malignancy.
E. They have a less than 20% chance of being malignant.

Radiologic Findings:

5-14. Figure 5–24 shows back-to-back craniocaudal views of the right breast obtained 1 year apart. In the interval a small spiculated mass has enlarged so as to become more apparent (*arrow*).

5-15. The mammogram of the patient in this case (Fig. 5–25) shows a cluster of microcalcifications posteriorly in the central aspect of the breast. Previous mammograms have been normal.

5-16. Magnification view of a portion of the breast of the patient in this case (Fig. 5–26) shows coarse calcifications, some of which are rounded or ring-like.

Discussion:

Case 5-14 (Fig. 5–24) illustrates the concept of developing density. A developing density is any opacity that increases in size or density over time. All such opacities should be evaluated critically, because they can be signs of carcinoma. This concept is based on the natural behavior of breast cancer, which generally grows slowly. With periodic screening, the early tumor will be imaged but unrecognized on early images and may not be detected until 1, 2, 3, or more years later. Tumors 5 mm or smaller are very difficult to differentiate from normal breast tissue, but masses larger than 1 cm are more easily detected. The typical breast cancer has been present for several years by the time it is 1 cm in size.

Therefore, breast cancers are routinely visible in retrospect on previous mammograms if the patient has had frequent screening. This does not mean, however, that malpractice has occurred. If the cancer is still small, no harm has been done and more harm could potentially be done by biopsying all such tiny densities, because most of them would be normal breast. (Statement *C* is true.) Being suspicious but judicious with any developing density, therefore, is necessary to detect breast cancer early without unnecessary biopsy.

This patient has a small (about 1-cm) spiculated mass in the central part of the breast. (Statement *A* is true.) It has increased slightly in size over 1 year, with a growth rate typical for breast carcinoma. (Statement *B* is false and is the correct answer to Question 5-14.) Being so small in a medium-sized breast, it is unlikely to be palpable (statement *D* is true) and, therefore, would require imaging guidance for any biopsy. The spiculated margins, the rate of growth, and the patient's age group all make this a very suspicious lesion, and biopsy is warranted. (Statement *E* is true.) This lesion was an infiltrating ductal carcinoma.

Case 5-15 illustrates a new finding after a previous normal screening. Figure 5–25 shows a cluster of microcalcifications in the central area. Note that the calcifications are small and irregular, but we do not see their configuration exquisitely; nor can we be confident of the extent of disease, since there may be other smaller calcifications that we do not see. The patient, therefore, requires recall for magnification mammography (Fig. 5–27). (Statement *E* is true.) On magnification, we can appreciate that the calcifications are of many different sizes and shapes (i.e., pleomorphic). (Statement *A* is true.) Malignant microcalcifications are usually less than 0.5 mm in size, and the very coarse calcifications are classically benign. However, there is significant overlap, and configuration is generally a more helpful sign. Malignant calcifications are usually either granular or linear and branching.

These granular, linear, and branching calcifications are typical of intraductal carcinoma. The aggressive type of intraductal carcinoma, comedo or high-nuclear-grade carcinoma, causes necrosis in the cancerous mammary duct walls. Calcifications form in areas of necrosis forming a "cast" of the duct. This process results in the linear and branching forms of calcification. (Statements *C* and *D* are true.) Pathologic analysis of this tissue showed intraductal carcinoma of the comedo type.

Lesser degrees of necrosis result in smaller, more granular calcifications, whereas extensive necrosis yields rather large rod-shaped or branched calcifications. Statement *B* is false because, although large calcifications alone are usually benign, the mixture of tiny irregular calcifications with the coarse casting calcifications remains very suspicious for malignancy. (Statement *B* is false and is the correct answer to Question 5-15.)

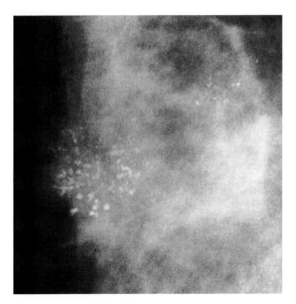

Fig. 5–27. Magnification view of microcalcifications seen on a screening mammogram of the patient in Case 5-15. Note the pleomorphism of the microcalcifications. The size varies from very fine to coarse, and shapes are bizarre. This appearance is typical of comedocarcinoma.

In Case 5-16 the mammogram detail (Fig. 5–26) shows typical benign calcifications. Benign calcifications take many forms, but if we see rings with lucent centers, as in this case, we can rest assured that they are benign. These rings are calcifying microcystic areas of fat necrosis. This is a very common benign finding. Punctate, or dot-like, calcifications are also usually benign if uniform

and smooth. Granular calcifications are more angular, like broken needle tips, and would be more suspicious. (Statement *A* is false.)

Benign calcifying processes such as fibroadenoma, sclerosing adenosis, and fat necrosis can all be unifocal, or regional, as well as multifocal or diffuse; therefore, distribution alone does not make calcifications suspicious. (Statement *B* is false.)

Benign processes of many types do present in adulthood and, therefore, may appear de novo after a previously normal screening examination. Again, the configuration of calcifications is more helpful. (Statement *D* is false.)

For obviously benign calcifications such as these, routine follow-up alone is adequate. (Statement *C* is false.) Some calcifications are obviously malignant as in Case 5-15. A third group of calcifications is classified as indeterminate, and these require further evaluation, either close mammographic follow-up or some type of biopsy. Taken as a group, biopsied microcalcifications historically have had a rate of malignancy of only 20%. Therefore, statement *E* is true, since these ringlike calcifications have a better-than-average chance of being benign. (Statement *E* is true and is the correct answer to Question 5-16.)

BIBLIOGRAPHY

Hayes DF. *Atlas of Breast Cancer.* London: Wolfe; 1993.

Kopans DB. *Breast Imaging.* 2nd ed. Philadelphia: Lippincott-Raven; 1998.

Love SM. *Dr. Susan Love's Breast Book.* Reading, Mass: Addison-Wesley; 1990.

Smith RA, Cokkinides V, Fyre HJ. American Cancer Society guidelines for the early detection of cancer, 2003. *CA Cancer J Clin* 2003;53:27–43.

Svane G, Potchen EJ, Sierra A, Azavedo E. *Screening Mammography.* St. Louis: Mosby; 1993.

PART 3

Bones and Joints

Musculoskeletal Imaging

Tamara Miner Haygood & Sam T. Auringer

INTRODUCTION

When Wilhelm Conrad Roentgen discovered the x-ray in November 1895, he investigated it thoroughly, testing its ability to penetrate various inanimate objects and observing its effects on fluorescent screens and photographic film. He gazed in amazement at the image of the bones of his own hand as he allowed the new rays to penetrate his flesh. He made a photographic x-ray image of a hand (reportedly his wife's) and sent prints of it together with his paper describing the new phenomenon to a carefully selected list of scientific colleagues.

By mid-February 1896 Rontgen's paper had not only been published but also reprinted in other scientific journals including the American journal *Science*. Scientists everywhere repeated Rontgen's simple experiments and confirmed the truth of his discovery. Within a year x-rays were in widespread use for medical purposes—chiefly for imaging of the skeleton.

Since Rontgen's time many new imaging techniques have been developed that allow radiologists to see the muscles and other soft tissues of the musculoskeletal system as well as the bones. These techniques make skeletal imaging a very exciting area of radiology and one that can enhance patients' quality of life. They can also be very expensive, however. This chapter is intended to introduce you to musculoskeletal imaging techniques and to suggest efficient ways to use them that will help you not only to make correct diagnoses but also to do so without excessive cost. Naturally, the suggestions made in these pages must be tailored to the needs of individual patients.

TECHNIQUES

Conventional Radiography

Conventional radiographs, or *plain films,* as they are often called, are the most frequently obtained imaging studies. They are chiefly useful for evaluation of the bones, but useful information about the adjacent soft tissues may also be obtained. Gas may be seen within the soft tissues and may be a clue to an open wound, ulcer, or infection with a gas-producing organism. Calcifications within the soft tissues can indicate a tumor,

myositis ossificans, or systemic disorders such as scleroderma or hyperparathyroidism.

To get the most information possible from conventional radiographs, you should carefully choose the study to be ordered. At most hospitals and clinics standardized sets of views have been developed that are routinely obtained for evaluation of specific body areas in certain clinical settings. It is useful to know what will routinely be obtained when a certain set of films is ordered. Radiographs of the ankle, for example, usually include a straight frontal view of the ankle, a frontal view

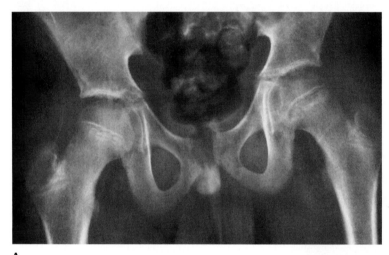

A

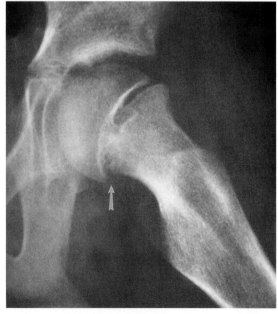

B

Fig. 6–1. Slipped capital femoral epiphysis. **A** AP radiograph of the pelvis. There are signs of a fracture through the physis of the left proximal femur: That femoral epiphysis is less well mineralized than the one on the right, the lucent line demarcating the physis is slightly widened, and the alignment of the edges of the epiphysis and metaphysis is abnormal. These signs are relatively subtle and could easily be missed. **B** Frog-leg lateral view of the left hip. This view, a lateral of the proximal femur, is much more obviously abnormal. Along the posterior edge of the femur, the cortices of the epiphysis and metaphysis should be flush but are instead offset by approximately 5 mm (*arrow*).

obtained with approximately 15 degrees internal rotation of the ankle (the mortise view), and a lateral view. There will be some variation among institutions, however. At a minimum, two views at right angles to one another should be obtained when a fracture or dislocation is suspected, because such injuries are notorious for being very subtle or even invisible in one projection, even when they are glaringly obvious in another view (Fig. 6–1). Radiographs should be focused on the anatomic area being evaluated, free of overlapping, extraneous anatomy (Fig. 6–2). If the knee is the site of trouble, do not order views of the entire tibia and fibula; you will be disappointed with the visualization of the knee. This principle must be abandoned more or less in young children and individuals with mental impairments who may not be able to localize their symptoms well and also in trauma victims with so many injuries that the relatively minor ones may be overlooked.

In addition, when the radiographs will be studied by a consulting radiologist, it is helpful to provide a succinct yet accurate history pinpointing your clinical concerns.

Simply indicating the site of injury will improve the likelihood that a subtle fracture will be discovered.

A conventional radiograph of a normal bone will show a smooth, homogeneous cortex surrounding the medullary space. The cortex will be thicker along the shaft (diaphysis) of long bones and thinner in small, irregular bones such as the carpal and tarsal bones and at the ends of long bones (Fig. 6–3). Exceptions are the normal roughening of the cortex at tendon and ligament insertion sites and the normal interruption of the cortex at the site of the nutrient arteries. Naturally these occur at predictable places that differ from bone to bone. Within the medullary space of a normal bone are trabeculae. These are visible in radiographs as thin, crisp white lines that are arranged not randomly but in predictable patterns that enhance the stress-bearing capability of the bone. It is beyond the scope of this chapter to address the appearance of each bone.

When questions arise concerning whether a particular appearance is normal or abnormal, several solutions are possible. Two books, Keats' *Normal Variants* and

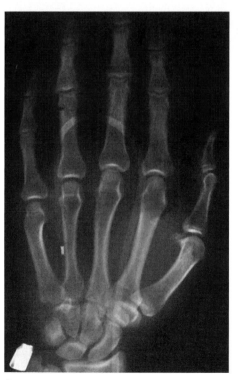
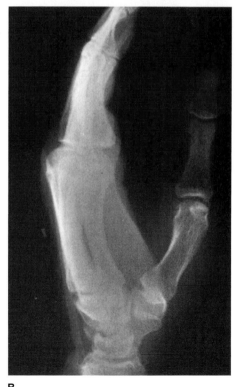

A　　　　　　　　　　　　　　　**B**

Fig. 6–2. **A, B** Phalangeal fracture. AP and lateral radiographs of the hand. This young man was first evaluated for trauma to the ring finger with frontal and lateral views of the whole hand. On the lateral view all fingers other than the thumb are overlapped. No fracture was found.

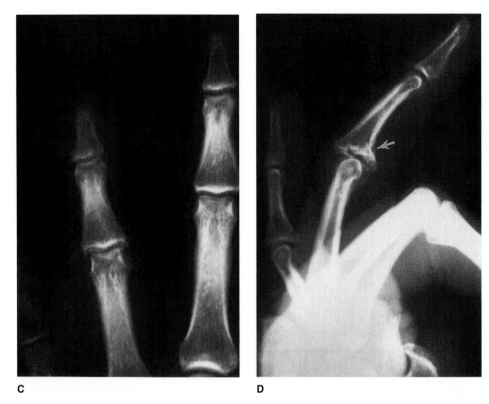

C   D

Fig. 6–2. **C, D.** AP and lateral radiographs of the finger. The patient returned 2¹/₂ months later, complaining that his finger still hurt. This time radiographs were coned more closely to the finger and care was taken on the lateral view to image the ring finger separately from the others. In that view the intra-articular fracture of the proximal aspect of the middle phalanx is quite obvious (*arrow*). It is far more subtle on the frontal view.

Kohler's *Borderlands* (see Bibliography), are very useful in helping to distinguish the normal from the abnormal. Correlation with the results of the history and physical examination may also be helpful. Finally, comparison with the patient's prior plain radiographs or with a radiograph of the opposite extremity may also help (Fig. 6–4). Comparison views of the opposite extremity are especially helpful in children, in whom the open physes and accessory centers of ossification may vary a surprising amount from individual to individual.

Mammographic Techniques

Any soft-tissue area that can be pulled away from the skeleton and placed between the compression paddle and film may be imaged with the mammographic technique. In extremity imaging, the mammographic technique is occasionally used to search for small calcifications or foreign bodies in the soft tissues.

Fluoroscopy

Fluoroscopy plays an important role in evaluation of joint motion. It is often used by orthopedic surgeons to monitor placement of hardware. It may also be of assistance in positioning patients for unusual conventional radiographic views.

Computed Tomography

Tomography has two major uses in skeletal imaging. The first is evaluation of fracture fragment position. CT with good multiplanar reconstruction provides excellent delineation of fractures (Fig. 6–5). With multiplanar reconstruction, fracture may be evaluated in planes of section that cannot be achieved in the primary view (Fig. 6–6). Even with multiplanar reconstruction, MR imaging may give better results for fractures running primarily in the axial plane. The decision to use advanced imaging

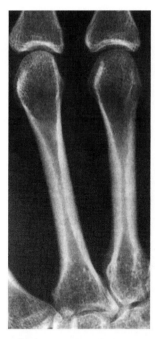

Fig. 6–3. Normal metacarpals. PA radiograph of the second and third metacarpals of a 36-year-old woman. The cortex is thick and homogeneously white in the midshaft of the metacarpal. It becomes progressively thinner as it approaches the ends of the bones. At the articular surfaces the cortex has been reduced to a thin, yet distinct, white line.

beyond conventional radiographs should be based on whether the study will change treatment or will be of sufficient help in operative planning to justify the additional radiation and expense. Scapular fractures, for example, are often treated conservatively, but orthopedic surgeons differ on the treatment of fractures that extend into the glenoid or involve the scapular spine. Some believe these benefit from internal fixation; others do not. Tomographic evaluation of these structures will be more useful to a surgeon who would use internal fixation selectively than to one who would use conservative therapy on all scapular fractures.

Three-dimensional reconstruction is available with many CT scanners. Extra technologist time is required to perform the scan and more films as well, so there is usually an extra charge. This may be justified if it helps the orthopedic surgeon to plan operative intervention and thus decrease the time required for surgery. Three-dimensional images are also useful for teaching purposes, because they can often be understood by less experienced individuals. They do not, however, contain information beyond that available in tomographic images.

The second major use of CT is in evaluation of bone tumors or tumor-like diseases. For this purpose, MR imaging is the principal competing technique. CT is more sensitive than MR imaging in demonstrating small amounts of calcium and can show early periosteal new bone formation or small amounts of matrix calcification before they may be seen with conventional radiography. This finding can be helpful in narrowing the differential

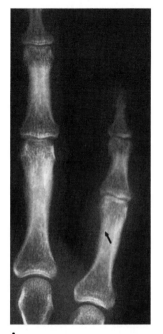

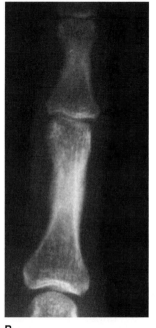

Fig. 6–4. Nutrient canal. **A** PA radiographs of the small finger. The smooth white cortex of the radial side of the proximal phalanx of the small finger is interrupted by a thin, obliquely oriented dark line (*arrow*). The soft tissues are swollen, and there is tenderness in this area. How can you distinguish this nutrient canal from a fracture? It is in a typical location for a nutrient canal. Its borders are smooth and sclerotic, not jagged. For definitive proof, delve into the patient's film folder. **B** The same lucency was present 2¹/₂ years earlier. In this case, the soft-tissue swelling was due to cellulites after a cat bite.

A   B

Fig. 6–5. Calcaneal fracture. **A** Lateral radiograph of the foot. The calcaneus of this 27-year-old man has comminuted fracture that can easily be diagnosed with this conventional radiograph, but the degree of involvement of the articular surfaces is difficult to appreciate.
B Direct coronal CT image through the posterior and middle subtalar joints demonstrates obliquely oriented fracture lines entering the posterior facet (*arrows*). There is a gap of approximately 8 mm between the fracture margins, and the lateral fragment has been rotated outward. **C** Axial CT image demonstrates a comminuted fracture of the inferior aspect of the calcaneocuboid joint.

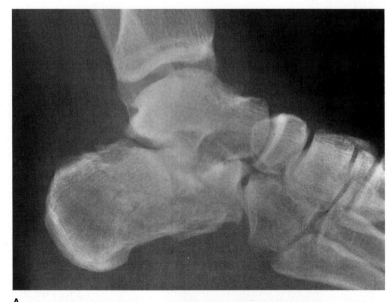

A

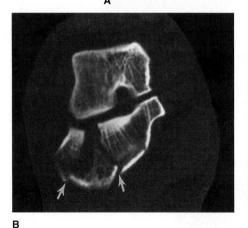

B

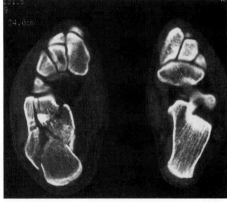

C

diagnosis of a tumor. Before MR imaging was developed, CT was also used widely for determining the extent of bone and soft-tissue tumors. MR imaging, however, is now more often used for staging. Its superior contrast resolution greatly eases the task of determining tumor extent within bone marrow and muscle or other soft tissues (Fig. 6–7).

Magnetic Resonance Imaging

The exquisite contrast of MR imaging makes it ideal for evaluation of soft tissues. Its most frequent use in skeletal imaging, therefore, is for diagnosis of injuries to muscles, tendons, or ligaments about joints. This superb contrast resolution also makes it very useful for

evaluating disorders of the bone marrow including neoplasm, marrow-packing diseases such as Gaucher's disease, osteomyelitis, fractures that are occult on conventional radiographs, and avascular necrosis. Unfortunately, although MR imaging is very sensitive to these abnormalities, it is also very nonspecific. Many diseases of marrow cause similar signal alterations. One must then narrow the differential diagnosis based on the distribution of the abnormalities together with the clinical history.

Nuclear Medicine

Several nuclear medicine studies are used for skeletal disease. The two most common are the technetium

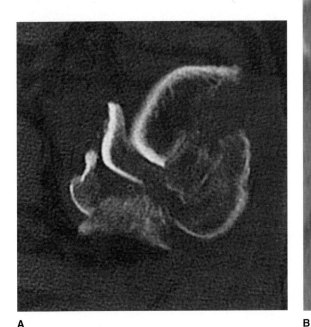

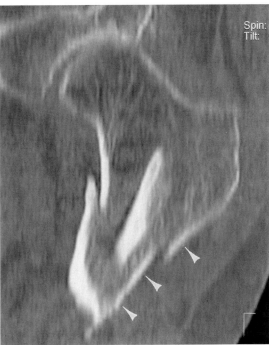

A

B

Fig. 6–6. **A** Axial and reconstructed coronal CT images of the left proximal femur. The axial image obtained through the level of the intertrochanteric left proximal femur demonstrates a comminuted fracture with 1- to 2-cm displacement of the fracture fragments with respect to one another. **B** Examination was accomplished with a helical technique, allowing reconstruction in the coronal plane that clearly demonstrates a shard of cortical bone that has been driven into the central marrow cavity. The reconstruction is quite smooth, differing from a directly acquired image such as the axial image primarily in the presence of tiny stairstep artifacts along some edges (*arrowheads*).

bone scan and the technetium- or indium-labeled white blood cell scan. One of several phosphate compounds of ^{99m}Tc is selected for use in a bone scan. Methylene diphosphonate is used most frequently. If there is a specific anatomic area of interest, images may be acquired over that area at the time the radionuclide is injected, as well as 3 to 4 hours later. The immediate images reflect the amount of blood flow to the area; the delayed images reflect the amount of bone remodeling occurring there.

Bone scintigraphy is a sensitive but nonspecific technique. Most osseous abnormalities of clinical significance will cause an increase in radiolabeling. Exceptions are destructive lesions that incite little reparative reaction in the host bone or that destroy bone so quickly that it cannot remodel.

Because of their sensitivity and because they provide physiologic rather than anatomic information, bone scans can be used to find abnormalities before they are detectable by conventional radiography. In particular,

they are often used for screening for bone metastases in patients with known malignancy. Both multiple myeloma in adults and Langerhans' cell histiocytosis in children, however, are notorious for causing no increased accumulation on bone scans. Therefore, in these diseases conventional radiographs or skeletal surveys are better than bone scans for screening for osseous involvement. MR imaging is sometimes also used for screening for metastatic disease.

Early detection of avascular necrosis, historically an indication for bone scanning, has largely been usurped by MR imaging because it is more sensitive and provides greater anatomic detail. Legg-Calvé-Perthes disease (spontaneous avascular necrosis of the capital femoral epiphysis) in children is an exception, however; in this diagnosis, bone scans may be more sensitive than MR imaging.

White cell scans vie with MR imaging and bone scans as a method of detecting osteomyelitis. Which technique or combination of techniques is best is far from certain.

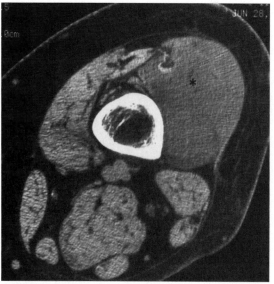

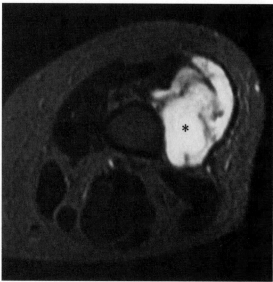

A

B

Fig. 6–7. A Axial CT image of the distal thigh. This 49-year-old woman complained of a palpable mass in her thigh. It had been present for a year and was painless. The internal architecture of the vastus lateralis muscle (*) is disrupted. The interdigitated fat and muscle tissue evident in the patient's other muscles has been replaced with a more homogeneous mass of decreased attenuation. There is no apparent associated calcification. The mass closely approximates the femur but is not causing osseous destruction. **B** T_2-weighted (2500/80) MR image of the thigh at approximately the same level. While this tumor (*) could be seen on the CT scan, on the MR image it is far more obvious and more easily distinguished from normal tissue. The superiority of MR imaging in detecting soft-tissue neoplasms makes it excellent for determining the extent of primary soft-tissue tumors like this myxoid liposarcoma as well as for evaluating the spread of primary bone tumors into adjacent soft tissues.

Some studies have favored nuclear medicine; others have favored MR imaging. Both bone scan and MR imaging are sensitive but lack specificity. White cell scans are relatively specific for infection but often cannot distinguish cellulitis from osteomyelitis with certainty.

Biopsy

When tumor or infection is suspected, it is often useful to obtain a tissue sample for cytologic or histologic analysis or for culture. This may be accomplished by means of an "open" procedure in the operating room or a percutaneous needle puncture of the lesion to obtain a cellular aspirate or slender core of tissue. Needle biopsies of palpable lesions need no radiologic intervention. When the lesion is not palpable, however, biopsy may be accomplished under fluoroscopic, CT, or sometimes ultrasound guidance.

When a skeletal lesion should be biopsied and by whom are important questions that can have a tremendous impact on the patient's outcome. For example, sarcomas have been reported to grow along the surgical or needle tracks after diagnostic biopsies. Therefore, when planning biopsies of suspected musculoskeletal sarcomas great care must be taken to approach the lesion through a track that can be resected en bloc with the tumor at the time of ultimate excision. These biopsies should be carried out in close consultation with the surgeon who will be performing the definitive surgery.

When systemic disease such as metastatic carcinoma is the primary consideration, percutaneous needle biopsy is the most efficacious means of making a diagnosis if the lesion is amenable to this procedure. In this setting, the yield of needle biopsy is very good (90% or more of such biopsies yield a positive diagnosis when tumor is truly present) and a negative result is less likely to lead to open biopsy than it would in some suspected primary tumors. Nonetheless, biopsy should still be performed in consultation with the oncologist or other physician giving overall care.

TECHNIQUE SELECTION

In general, as in most other organ systems, the radiograph is the initial imaging test after history and physical examination. The selection of subsequent (often more expensive) imaging tests depends not only on medical need but also on a variety of other factors, including availability, expense, and the preferences of the radiologist, clinician, and patient.

Trauma

Rely primarily on conventional radiography. When a strongly suspected fracture is not identified, you may choose among repetition of conventional radiographs in 7 to 10 days, nuclear medicine bone scanning, and MR imaging. If a fracture is noticed and more information is needed concerning the location of fragments, CT is useful.

Bone or Soft-Tissue Tumors

For local staging of both bone and soft-tissue neoplasms, MR imaging is the best technique. When a bone tumor is suspected but is not discovered with conventional radiographs, MR imaging is a useful secondary screening tool.

Metastatic Tumors

Symptomatic sites suspected of being involved by metastatic neoplasm are best evaluated initially with radiographs. An overall survey for osseous metastases may be performed by nuclear medicine bone scan. Conventional radiography is then used to evaluate sites of possible tumor involvement. Suspected soft-tissue metastases are best evaluated by MR imaging.

Osteomyelitis

Conventional radiographs should be obtained first. If these are normal or inconclusive, MR imaging, nuclear medicine bone scan, or white blood cell scanning may be helpful.

EXERCISES

EXERCISE 6–1: TRAUMA

Clinical Histories:

Case 6-1. On the first day of your medical school rotation in orthopedic surgery, the resident and attending physician send you to the emergency room to see a 26-year-old man with a broken leg (Fig. 6–8).

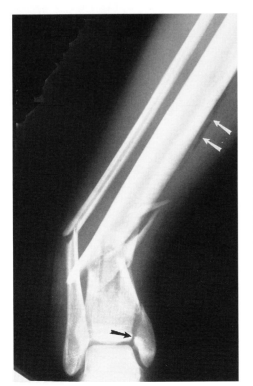
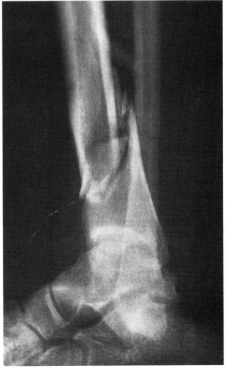

A

B

Fig. 6–8. AP and lateral views of the distal tibia and fibula.

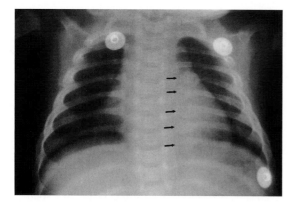

Fig. 6–9. Frontal view of the chest.

Case 6-2. Infant with low-grade fever. You obtain a chest radiograph to "rule out pneumonia" (Fig. 6–9).

Case 6-3. While moonlighting in the emergency department of a small community hospital you examine a 25-year-old man who fell on an outstretched hand and now complains of elbow pain. You obtain a lateral view of his elbow (Fig. 6–10).

Case 6-4. A week later you are once again moonlighting in the same small emergency department when a 29-year-old man is carried in complaining of ankle pain after a twisting injury. His ankle is swollen and ecchymotic, and he is tender to palpation along the medial malleolus. He has no other complaints. You order frontal, lateral, and oblique views of the ankle (Fig. 6–11).

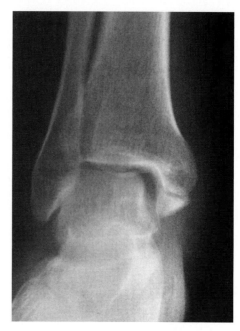

Fig. 6–11. AP view of the ankle.

Case 6-5. A 15-year-old boy complains of ankle pain after a fall (Fig. 6–12).

Questions:

6-1. You are supposed to look at the radiographs (Fig. 6–8) and call your colleagues in the operating room to describe the fracture. Which of the following statements concerning the fracture would you not wish to make?

A. The distal tibial fragment is displaced 1 cm posteriorly.

B. There is comminution of the metaphyseal component of the tibial fracture.

C. There is slight valgus angulation of the distal tibial fragment.

D. A tibial fracture line extends to the articular surface.

E. This is an open fracture.

6-2. You interpret the chest radiograph (Fig. 6–9) and render the following diagnosis:

A. Normal chest radiograph

B. Round pneumonia

C. Viral pneumonia

D. Multiple healing rib fractures

E. Pneumothorax

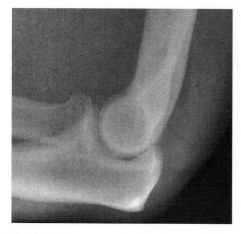

Fig. 6–10. Lateral view of the elbow.

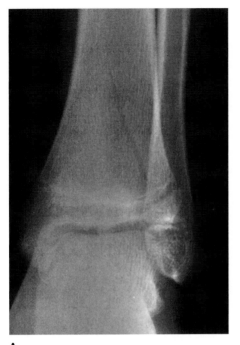
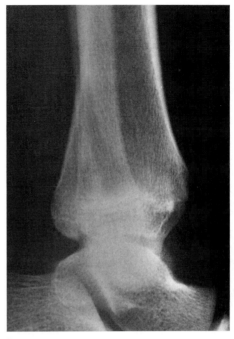

A   **B**

Fig. 6–12. AP and lateral views of the ankle.

6-3. You first examine the lateral view of the elbow. You find
    A. A lytic lesion in the distal humerus.
    B. A fracture through the proximal ulna.
    C. Displacement of the anterior and posterior fat pads of the elbow.
    D. Dislocation of the elbow.

6-4. You examine the radiographs. Only the AP view is shown here (Fig. 6–11). You tell the patient he has broken his ankle but you want to get one more study:
    A. Contralateral ankle, for comparison purposes
    B. Ipsilateral foot, to exclude a fracture of the fifth metatarsal
    C. Remainder of the ipsilateral tibia and fibula, to exclude more proximal fractures
    D. CT, for more precise evaluation of the alignment of the fracture

6-5. What is the abnormality in Fig. 6–12?
    A. Ankle sprain
    B. Fracture of the distal fibula
    C. Stress fracture of the talus
    D. Triplane fracture of the distal tibia
    E. Avascular necrosis of the talus

Radiologic Findings:

6-1. Figure 6–8 shows comminuted fractures of the distal tibia and fibula with intra-articular extension of the tibial fracture. Gas density (*white arrows*) indicates that air has penetrated into the soft tissues through a skin wound, so this is an open fracture. A fracture line extends to the tibial articular surface (*black arrow*).

6-2. In Fig. 6–9 a row of rounded opacities (*arrows*) in the left chest represents posterior healing rib fractures.

6-3. This patient's anterior fat pad is pushed away from the bone, creating a small triangular "sail" (Fig. 6–13, *arrowheads*). The posterior fat pad (*arrow*) is visible when it should not normally be visible at all. There is no visible fracture or dislocation.

6-4. Figure 6–11 indicates a transverse fracture of the distal medial malleolus with widening of the medial aspect of the ankle joint.

6-5. Abnormal lucencies run vertically through the epiphysis on the frontal view (Fig. 6–12) and obliquely through the metaphysis on both the frontal and lateral views. The lateral aspect of the distal tibial physis or growth plate is widened.

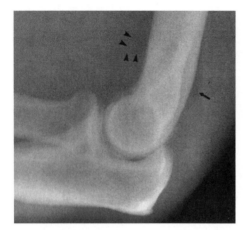

Fig. 6–13. Lateral view of the elbow with anterior (*arrowheads*) and posterior (*arrow*) fat pad signs.

Discussion:

Your mission on Case 6-1 is to describe accurately and succinctly the features of this fracture that will affect treatment and outcome. You should discuss the alignment of the largest tibial and fibular fragments. Address both displacement and angulation. Displacement is always described in terms of the position of the distal fragment relative to that of the proximal fragment. The lateral view shows that the distal tibial fragment is displaced 1 cm posteriorly.

On the frontal view there is obvious angulation (Fig. 6–8A). Angulation may be described either in terms of the direction of shift of the distal fragment or in terms of the direction in which the apex of the angle points. In either case, it is better to give a measurement than to use subjective modifiers like "slight" or "moderate." This angulation may correctly be described as "30 degrees of varus angulation of the distal fragment" or "30 degrees lateral apical angulation" (Fig. 6–14). (*C* is an incorrect statement and therefore the correct answer to Question 6-1.)

In Case 6-2, rib fractures in a young child suggest child abuse. (*D* is the correct answer to Question 6-2.) Because most rib fractures in infants are caused by nonaccidental injury, you should reexamine the child for other stigmata of child abuse, such as bruises, welts, burns, or retinal hemorrhages; notify protective services; and obtain a skeletal survey. If you are unsure of your diagnosis or desire confirmation of the radiographic findings, you should obtain a radiology consult. Discharging the patient could place the child in serious danger.

Figure 6–15 from the skeletal survey reveals the classic metaphyseal "corner" (*large arrows*) and "bucket handle" (*small arrows*) fractures virtually pathognomonic of infant abuse. The astute observer will also note a healing fracture of the superior pubic ramus. In summary, radiologic findings with moderate to high specificity for infant abuse include posterior rib fractures, metaphyseal fractures, multiple fractures, and fractures at differing stages of healing.

When examining a radiograph for a suspected fracture, as in Case 6-3, it is important to evaluate not only

Fig. 6–14. Varus and valgus angulation. In **A** the distal tibial fragment has shifted laterally with respect to the proximal tibia. This is valgus angulation. In **B** the distal tibial fragment has shifted medially with respect to the proximal fragment. This is varus angulation.

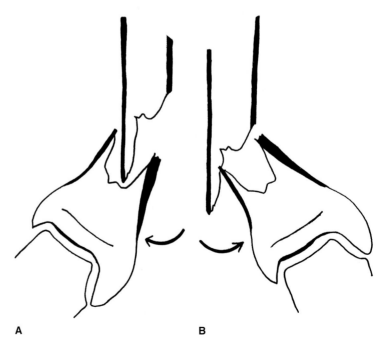

A

B

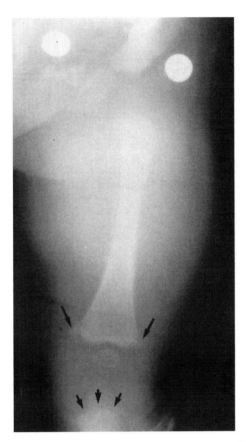

Fig. 6-15. AP view of the distal femur and proximal tibia. There are metaphyseal fractures of both the femur (*large arrows*) and the tibia (*small arrows*).

Transverse medial malleolar fracture (Case 6-4) usually accompanies eversion of the ankle and is often associated with a fibular fracture. The fibular injury may occur at any level from the ankle to the knee. When there is no apparent distal fibular fracture, the remainder of the bone should be imaged. (*C* is the correct answer to Question 6-4.) In this case, there is, indeed, a fracture of the proximal fibula (Fig. 6–16.) This fracture indicates rupture of the intraosseous membrane all along its course from the ankle to the fibular fracture, so this is an unstable injury that many orthopedic surgeons will treat with open reduction and internal fixation of the malleolar component and of the syndesmosis.

Fractures of the proximal fifth metatarsal may accompany ankle inversion and may be difficult to distinguish clinically from other ankle injuries; therefore, that part of the foot should always be included on at least one view of the ankle. If it is not, then it is prudent when possible to obtain one more view, but this should not ordinarily be considered a separate study or incur an additional charge. CT is not necessary in this case.

The adolescent patient of Case 6-5 has suffered a relatively common growth plate injury with a typical but somewhat complex fracture pattern. It is called a *triplane* fracture because it has components that run, more or less, in all three primary planes of section. It travels in the sagittal plane through the epiphysis, in the axial plane through the unfused portion of the physis or growth plate, and in the coronal plane through the metaphysis. (*D* is the correct

the bones themselves but also the adjacent soft tissues. In a number of areas of the body there are normal deposits of fat, termed *fat pads*, which may be displaced by accumulation of blood or fluid in the underlying tissues. The fat pads of the elbow are particularly helpful. (C is the correct answer to Question 6-3.)

Displacement of the elbow fat pad is a nonspecific sign that indicates distension of the joint. Effusions due to rheumatoid arthritis, an infected joint, or hemorrhage, especially in a patient with a bleeding disorder, could all cause the "fat pad sign" seen in this patient. In an otherwise healthy person who has suffered trauma, however, a radial head fracture should be suspected since it is the most common elbow fracture in an adult. This patient's frontal view did actually demonstrate a small lucent fracture line in the radial head. Even without that, however, the most prudent course is to treat the patient as though he had a radial head fracture and also arrange for follow-up care with a physician accustomed to caring for fractures.

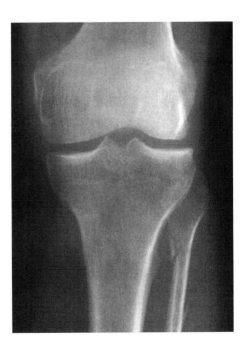

Fig. 6-16. AP view of the knee. The proximal fibula is fractured.

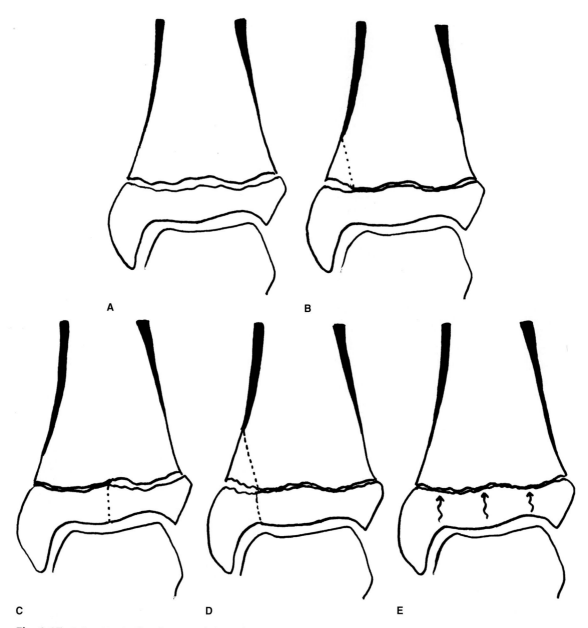

Fig. 6-17. Salter-Harris Classification of Physeal Injuries. This is a commonly used method of describing fractures through the physis of skeletally immature individuals. Outcome worsens as the number describing the fracture increases. **A** Salter-Harris type I fractures are through the physis or growth plate without involvement of the bone of the epiphysis or metaphysis. The slipped femoral capital epiphysis shown in Fig. 6–1 is a type of Salter-Harris I fracture. **B** Salter-Harris type II fractures involve part of the metaphysis (often only a small flake) and extend to the physis. **C** Salter-Harris type III fractures involve the epiphysis and extend to the physis. The Salter-Harris type III fracture illustrated here is similar to the epiphyseal and physeal components of the triplane fracture without extension to the metaphysis. It also is a fairly common injury pattern. **D** The Salter-Harris type IV fracture involves both the metaphysis and epiphysis. **E.** The Salter-Harris type V injury involves only the physis and is a compressive injury secondary to axial loading forces.

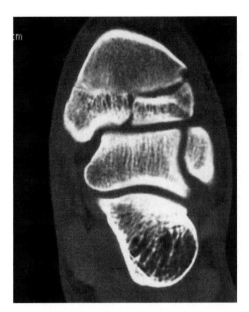

Fig. 6–18. Coronal CT scan of the ankle. This image was obtained with direct coronal technique. The patient was positioned with his feet on the CT table and knees bent. Images were then obtained about 15 degrees from a true coronal through the tibiotalar joint. Putting together the information on multiple such images allows more precise evaluation of fracture fragment position than is possible with conventional radiographs. This image demonstrates widening of the physis laterally and the sagittal split through the epiphysis.

answer to Question 6-5.) It is a Salter-Harris type IV fracture (Fig. 6–17). It can be easily diagnosed on the conventional radiographs. Overlapping of several bones in the ankle region, together with the inferiorly concave shape of the articular surface of the distal tibia, the tibial plafond, complicates evaluation of fracture fragment position, and so a CT scan was obtained (Fig. 6–18).

EXERCISE 6-2: LOCAL DISEASE

Clinical Histories:

Case 6-6. A 12-year-old girl comes to your pediatrics office complaining of 2 weeks of knee pain. There is no history of trauma. Her proximal fibula is slightly swollen, tender, and erythematous. You obtain frontal and lateral views of the tibia and fibula (Fig. 6–19).

Case 6-7. This 5-year-old girl has been limping off and on for 2 months. Her knee is warm and swollen (Fig. 6–20).

Case 6-8. A 35-year-old man complains of a lump in the soft tissues of the right arm. He first noticed the lump 6 months ago after hurting his arm in a fall from a bicycle (Fig. 6–21).

Case 6-9. A 10-year-old girl complains of a lump on the inside of her thigh near the knee. It has been there as long as she can remember but has been annoying her since she recently took up horseback riding (Fig. 6–22).

Questions:

6-6. Based on the history, physical examination, and radiographs (Fig. 6–19), which of the following choices is the best working diagnosis?
   A. A bone tumor, most likely benign
   B. A bone tumor, most likely malignant
   C. Osteomyelitis
   D. A stress fracture of the proximal fibula

6-7. What is the most likely diagnosis for the patient in Case 6-7 (Fig. 6–20)?
   A. Osteomyelitis
   B. A bone tumor, most likely malignant
   C. A Salter-Harris type IV fracture
   D. Langerhans' cell histiocytosis (eosinophilic granuloma)

6-8. What should you do about the calcified lump in this patient's arm (Fig. 6–21)?
   A. Needle biopsy
   B. Open excisional biopsy
   C. Reassure the patient
   D. Bone scan

6-9. What is the lump in Fig. 6–22?
   A. An osteosarcoma
   B. An osteochondroma
   C. A normal variant
   D. A soft-tissue sarcoma

Radiologic Findings:

6-6. Focal lytic lesion in the proximal fibular metadiaphysis with an intact shell of new cortex and a well-defined, short zone of transition between itself and adjacent normal bone (Fig. 6–19).

6-7. Figure 6–20 shows a well-defined lytic lesion in the proximal tibia. Its edges are slightly sclerotic. It extends across the physis to involve portions of both the metaphysis and epiphysis.

6-8. A well-defined ossified mass projects in the musculature of the posterolateral arm (Fig. 6–21). It has a thin but distinct cortex (*arrows*) surrounding trabeculae.

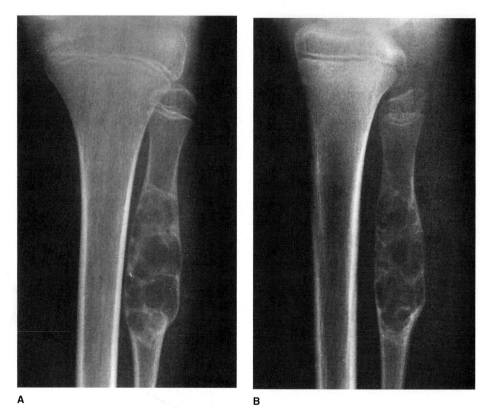

Fig. 6–19. AP and lateral views of the proximal tibia and fibula.

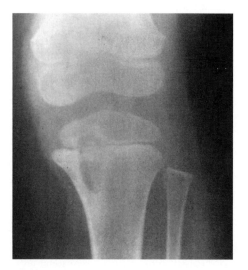

Fig. 6–20. AP view of the knee. *Case courtesy of Murray K. Dalinka, M.D.*

6-9. Arising from the medial cortex of the femur is an ossified mass topped by a cauliflower-like thin shell of cortex (Fig. 6–22). The cortex of the remainder of the femur is continuous with the cortex of the tumor (*arrowheads*), and the trabecular bone of the femoral metaphysis blends imperceptibly with that of the mass. The mass has grown away from its metaphyseal place of origin and points toward the diaphysis and away from the joint.

Discussion:

The radiographs of Case 6-6 (Fig. 6–19) demonstrate a focal lytic lesion in the proximal fibular metadiaphysis. The cortex appears intact around the lesion, and the bone is widened. Cortex is not pliable; it will not stretch to accommodate a growing lesion. Instead it will slowly remodel by resorption of endosteal bone and deposition of periosteal new bone. The intact cortex implies a slow growth rate for this lesion. Another indication of a slow growth rate is the sharp demarcation or short zone of transition between the lesion and adjacent normal bone.

In general, osteomyelitis will not cause apparent expansion of bone the way this lesion has. Stress fractures are usually linear lesions and usually are oriented transversely across the bone, though there are exceptions. Stress fractures may be lucent, if a gap in cortical bone is their primary manifestation, or sclerotic, either due to compression of trabeculae with resultant overlap or to healing. The periosteal reaction that they engender may cause them to be mistaken for bone tumors, but they will not look like this particular lesion (Fig. 6–23).

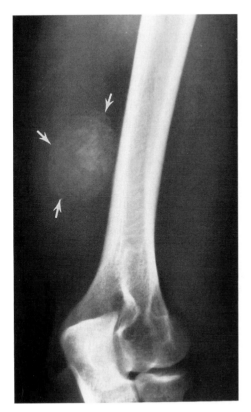

Fig. 6–21. AP view of the arm.

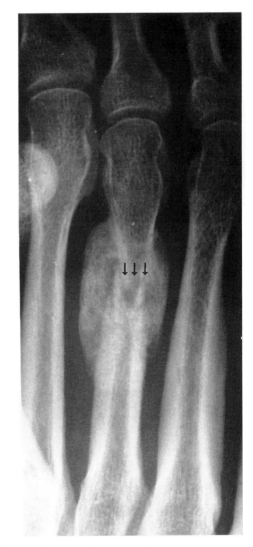

Fig. 6–23. Stress fracture. Oblique view of the third metatarsal. This typical healing stress fracture demonstrates both a transverse fracture oriented perpendicular to the shaft (*arrows*) and abundant callus formation.

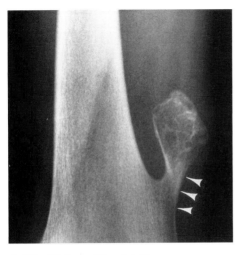

Fig. 6–22. AP view of the distal femur.

Of the choices given in the question, the remaining ones are benign and malignant bone tumor. For the most part, malignant bone tumors in children have a rapid growth rate. This will cause them to have poorly defined borders. In addition, where they destroy cortex, the periosteum will be unable to contain them with solidly mineralized new bone, as has occurred here. There may be gaps in the cortex where tumor has broken through (Fig. 6–24). The periosteal new bone may mineralize at 90-degree angles to the diaphysis or may be lamellated (like onion-skin) or incomplete. The intact shell of periosteal new bone seen in this patient and the short zone of transition are more typical of a benign than a malignant tumor. (*A* is the correct answer to the Question 6-6.)

A primary bone tumor, no matter how benign its appearance, is most appropriately handled by an orthopedic

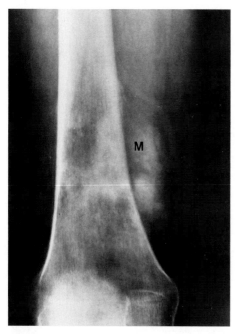

Fig. 6–24. AP view of the distal femur. Many of the radiographic features of this osteosarcoma mark it as a malignant tumor. The abnormal area of mottled lucent and sclerotic tumor in the metaphysis fades gradually into the shadows of surrounding normal bone. It is difficult to see where the tumor begins and ends. There is a large soft-tissue mass adjacent to the bone (M). The periosteum has been unable to maintain a shell of mineralized new bone around this mass. The sclerotic areas within the bone and the mineralized portions of the soft tissue mass both have a relatively amorphous, smudged appearance that is seen with calcified osteoid matrix.

surgeon experienced with tumor patients. Because the question stipulates that you are a pediatrician, the patient should be sent to an orthopedic surgeon who specializes in treatment of tumors.

Performing a percutaneous needle biopsy has the potential to cause great harm if a poorly chosen route is taken. For example, if the needle passed close to the common peroneal nerve and then the lesion proved unexpectedly to be malignant, the nerve might have to be sacrificed in order to obtain a curative resection.

Obtaining additional imaging studies to evaluate this lesion further is not a bad idea. It is better, however, to allow the orthopedic surgeon to whom the patient will be referred (in consultation with the radiologist) to decide which imaging tests are most appropriate to evaluate the lesion more thoroughly before ordering additional tests.

The edges of malignant tumors are usually not as well defined as those of the lesion shown in Case 6-7 (Fig. 6–20). Malignant tumors may extend across the growth plate, but it is uncommon for them to do so while they are still as small as this lesion.

Osteomyelitis, on the other hand, often breaches the growth plate. (*A* is the correct answer to Question 6-7.) The most common organisms to cause osteomyelitis are species of *Staphylococcus* and *Streptococcus* (Fig. 6–25). The relatively long history of limping, however, should suggest a more indolent organism such as *Mycobacterium tuberculosis*. Skeletal tuberculosis is uncommon and thus often is overlooked as a diagnostic possibility. Because it is curable yet responds to very different drugs than would be used for pyogenic osteomyelitis, it is important to keep it in mind. It may occur at any site, but it is most common in the spine. In the extremities it most often occurs in or near the hip and knee.

Langerhans' cell histiocytosis (eosinophilic granuloma) is much less common than osteomyelitis and is thus not as likely a diagnosis. When it does occur, its favorite location is the skull.

The ossified mass of Case 6-8 (Fig. 6–21) represents myositis ossificans, also known as heterotopic new bone formation. Though often associated with trauma, it may also be seen in patients without a distinct history of trauma. When it resembles mature bone as closely as in this patient, it is not a diagnostic dilemma, and you may reassure the patient that there is a benign cause for his lump. (*C* is the correct answer to Question 6-8.)

Occasionally myositis ossificans warrants excision on the basis of mechanical interference with the use of a muscle or joint. Recurrence is less likely if excision is performed after the lesion has matured. A bone scan may help to distinguish between mature and immature lesions. An immature lesion that is still undergoing ossification will exhibit marked radionuclide uptake. Once ossification is complete, radionuclide accumulation will resemble that of other bones.

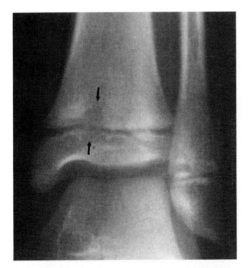

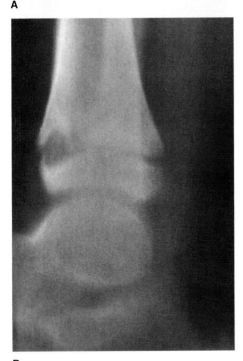

Myositis ossificans may be diagnosed more confidently with radiography than with histology. An immature lesion will be full of immature, rapidly proliferating cells that may be mistaken for a sarcoma by the pathologist. Radiologically, however, there is a distinct difference between the two. Myositis ossificans ossifies from the outside in. Sarcomas ossify from the inside out. (See Fig. 6–24 and notice that the central portion of the soft-tissue mass of the osteosarcoma is ossified, whereas the outer portion is not.) If it is not entirely clear from conventional radiographs where and how the ossification is occurring, a CT scan is the test of choice because of its sensitivity to calcium.

The mass of Case 6-9 (Fig. 6–22) has the characteristic appearance of an osteochondroma, the most common of all benign, cartilaginous neoplasms. Osteochondromas may be very large or very small, pedunculated or sessile (Fig. 6–26). They grow as the child grows and should cease growth by adulthood. Often asymptomatic, they may be an incidental finding. They may, however, cause a

Fig. 6–25. **A** AP view and **B** sagittal tomogram of the ankle. This focus of osteomyelitis (*arrows*), occurring in a 5-year-old boy, also crosses the growth plate. It is radiographically indistinguishable from the case of tuberculous osteomyelitis, yet it was due to *Staphylococcus*. The distinction between pyogenic and tuberculous osteomyelitis must be made on clinical grounds and proven by biopsy.

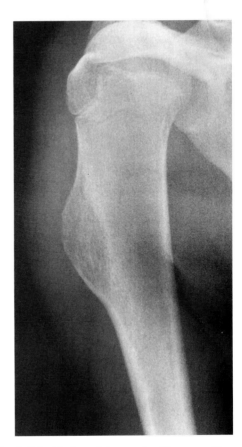

Fig. 6–26. AP view of the proximal humerus. There is a sessile osteochondroma on the lateral aspect of this child's humerus.

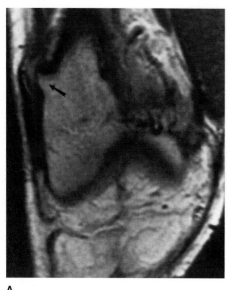
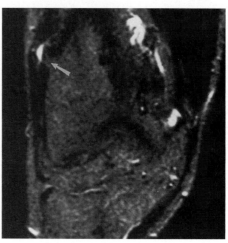

A   **B**

Fig. 6–27. **A** Proton-density and **B** T$_2$-weighted coronal MR image of the knee. A very tiny osteochondroma arises from the lateral metaphysis of the distal femur (*arrow*). Notice that the signal intensity (shade of gray) inside this diminutive tumor is the same as that of the adjoining marrow space. The bright area (*arrow*) over the osteochondroma in part *B* represents a small, fluid-filled bursa. This patient complained of a snapping sensation, which most likely was due to movement of the iliotibial band back and forth over the osteochondroma.

wide range of symptoms. The most common complaint is that they interfere with activities or with wearing certain clothes, such as tight blue jeans. They may be painful as a result of irritation of an overlying bursa (Fig. 6–27), and they are subject to fracture. An uncommon (1% or less) but feared complication is malignant transformation, usually resulting in a chondrosarcoma. Signs of such transformation include enlargement of the osteochondroma in an adult, thickening of the cartilaginous cap that covers the tumor, development of a soft tissue mass, and destruction of bone.

When further radiologic studies are needed, MR imaging is probably the most useful modality. It can demonstrate the cartilage cap and any associated soft-tissue mass. When the diagnosis is not as obvious as in this case by conventional radiography, MR imaging can assist in confirming the identity of the tumor by demonstrating continuity between the cortices and medullary spaces of the tumor and the host bone.

EXERCISE 6-3: SYSTEMIC DISEASE

Case Histories:

Case 6-10. As a medical student on the oncology team, you see in clinic a 45-year-old woman with a history of breast cancer diagnosed 5 years previously. She underwent surgery and since that time has been free of disease. She has come for her routine follow-up appointment and complains only of vague, aching discomfort in her left hip (no figure).

Case 6-11. A 40-year-old man complains of knee pain and swelling of 3 weeks' duration. He has no other known disease. You order conventional radiographs of the knees. You notice some periosteal elevation on both femurs and tibiae (Fig. 6–28).

Case 6-12. This chest radiograph was obtained to exclude pneumonia in a chronically ill 26-year-old woman (Fig. 6–29).

Case 6-13. In a 50-year-old man with diabetes, radiographs of the hand were obtained to exclude fracture after a fall (Fig. 6–30).

Questions:

6-10. Which of the following studies do you not want to order today?
  A. Chest x-ray
  B. Conventional radiographs of the left hip and pelvis

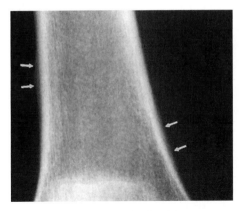

Fig. 6–28. AP view of the right distal femur.

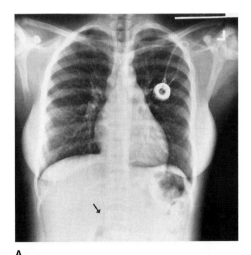

A

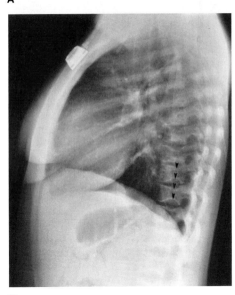

B

Fig. 6–29. PA and lateral views of the chest.

C.   Bone scan
D.   Skeletal survey
E.   Mammography

6-11.   What is the next study you should order after reviewing Fig. 6–28?
A.   Bone scan
B.   MR imaging of the knees
C.   Hand films
D.   Chest radiograph

6-12.   There is no evidence of pneumonia in Fig. 6–29, but there are several abnormalities that are clues to the nature of this patient's chronic illness. Which finding listed below is not such a clue?
A.   Surgical clips in the gallbladder bed
B.   Enlargement of the pulmonary artery segment of the mediastinum
C.   Depressions in the endplates of numerous vertebrae
D.   Irregular sclerosis of both humeral heads

6-13.   Which of the following statements about Case 6-13 (Fig. 6–30) is most likely to be correct?
A.   The patient has not suffered a fracture.
B.   A metastatic tumor is destroying the distal phalanx of the index finger.
C.   The bones are normally mineralized.
D.   The patient has renal failure.

Radiologic Findings:

6-11.   A thin rim of calcium added to the bony contour of both sides of the right femoral metaphysis (Fig. 6–28 *arrows*) is due to periosteal elevation. Similar findings were present on the left femur and both tibiae.

6-12.   Figure 6–29 shows surgical changes (*arrow*) in the right upper quadrant. The humeral heads have an abnormal, mottled, sclerotic appearance. Many vertebral bodies, as best appreciated in the lateral view, are shaped like the letter H (*arrowheads*), with central depressions in the superior and inferior endplates.

6-13.   In Fig. 6–30, the distal interphalangeal joint of the middle finger is held in slight flexion. A small triangular chip (*arrow*) of bone projects in the soft tissues dorsally and a few millimeters proximally to the proximal aspect of the distal

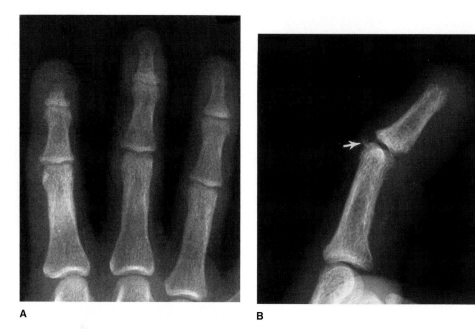

A

B

***Fig. 6–30.* A** AP views of the index, middle, and ring fingers. **B** Lateral view of the index finger.

phalanx representing an avulsion fracture of the attachment site of the extensor tendon. The tufts of all fingers are abnormal. This patient's distal phalanges are too short and too narrow at their tips. The cortex has been resorbed in many places. It is difficult to decide exactly where the edge of the bone is. Besides resorption of the most distal portion of the tuft of the index finger, there is also irregular resorption or destruction of the central portion of the distal phalanx.

Discussion:

In Case 6-10, options *A,* a chest radiograph, and *E,* mammography, are both reasonable screening examinations often obtained yearly in asymptomatic cancer patients. These would be good tests to order for this patient even without new symptoms. Indeed, mammography should be obtained in any woman of 45 years every year for screening purposes, irrespective of her history. Bone scans are also often ordered as screens for metastatic disease in asymptomatic breast cancer patients, particularly for the first 2 to 3 years after diagnosis. Because this patient is complaining of skeletal pain, both a bone scan (Fig. 6–31*A*) and conventional radiographs of the affected area (Fig. 6–31*B*) are indicated. A skeletal survey is not appropriate. (*D* is the correct answer to Question 6-10.) In general, a skeletal survey is utilized in oncology only for screening for multiple myeloma and Langerhans' cell histiocytosis.

In this patient's case, a bone scan revealed multiple areas of abnormally increased accumulation of radionuclide, including the left acetabulum (Fig. 6–31*A*). The multiplicity of lesions, together with the history of breast cancer (which often metastasizes to bone and may do so after a disease-free interval of many years), is very suggestive of metastatic disease. Some oncologists would choose to treat the patient for presumed metastatic disease on the basis of the bone scan, history, and current symptoms. Others would prefer a biopsy before proceeding to further treatment. This patient underwent a CT-guided needle aspiration of the acetabular lesion, which revealed metastatic tumor (Fig. 6–31*C*). To evaluate for possible impending pathologic fracture (Fig. 6–32), most oncologists would also request conventional radiographs of areas demonstrating increased activity on the bone scan, particularly those in weight-bearing bones.

Periosteal elevation (Case 6-11, Fig. 6–28) is a nonspecific finding that occurs with local disorders such as fracture, bone tumors, and osteomyelitis and also with systemic or multifocal disorders such as bone infarction (Fig. 6–33), venous stasis, and secondary hypertrophic osteoarthropathy. Because this finding is bilateral, it is more likely due to a systemic or multifocal disorder than to a local one.

Of all the systemic disorders that may be associated with periosteal new bone formation, secondary hypertrophic osteoarthropathy is the most important to exclude. At one time it was called *hypertrophic pulmonary*

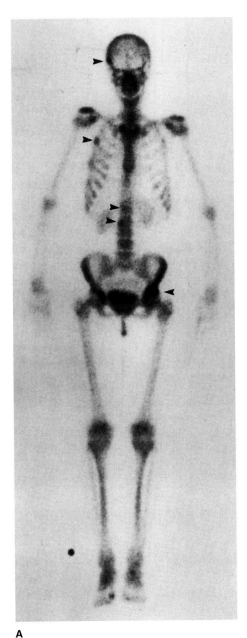

A

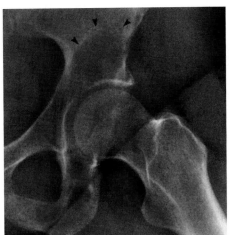

B

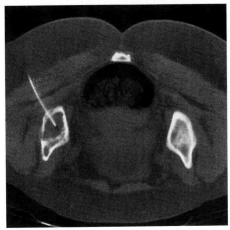

C

Fig. 6–31. **A** Anterior view from a ^{99m}Tc-MDP whole-body bone scan. In several areas more radionuclide has accumulated than in the remainder of the skeleton, and these areas appear darker: left acetabulum, two upper lumbar vertebrae, the lateral aspect of the right third rib, and the right side of the skull (*arrowheads*). Numerous foci of increased radioactivity, sprinkled somewhat haphazardly about the body but mostly involving the axial skeleton, are very typical of the appearance of metastatic cancer. **B** Frog-leg lateral view of the left hip. The ilium just above the acetabulum is too lucent, and a thin, irregular white line (*arrowheads*) demarcates the edge of the lucency. **C** Axial CT scan, obtained with the patient prone. The trabecular bone of the left ilium has been replaced by material of approximately the same density as the muscle. Using a percutaneous approach through the left buttock, a needle has been placed into the center of the lesion. Aspiration of cells yielded a diagnosis of metastatic breast carcinoma. The needle appears to be wholly embedded within the patient because it has traveled an oblique course. The rest of it would be apparent on adjacent sections.

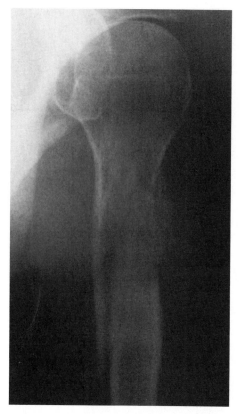

Fig. 6–32. AP view of the proximal left humerus. An acute fracture has occurred through an area of bone destruction caused by metastatic carcinoma. (The same radiographic appearance could be seen in a healing fracture through previously normal bone.) Conventional radiographs are used to identify bony metastases that have destroyed enough bone to make a pathologic fracture likely.

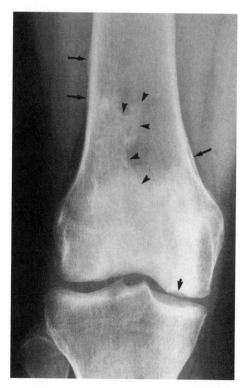

Fig. 6–33. AP view of the knee. This is an example of periosteal new bone formation (*arrows*) associated with bone infarction. The infarction is marked by an irregular sclerotic area in the metaphysis (*arrowheads*), as well as a small, rounded lucent defect in the articular surface of the medial femoral condyle (*short arrow*).

osteoarthropathy because it is usually caused by pulmonary disease. The designation *secondary hypertrophic osteoarthropathy* reflects current understanding that this disorder may also be due to nonpulmonary diseases such as inflammatory bowel disease or congenital cardiac anomalies. Nonetheless, pulmonary disease, specifically lung cancer, remains the most common cause. (*D* is the correct answer to Question 6-11.) This patient, in fact, had lung cancer (Fig. 6–34).

A bone scan could be useful if you did not notice the periosteal new bone or were not sure of its presence. Hand films could demonstrate clubbing, which may be seen with some of the same disorders that cause hypertrophic osteoarthropathy, but simple physical inspection of the patient's hands would accomplish the same thing. MR imaging of the knees will not be helpful in this case.

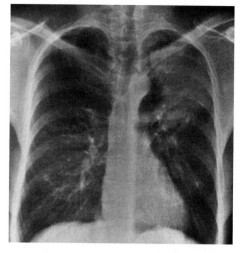

Fig. 6–34. PA view of the chest. A large mass in the left upper lobe represents a primary lung carcinoma.

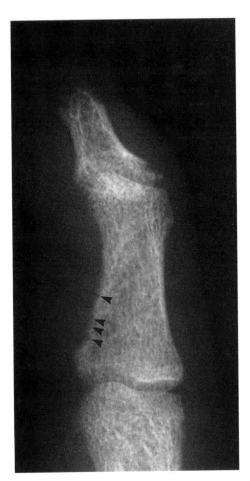

Fig. 6–35. Oblique view of the middle finger. Note the many tiny erosions of the cortex of the radial side of the middle phalanx (*arrowheads*). Contrast the pitted, irregular appearance of the radial cortex with the smooth ulnar cortex.

The patient in Case 6-12 (Fig. 6–29) has sickle cell disease. The surgical clips in the right upper quadrant of the abdomen are from a prior cholecystectomy. People with sickle cell disease are prone to early development of cholelithiasis.

The peculiar shape of multiple vertebral bodies is very characteristic of sickle cell anemia, though it may occasionally be seen in other diseases affecting the marrow cavity, particularly Gaucher's disease. It may be caused by infarction of bone beneath the end-plates, with remodeling of the cortex to produce the H shape.

When red cells sickle, they clump together and may block blood vessels. In bone this leads to avascular necrosis, which may be widespread, involving many bones simultaneously. The mottled appearance of the humeral heads is due to avascular necrosis and is a common finding in patients with sickle cell anemia.

Modest enlargement of the pulmonary artery, as seen in this patient, is so common in young women that it is considered normal in that population. (*B* is the correct answer to Question 6-12.)

Though it was not included among the possible answers to the question, another finding of interest on this examination involves the appearance of the left upper quadrant. The gas-filled splenic flexure of the colon occupies too much of the left upper quadrant on the frontal view. There is no room for a spleen of normal size. In sickle cell patients the spleen is often infarcted so that by the time they reach adulthood, it has shrunk to a small fraction of normal size.

The patient in Case 6-13 (Fig. 6–30) has many findings of hyperparathyroidism. Primary hyperparathyroidism usually results from a hyperfunctioning parathyroid adenoma, which is usually detected and removed before the osseous findings of hyperparathyroidism develop. Secondary hyperparathyroidism is most often associated with chronic renal failure, a common complication of diabetes mellitus. (*D* is the correct answer to Question 6-13.)

Parathormone stimulates the action of osteoclasts and thus causes resorption of bone. Acroosteolysis (resorption of the tufts of the fingers) is one manifestation of hyperparathyroidism. Two other places where such resorption

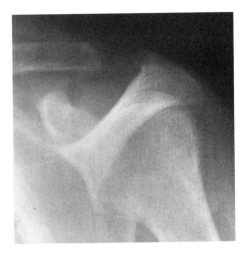

Fig. 6–36. Oblique view of the acromioclavicular joint. The clavicle is too short by approximately 1 cm, and the cortex of the distal end of this bone is fuzzy and ill defined.

often occurs are also seen in this patient's hands. One is intracortical, where resorption is causing longitudinal striation in the cortex. The other is subperiosteal. Notice that the cortex of the lateral or radial side of each of the the middle phalanges is finely serrated (Fig. 6–35). This is caused by resorption of bone in the troughs, and the peaks are areas where the cortex has maintained a more normal thickness. Subperiosteal resorption in this location is often the earliest radiographic sign of hyperparathyroidism. It is also nearly pathognomonic of this disorder. Another common site of bone resorption in hyperparathyroidism is the distal clavicle (Fig. 6–36).

Resorption of the central portion of the distal phalanx of the index finger may also be due to hyperparathy-roidism, but other causes such as osteomyelitis or tumor should also be considered. Of the two, osteomyelitis is more common and may occur in the fingers as a result of direct implantation of organisms from a puncture wound. Metastasis may occur in any bone but favors the axial skeleton and is uncommon in the hands.

BIBLIOGRAPHY

Keats TE, Anderson M. *Atlas of Normal Roentgen Variants That May Simulate Disease,* 7th ed. St. Louis: Mosby; 2001.

Schmidt H, Kohler A, Zimmer EA. *Borderlands of Normal and Early Pathologic Findings in Skeletal Radiography,* 4th ed. New York: Thieme Medical Publishers; 1993.

Imaging of Joints

Thomas L. Pope, Jr. & Johnny U. V. Monu

TECHNIQUES AND NORMAL ANATOMY

Radiography

Conventional radiography is the most commonly used imaging technique to evaluate the joints. This technique should always be the first imaging study performed in a patient suspected of having joint problems. Radiography has the following important advantages: It is almost universally available, is relatively inexpensive compared to other imaging studies, and delivers only a small radiation dose to the patient. In all instances, when possible, two images of the joint perpendicular to each other should be performed. These are usually a frontal projection either in the anteroposterior (AP) or posteroanterior (PA) directions and a lateral. In some instances oblique images may also be obtained depending on the preferences of the referring physician or radiologist or the clinical situation. In certain instances it may also be important to obtain images of the joint above and below an injury. Two examples of this scenario are in forearm and lower leg injuries (paired bones), because pathology may exist at either the proximal or distal joint. Because some ionizing radiation is present in radiography, it should be used only when absolutely necessary in pediatric patients and pregnant women.

Historically, radiographic images were printed on film but a gradual conversion to computed radiography is being made in which images are electronically processed and viewed on a computer workscreen. These images can then be transmitted via Ethernet or Internet anywhere.

Conventional Tomography

Conventional tomography is mentioned mainly for historical interest. High radiation dose, relatively poor image resolution, and imaging in only one plane were its major disadvantages. The technique has been almost totally replaced by other imaging tests, especially CT and MR imaging.

Arthrography

Arthrography is a technique in which contrast or contrast and air are injected into the joint. The joint is then imaged using radiography, CT, or MR imaging or a combination of these techniques. The injected contrast may be an iodine-containing water-soluble compound (e.g., Conray), which is then imaged with radiography or CT (Fig. 7–1). Alternatively, a paramagnetic compound (e.g., gadolinium pentazocine) may be injected and imaged with MR technique. MR arthrographic images of the joint may also be performed after intravenous injection of the paramagnetic contrast agent although this technique is not used very often today. MR

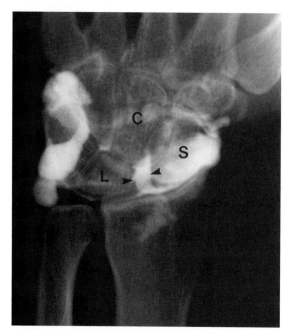

Fig. 7–1. Contrast arthrogram with radiography: AP wrist arthrogram view obtained after injection of contrast material into the radiocarpal joint shows contrast material passing through the scaphoid (S)–lunate (L) space from the radiocarpal joint into the midcarpal joint (*arrowheads*). This indicates a tear in the scapholunate ligament (C = capitate bone).

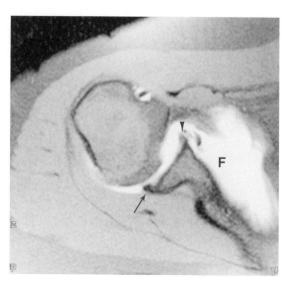

Fig. 7–2. Axial MR arthrogram shows marked joint distension with contrast (F) and the normal glenoid labrum anteriorly (*arrowhead*) and posteriorly (*arrow*). MR arthrography is used mainly to evaluate the shoulder for tears of the labrum and symptoms of instability.

arthrography is mainly used to evaluate the labra of the glenohumeral joint or hip but is also useful for evaluating the knee for meniscal tears in the patient who has had prior meniscal surgery (Fig. 7–2). CT arthrography and, less commonly, radiographic arthrography are most useful in the patient who cannot undergo MR imaging (Fig. 7–3).

Computed Tomography

Conventional computed tomography, a technique that makes individual axial (transverse) slices of the patient, uses the same ionizing radiation as radiography. CT technique has been vastly improved in the past few years. The recently developed "spiral" CT has major advantages over conventional CT. With the spiral CT technique, axial (transverse) images are acquired much more rapidly with dramatic decreases in radiation dose. For instance, a CT of the chest, abdomen, and pelvis can be performed in about 30 seconds. The CT data are stored in three-dimensional packets that can then be reconstructed and displayed on almost any other

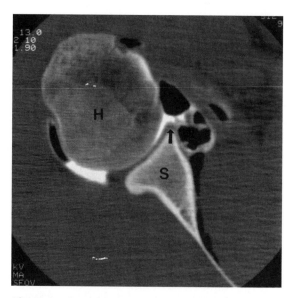

Fig. 7–3. Air-contrast arthrogram with CT. Axial (transverse) CT image of the shoulder of a patient after injection of air and contrast material into the joint. This so called "double-contrast" study shows the anterior glenoid labrum surrounded by contrast (*arrow*). Radiographic contrast material and air can be seen outlining the rest of the joint. H = humeral head, S = the glenoid process of scapula.

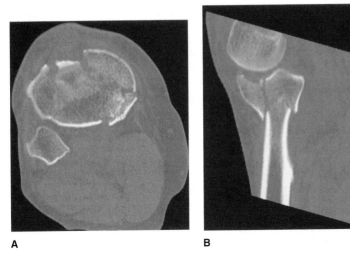

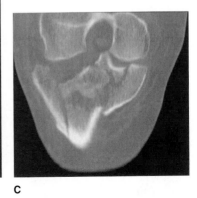

A   **B**   **C**

Fig. 7–4. **A** Axial spiral CT scan showing a comminuted fracture of the proximal tibia. **B** Sagittal reconstruction from the spiral CT again showing the comminuted tibial fracture. **C** Coronal reconstructed CT image showing the markedly comminuted fracture of the proximal tibia and the extension into joint. Spiral CT has the advantage of being able to be reconstructed in multiple planes.

plane. The most common images reconstructed from the axial plane are the sagittal and coronal planes (Fig. 7–4).

Magnetic Resonance Imaging

MR imaging has revolutionized the imaging evaluation of almost all body areas but particularly those of the central nervous system and musculoskeletal system. It has tremendous advantages over other imaging modalities in the evaluation of joints because of its excellent soft-tissue contrast, high resolution, and ability to image in every plane. This technique may show pathophysiologic events even before they are seen on x-ray, such as showing the very early changes of avascular necrosis (Fig. 7–5). Because of its exquisite soft-tissue contrast, MR imaging allows radiologists to visualize subtle differences in soft tissues that had never before been seen with other imaging modalities. For example, the subtle contrast between fat and muscle depicted on a radiograph or CT is dramatically highlighted with MR imaging because of their very different chemical compositions (Fig. 7–6). MR imaging can also depict subtle changes within the bone marrow cavity, an area difficult to evaluate with radiography or CT. Finally, this technique allows precise definition of almost each component within or surrounding the joint. Therefore, MR imaging is a tremendous aid to preoperative evaluation of any person who has unexplained joint pain or who has had trauma to a joint. In

fact, MR imaging should almost always be performed in patients with these symptoms before any invasive procedure is attempted. The major disadvantages of

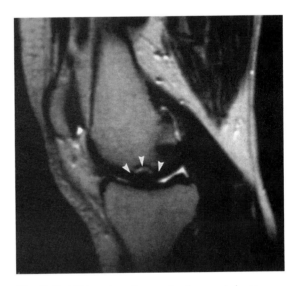

Fig. 7–5. MR imaging of avascular changes in bone. Sagittal MR image of the knee shows an area of bone infarct in the femur just below the cortex (*arrowheads*). This abnormality was not seen on the radiograph. MR imaging can also show these changes in the femoral head long before conventional film shows any abnormality.

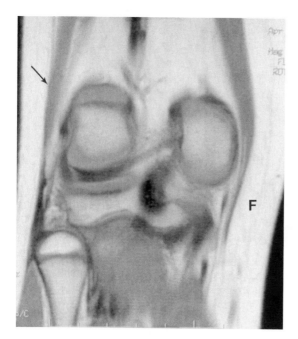

Fig. 7–6. Posterior coronal MR image of the knee shows the differentiation between the fat (F) and the biceps femoris muscle (*arrow*). MR can dramatically demonstrate small changes in density, one of its most effective advantages over other imaging techniques.

MR imaging are that some patients with claustrophobia cannot tolerate the small space of the magnet, and patients with metal in their bodies or who have certain heart valves or clips for vascular problems cannot be imaged.

Ultrasonography

Ultrasonography, first developed for use in World War II for detection of submarines, was adopted after the war for use in imaging. High-frequency transmission of sound can be used to evaluate the soft tissues, tendons, ligaments, and even the cartilage of the joint (Fig. 7–7). The ultrasound waves cannot be transmitted through cortical bone so the intramedullary cavity cannot be imaged with this technique. Ultrasound is used much more extensively in Europe than in the United States.

Radionuclide Imaging ("Bone Scans")

Radionuclide imaging uses radioactive materials that are injected intravenously so they can localize in regions of abnormally increased blood flow (hyperemia) or regions of increased osteoblastic or osteolytic changes or heightened metabolic activity. The major uses of bone scanning are in patients suspected of having metastatic disease or infection. Its primary use in suspected joint disease is limited.

Anatomy of the Normal Joint

The typical normal synovial joint consists of at least two articulating bones enclosed in a synovium-lined joint capsule. The apposing bony surfaces are covered by smooth articular cartilage (hyaline cartilage). On radiographs, the normal joint has a separation between the adjacent bones representing the region occupied by the hyaline or articular cartilage, meniscus, and joint fluid (the so-called "articular space") depending on which joint is imaged. These structures are not normally depicted on radiographs because of the limited soft-tissue contrast of the technique unless they are calcified (Fig. 7–8). However, MR imaging exquisitely shows the components of the normal joint (Fig. 7–9).

Joint Disease

The clinical signs and symptoms of joint disease are manifestations of abnormal function such as reduced mobility, hypermobility, and pain. Altered function may be due to pain, discomfort, apprehension, or instability.

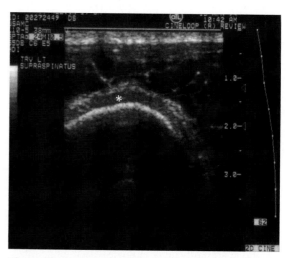

Fig. 7–7. Ultrasonography of the shoulder. An axial (transverse) ultrasonographic image of the shoulder shows an intact supraspinatus tendon (*), seen as a zone of hypoechogenicity (low-signal echoes) on the scan. This technique is very operator dependent.

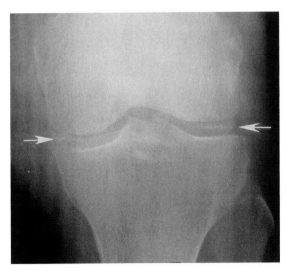

Fig. 7–8. Frontal views of 82-year-old woman showing chondrocalcinosis represented by calcification of the menisci (*arrows*). The menisci are not normally demonstrated on radiography unless they are calcified.

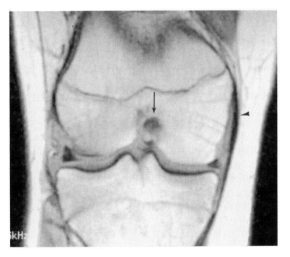

Fig. 7–9. Coronal MR image showing the normal components of the knee joint. Note the menisci, the posterior cruciate ligament (*arrow*), and the medial (tibial) collateral ligament (*arrowhead*).

The wide range of joint abnormalities is summarized below and many of these processes are discussed in the exercises. Any of these signs may occur singly or in combination with any others.

Radiographically, joint disease may be diagnosed by any of the following:

1. Incongruity of the articulating bone as is seen with dislocations, e.g., traumatic dislocation or dislocations caused by arthropathies such as lupus arthritis or rheumatoid arthritis

2. Irregularity of articulating bone ends and margins, as in erosions (e.g., in psoriasis or gout)

3. Increased density or sclerosis of articulating bone ends (also called *eburnation*), as in osteoarthritis

4. Bony outgrowth (proliferation) at bone ends, known as *osteophytes*

5. Diffuse reduced density of bone ends, described as juxta-articular or periarticular osteopenia (e.g., rheumatoid arthritis, tuberculous arthritis)

6. Focal areas of loss of medullary bone substance beneath the articular cortex, known as *subchondral cysts* or *geodes* (e.g., osteoarthritis, rheumatoid arthritis)

7. Loss of articular space from articular cartilage destruction (e.g., septic arthritis, osteoarthritis)

8. Accumulation of excess joint fluid within the joint (joint effusion) (Excess joint fluid is a common manifestation of joint disorders. The fluid may be synovial fluid, blood, or even pus, depending on the etiology of the joint disease.)

9. Calcification of articular (hyaline) cartilage or fibrocartilage (chondrocalcinosis), or intra-articular soft-tissue calcification such as that seen in scleroderma or polymyositis or dermatomyositis

10. Synovial proliferation or abnormal increase in the synovial lining, such as that seen with pigmented villonodular synovitis (PVNS).

TECHNIQUE SELECTION

Radiography should always be the initial imaging test to evaluate the joints and should only be obtained after the patient has had a thorough history and physical examination and there is a clear indication to obtain the study. Various projections may be used depending on the clinical indication or the situation, but at least two projections perpendicular to each other should be obtained. Often radiographs alone will confirm the clinical diagnosis or the findings will suggest an entirely different one. In many instances, however, it may be necessary to use other more expensive imaging techniques to clarify the x-ray findings or to evaluate significant clinical symptoms or signs or laboratory abnormalities if the radiographs are normal. The following paragraphs discuss the selection of the imaging techniques in a few common clinical scenarios.

Congenital Diseases

If the clinical situation of a suspected congenital anomaly or a pediatric joint abnormality or if a limp is present in a child, an x-ray film of the suspected joint should be obtained first. Because the joint structures are not well mineralized in the child, further evaluation of the joint with ultrasonography or MR imaging will often be required to make a more definitive diagnosis because, as discussed earlier, they are the best techniques to image nonmineralized structures. If MR imaging facilities are not available, the congenital abnormality may be investigated with a combination of conventional radiography, ultrasonography, conventional arthrography, and CT with or without intra-articular contrast injection.

Acute Trauma

In acute trauma, the first line of radiologic investigation is the radiograph. If fractures are identified, further imaging will depend on the needs of the clinician or subspecialist physician as dictated by the clinical situation. Generally, fractures that extend into the joint surface (intra-articular fractures) are treated very aggressively with the aim of reestablishing the integrity of the joint. Intra-articular fractures are frequently treated by operative reduction and internal fixation if the fracture fragments are severely displaced. CT examination of the involved limb and joints may also be performed preoperatively in selected cases for surgical planning. Postoperative CT may also be required to assess the results of surgical intervention. The advantages of CT are that it enables precise assessment of joint reconstitution and also confirms or excludes the presence of any intra-articular fragments that may interfere with proper reduction and healing (see Fig. 7–4).

Subacute and Remote Trauma

If the trauma is subacute or remote, the investigation should also begin with the radiograph. If the joint is normal and there is a strong clinical suspicion of injury, the patient may benefit from a radionuclide bone scan or more appropriately MR imaging because of its superior soft-tissue contrast and resolution. It is, therefore, particularly suited for investigation of the intra-articular and periarticular soft-tissue structures and subchondral bone (see Figs. 7–5 and 7–6).

Nontraumatic Cases

After an initial normal or unrevealing radiographic examination, MR imaging is the next modality of choice. If there is a joint effusion, it may be cost effec-tive to aspirate the fluid and analyze it for metabolic or infectious causes. If there is no obvious effusion at radiography, MR imaging is usually the next best and most cost-effective imaging test to evaluate injury to the intra-articular and periarticular structures of a joint.

EXERCISES

EXERCISE 7-1: CONGENITAL JOINT DISORDERS

Clinical Histories:

Case 7-1. This 25-year-old woman had hip pain that had become unbearable. She always walked abnormally and had some discomfort for as long as she could remember. Her pelvis radiograph is shown in Fig. 7–10.

Case 7-2. This child was examined by a pediatrician because of developmental delay. He has not attempted walking and is still crawling at 2 years. Several radiographs were performed. Figure 7–11 is a radiograph of the pelvis.

Case 7-3. This young boy was examined by a pediatrician because "he walks funny," according to his mother. He denies any pain. A film of the tibia and fibula is shown in Fig. 7–12.

Questions:

7-1. The most likely diagnosis in Fig. 7–10 is
   A. bilateral developmental dysplasia of the hips (DDH).
   B. Legg-Calvé-Perthes disease.
   C. proximal focal femoral deficiency syndrome.
   D. neuropathic joint disease.

7-2. In Case 7-2, the next best imaging test would be
   A. tomography of both hips.
   B. MR imaging of the hips.
   C. radionuclide bone scan of the pelvis.
   D. CT of the hips.

7-3. The patient whose film is shown in Fig. 7–12 has congenital insensitivity to pain (asymbolia). These patients may develop neuropathic joint disease. The signs of a neuropathic joint disease include
   A. multiple fractures.
   B. soft-tissue swelling.
   C. joint disorganization.
   D. all of the above.

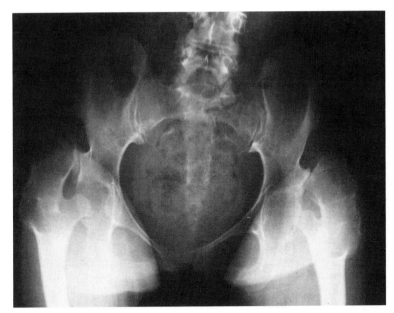

Fig. 7–10.

Radiologic Findings:

7-1. Both hips in the patient in this case (Fig. 7–10) are abnormal. The femoral heads and necks are malformed and dislocated from the acetabula fossae superiorly. The acetabulae are also malformed and oriented more vertically than normal. The patient had bilateral congenital dislocation of the hips that had been ignored by her parents. (*A* is the correct answer to Question 7-1.) This diagnosis should have been made at birth or shortly thereafter so that corrective therapy could have been instituted.

7-2. In this case (Fig. 7–11), the capital femoral epiphysis on the right (*arrow*) is laterally displaced and

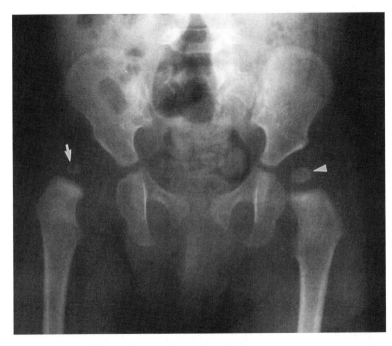

Fig. 7–11.

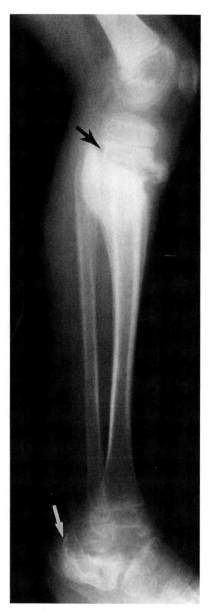

Fig. 7–12.

next most appropriate imaging test. (*B* is the correct answer to Question 7-2.)

7-3. In this case (Fig. 7–12), the calcaneus is deformed (*white arrow*). The talus is poorly visualized because of its complete dislocation from its normal position below the tibia and there are subluxations at the tibiotalar, talocalcaneal, and talonavicular joints. There is overall frank disorganization of this ankle joint, and clinically there was diffuse soft-tissue swelling around the ankle (not appreciated on this lateral film). There is also a metaphyseal fracture of the proximal tibia with exuberant periosteal/callus formation (*black arrow*). All of these findings in this patient are caused by chronic repetitive trauma in a patient with congenital insensitivity to pain. (*D* is the correct answer to Question 7-3.)

Discussion:

Congenital joint disorders are uncommonly encountered but they should be diagnosed as early as possible after birth because delayed diagnosis complicates management. Some of the more common congenital joint disorders include

1. Congenital dislocation of the hips, which is actually a bone dysplasia manifesting as a joint disorder
2. Arthrogryposis multiplex congenita
3. Congenital insensitivity to pain (asymbolia)

Congenital hip dislocation is actually a bone dysplasia. The femoral head is dysplastic and does not provide adequate stimulation for proper development of the acetabulum. Usually the femoral head is displaced laterally out of an unusually shallow (i.e., more vertically oriented) acetabulum (Fig. 7–11). Once the diagnosis of DDH is confirmed, treatment should begin at birth or in the perinatal period to minimize complications.

Historically, hip arthrograms were used to define the location of the femoral head in the neonate because the structure is cartilaginous at birth and therefore radiolucent on radiographs. Ultrasonography is an excellent test to assist in the diagnosis of DDH *in utero* and in the neonatal period because it requires no ionizing radiation. However, the interpretation of ultrasound is very observer dependent. The diagnosis and clarification of DDH can be difficult at times. MR imaging can show the soft-tissue structures, the osseous structures, and the articular cartilage well and is at present the modality of choice in the evaluation of DDH. If patients are not treated or poorly treated they will eventually develop secondary osteoarthritic changes. However, MR imaging is of no diagnostic value at this stage because the advanced nature of the disease can be ascertained just as well from radiographs.

Proximal focal femoral deficiency is a disease of uncertain etiology that is characterized by congenital absence of a segment or all of the proximal third of the

smaller than the left epiphysis (*arrowhead*). The acetabular fossa on the right side is also malformed and more vertical than the one on the left. The normal development of the acetabulum depends on a normally located femoral head and this is the explanation for this abnormality. These findings are the classical radiographic features of developmental dysplasia of the hip (DDH). When this finding is encountered, MR imaging is the femur. The incidence is higher in children of diabetic mothers and there is also an association with congenital hip dysplasia. MR imaging is also the imaging modality of choice in evaluating children with these disorders.

Arthrogryposis multiplex congenita is a noninheritable congenital disease of uncertain etiology characterized by multiple joint contractures. It is believed to be due to neuromuscular events occurring *in utero*. The joints of the lower limb are almost invariably affected. There may be other associated extraskeletal congenital anomalies.

A neuropathic joint is caused by chronic repetitive trauma in the setting of impaired or absent sensation. The characteristic features of neuropathic joint include soft-tissue swelling, fragmentation of the bony structures, and general disorganization of the joint. Joint effusion is often present. The more common causes of neuropathic joints in the lower extremities include diabetes mellitus and tabes dorsalis (neurosyphilis). Asymbolia or congenital insensitivity to pain, as exhibited in Case 7-3 (Fig. 7–12), is a group of uncommon congenital disorders in which there is a variable degree of loss of pain sensation and is an unusual cause of neuropathic joint. Patients with asymbolia almost always acquire deformities of the extremities after repeated trauma. This diagnosis should be considered in the young patient with multiple healing fractures and without suspicion of child abuse syndrome.

EXERCISE 7-2: JOINT TRAUMA

Clinical Histories:

Case 7-4. A 25-year-old man fell on his outstretched hand. AP and lateral radiographs of his wrist are shown in Fig. 7–13.

Case 7-5. A 30-year-old basketball player fell in practice and Fig. 7–14 shows AP and axillary views of radiographs from his shoulder.

Case 7-6. A 34-year-old anesthesiologist was injured in a basketball game. Figure 7–15 is a sagittal MR image from his knee study.

Case 7-7. A 40-year-old squash player was having shoulder pain and was referred for an MR scan. Figure 7–16 is an oblique coronal MR image from his study.

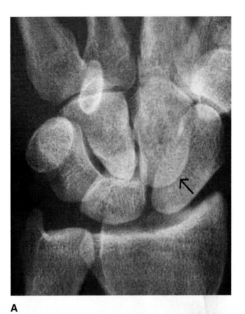

A

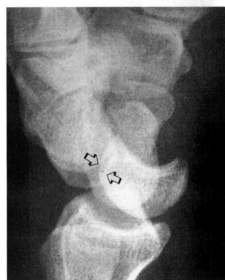

B

Fig. 7–13.

Questions:

7-4. In Fig. 7–13, the most likely diagnosis is
- **A.** lunate dislocation.
- **B.** perilunate dislocation.
- **C.** transcaphoid fracture-dislocation.
- **D.** none of the above.

7-5. The basketball player in Fig. 7–14 shows which of the following injuries?
- **A.** Fracture
- **B.** Dislocation
- **C.** Osteoarthritis
- **D.** None of the above

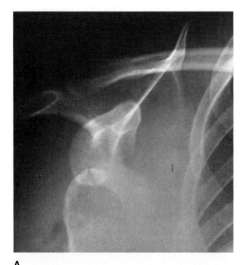

A

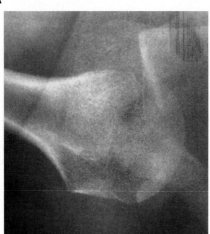

B

Fig. 7–14.

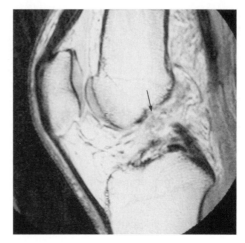

Fig. 7–15.

Radiologic Findings:

7-4. In the frontal projection (Fig. 7–13*A*), there is disorganization of the carpal arcs. The capitate is no longer articulating with the lunate and partly overlaps the scaphoid (*arrow*). The scaphoid is elongated on this view but not fractured. On the lateral projection (Fig. 7–13*B*), the lunate is still in line with the distal radius but the capitate has been dislocated dorsally (*open arrows*). Therefore, the patient has a dorsal perilunate dislocation. (*B* is the correct answer to Question 7-4.)

7-5. The AP radiograph of the shoulder of the basketball player (Fig. 7–14*A*) shows inferior displacement of the humeral head out of its normal position within

7-6. The anesthesiologist playing basketball in Fig. 7–15 has which type of abnormality on the MR image?
   A. Tendon injury
   B. Muscle injury
   C. Ligament injury
   D. Cartilage injury

7-7. The MR image in Fig. 7–16 shows which abnormality?
   A. Muscle injury
   B. Ligament injury
   C. Tendon injury
   D. Cartilage injury

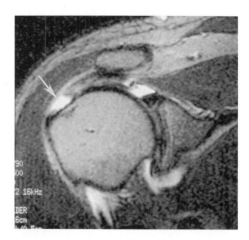

Fig. 7–16.

the glenoid. The axillary view of the shoulder (Fig. 7–14B) shows that the humeral head is dislocated anteriorly in relation to the glenoid, thus representing an anterior shoulder dislocation. This is the classic appearance of an anterior dislocation of the shoulder. (*B* is the correct answer to Question 7-5.)

7-6. The sagittal MR image shows the advantage of MR imaging in this clinical setting. Figure 7–15 shows a tear of the anterior cruciate ligament (ACL) (*arrow*). (*C* is the correct answer to Question 7-6.)

7-7. Figure 7–16 shows a torn supraspinatus tendon (*arrow*) in the squash player. (*C* is the correct answer to Question 7-7.)

Discussion:

Dislocation or subluxation: The terms *subluxation* and *dislocation* are often used interchangeably. However, *subluxation* refers to partial loss of congruity between the articulating ends of bones, whereas *dislocation* denotes complete loss of congruity. Disruption or loss of the integrity of the restraining ligaments around the joint leads to instability and thus permits dislocation to occur. Severe hyperflexion or hyperextension forces often cause traumatic dislocations. Fractures are frequently associated with traumatic dislocations.

CARPAL DISLOCATION

The normal arrangement of the carpal bones of the wrist is seen on the AP view of the wrist (Fig. 7–17A). Note the three smooth, parallel arcs in the proximal and midcarpal rows. The lateral view of the wrist (Fig. 7–17B) shows that the radius, lunate, and capitate are in an almost straight line. The two major types of wrist carpal dislocation are *perilunate* and *lunate*. In a perilunate dislocation, the lateral film shows that the lunate maintains its normal articulation with the radius and the capitate is displaced dorsally. In a lunate dislocation, the lunate has a triangular shape on the frontal projection (Fig. 7–18A) and is displaced from its normal articulation, and the radius and capitate maintain a linear relationship (Fig. 7–18B). Carpal dislocations are usually produced by a fall on the outstretched hand and are more common in young adults. The diagnosis is usually made by radiographic examination, although CT may be used after reduction to evaluate the wrist for joint congruity and for the presence of loose bodies (intra-articular fracture fragments).

SHOULDER DISLOCATION

The two main types of shoulder dislocation are anterior and posterior dislocations. Anterior dislocation, usually caused by falls, is most common and is seen in about 95% of cases. In an anterior dislocation, the humeral head is displaced anteriorly and inferiorly to the scapular

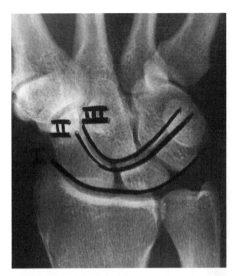

A

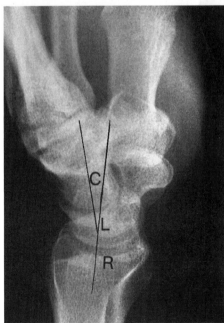

B

Fig. 7–17. **A** AP view of the normal wrist showing the three parallel arcs of the radiocarpal joint (I) and the midcarpal joint (II and III) (From Poeling G et al. *Arthroscopy of the Wrist and Elbow.* New York: Raven Press; 1994; used with permission.) **B** Lateral view of the normal wrist showing the almost linear arrangement (*straight lines*) of the distal radius (R), lunate (L), and capitate (C).

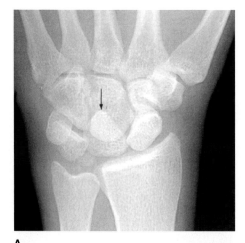

A

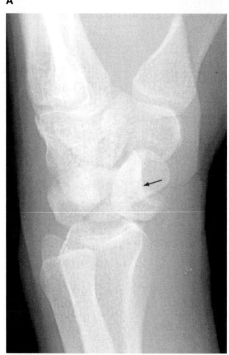

B

Fig. 7–18. **A** Frontal radiograph of a person who fell on an outstretched hand shows the triangular shape of the lunate (*arrow*) seen with lunate dislocation. **B** Lateral radiograph shows the displacement of the lunate volarly (*arrow*) with maintenance of the normal linear relationship between the distal radius and capitate.

glenoid fossa. There are various subtypes of anterior dislocation: subglenoid, subcoracoid, and medial. These subtypes are based on the location of the humeral head relative to the glenoid fossa and coracoid process.

Posterior dislocation is relatively uncommon. It is produced by severe contraction of the muscles of the shoulder girdle, which may occur in electric shock or convulsions. A diagnosis of posterior dislocation in one shoulder should prompt investigation of the other shoulder, since the injury is often bilateral.

If the postreduction radiographs are normal after a single instance of dislocation, there is usually no need for another imaging study in the acute setting. However, if there is a recurrence of dislocation or if the patient remains chronically symptomatic, MR imaging or CT arthrography of the shoulder should be obtained to search for the cause of the dislocations and any associated shoulder abnormalities resulting from the dislocation.

CT arthrography and MR imaging are used to investigate the shoulder for cartilage and soft-tissue injuries resulting from shoulder dislocation. After an anterior dislocation there is frequently associated injury to the anterior glenoid labrum. This is produced by the impaction of the posterior and lateral aspect of the humeral head beneath the anterior and inferior glenoid process. There may also be an accompanying compression fracture of the humeral head, referred to as the *Hill-Sachs deformity.*

Hip Dislocation

The hip is a relatively stable joint because of the surrounding strong muscles and joint capsule and significant trauma is required for dislocations to occur. A common mechanism causing hip dislocation is the "dashboard injury" where the knee is impacted on the dashboard and the femoral head is driven posteriorly in relation to the acetabulum. The most common dislocating direction of the femur is posterior and when this occurs the femoral head often ends up superior and lateral to the acetabulum. In posterior dislocations, there is almost always an associated fracture of the posterior aspect of the acetabular rim or the femoral head (Fig. 7–19). Anterior hip dislocation is uncommon and is produced by a blow to the hip when the femur is internally rotated and abducted. Central dislocation of the hip usually occurs with direct lateral forces and there is an associated fracture of the quadrilateral plate (medial aspect) of the acetabulum.

KNEE LIGAMENT TEARS

Tears of the ligaments of the knee are commonly seen in athletic individuals. The function of the anterior cruciate ligament (ACL) is to limit the anterior translation of the tibia in relation to the femur. Any sport that requires

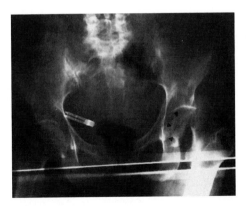

Fig. 7–19. AP radiograph of the pelvis in a person who had been involved in an automobile accident. It shows the left femoral head displaced superiorly and laterally to the acetabulum representing a left posterior hip dislocation. The *arrowheads* show a semilunar piece of bone (part of the femoral head) still within the acetabulum that was sheared off during the posterior dislocation.

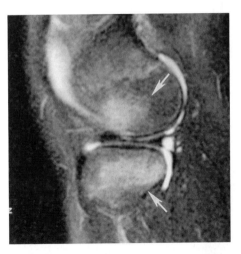

Fig. 7–21. Sagittal MR image in a patient with an ACL tear shows the classic "kissing contusions" of the lateral femoral condyle and the lateral tibial plateau (*arrows*). They are caused by the transient dislocation of the knee that occurs during this injury and these areas of edema are classically associated with an ACL tear.

pivoting and planting of the feet places an enormous stress on the ACL and may cause injury to it. The normal ACL originates on the inner aspect of the lateral femoral condyle and extends anteriorly and slightly obliquely to insert adjacent to the anterior tibial spine. The normal ACL has a fascicular arrangement with individual bands that can easily be seen by MR (Fig. 7–20). The most common mechanism of injury to the ACL is the "clipping" injury with valgus stress. On MR, the injured ACL is diagnosed by high signal intensity within the substance of the ligament (the so-called "pseudomass"). There may

also be other associated abnormalities such as bone contusions (usually on the posterolateral aspect of the tibia and the anterolateral aspect of the femur from the transient dislocation that occurs at the time of injury) and medial collateral ligament injury from the valgus stress (Fig. 7–21). There may also be associated meniscal tears, usually vertical tears in the acute setting (Fig. 7–22).

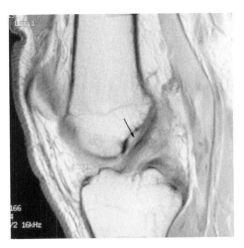

Fig. 7–20. Sagittal MR image showing a normal ACL (*arrow*). Notice the fascicular arrangement.

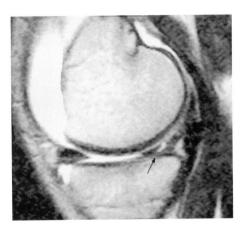

Fig. 7–22. Sagittal MR image in a patient with an ACL tear showing a vertical tear of the posterior horn of the medial meniscus (*arrow*). These vertical tears are often seen in the acute setting.

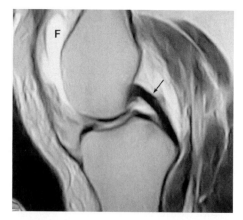

Fig. 7–23. Sagittal MR image of the knee showing the normal homogeneously low-signal-intensity PCL (*arrow*). Incidentally noted is a suprapatellar joint effusion anteriorly (F) (*white area of high signal intensity*).

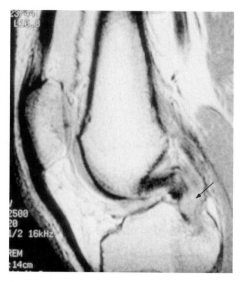

Fig. 7–24. Tear of PCL. MR imaging shows a typical example of a tear of the posterior cruciate ligamant (*arrow*).

The posterior cruciate ligament (PCL) serves to limit the posterior translation of the tibia in relation to the femur. The PCL is commonly injured in kicking sports such as soccer and is also injured in automobile accidents if the tibia impacts on the dashboard and is translated posteriorly in relation to the femur in the flexed knee.

The normal PCL on MR is a homogeneous structure that originates from the inner aspect of the medial femoral condyle and extends far posteriorly to insert onto the posterior aspect of the tibia (Fig. 7–23). The PCL should easily be seen on all knee MR studies. Tears of the PCL are diagnosed at MR imaging by increased signal within the ligament and swelling (partial tears), and a complete tear of the ligament is diagnosed by complete separation of the ligament at some point along its course (Fig. 7–24). MR imaging is extremely important in the evaluation of the knee of the injured athlete and is used frequently in this setting.

SUPRASPINATUS TENDON TEARS

The supraspinatus, infraspinatus, teres minor, and subscapularis muscles (SITS muscles) comprise the rotator cuff. The shoulder is the most unstable joint in the body and these muscles serve to help stabilize it. The most commonly torn tendon in the shoulder is the supraspinatus, and it usually tears approximately 1 cm proximal to its insertion onto the greater tuberosity of the humeral head. The supraspinatus tendon is easily seen on MR imaging as a low-signal-intensity structure, and tears of the supraspinatus tendon are easily and nicely demonstrated on MR. Fig. 7–16 is a typical

example of a supraspinatus tendon tear with fluid within the tendon. The most common causes of supraspinatus tendon tears are aging and impingement. Acute rotator cuff tears are unusual. MR imaging is vital in the preoperative evaluation of the patient suspected of having a rotator cuff tear because the morphology of the tendons, the size of the tear if there is one, and other associated abnormalities of the joint including pathology of the glenoid labrum can be diagnosed with this technique.

ACHILLES TENDON RUPTURE

The injury of achilles tendon rupture occurs most frequently in patients in the fourth and fifth decades of life. Although the injury may occur in any person, individuals who do not exercise regularly (the so-called "weekend warriors") are more susceptible to this tear.

The clinical history and physical findings are often enough to make a diagnosis of Achilles tendon rupture. Radiographic stress views should not be performed in the setting of a suspected Achilles tendon rupture because the stress may actually make the tear worse. Any question of whether the tear is partial or complete should usually be resolved, because the treatment for each of these is different. Moreover, the clinician needs to know the level of injury and how far the tendon fragments are separated. MR imaging is currently the imaging technique of choice to evaluate the Achilles tendon. The whole length of the tendon, including its insertion on the calcaneus, and any associated injuries can be shown in detail. In cases of complete rupture of the

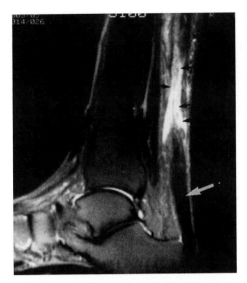

Fig. 7–25. A sagittal T2-weighted MR image of the ankle shows complete disruption of the Achilles tendon with high-signal-intensity hemorrhage and edema (*short arrows*) interposed between the tendon fragment. The *white arrow* points out the distal Achilles tendon.

tendon, the MR images show separation of the normally low-signal-intensity fibers of the Achilles tendon by high-signal-intensity edema and hemorrhage (Fig. 7–25). The frayed ends of each of the separated fragments may also be seen. In partial tears, areas of intermediate to high signal representing regions of partial disruption are seen within the normally low-signal-intensity tendon and some of the fibers of the tendon remain intact. Ultrasound may also be used to evaluate the Achilles tendon and color Doppler examination may be used to follow the process of revascularization and healing of a partially torn tendon, although musculoskeletal ultrasound is not widely practiced in the United States at this time.

EXERCISE 7-3: JOINT INSTABILITY

Clinical Histories:

Case 7-8. A 45-year-old former baseball pitcher had recurrent dislocations of the shoulder, pain, and inability to reach around to his back pocket. He also feels a click and catching sensation when he moves his arm. Radiographs of his shoulder are normal. He is referred by his orthopedist for MR imaging. A selected axial image from his study is shown in Figure 7–26.

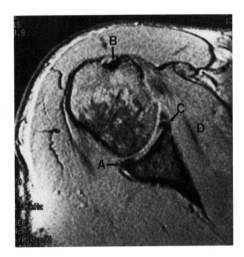

Fig. 7–26.

Case 7-9. A 20-year-old football player was examined in the emergency department after being tackled particularly hard. A radiograph was obtained first (Fig. 7–27).

Case 7-10. A little girl was running through her house and tripped on an electrical cord. Intense pain ensued and she was referred for an MR examination. A selected axial image from her MR study is shown in Fig. 7–28.

Case 7-11. A college football player was injured and was thought to have transiently subluxed his knee when he was hit on the lateral side of the leg. His orthopedic sports medicine physician noted medial laxity and referred him for an MR scan. A coronal MR image from his study is shown in Fig. 7–29.

Questions:

7-8. The most likely diagnosis in Fig. 7–26 is
  A. dislocation of the shoulder.
  B. myositis ossificans.
  C. tear of the anterior glenoid labrum.
  D. rotator cuff tear.

7-9. Regarding Fig. 7–27, the *arrowheads* indicate a
  A. fracture of the patella.
  B. lipohemarthrosis.
  C. tear of the anterior cruciate ligament.
  D. all of the above.
  E. none of the above.

7-10. The axial MR image on the little girl injured by tripping on the electrical cord (Fig. 7–28) shows a

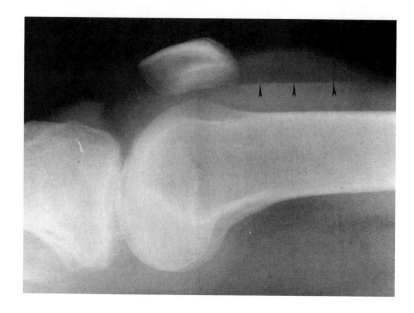

Fig. 7–27.

A. meniscal tear.
B. tendon injury.
C. medial retinacular injury.
D. ligament strain.

7-11. The medial pain in the soccer player was most likely caused by (*arrow* in Fig. 7–29)
A. a medial collateral ligament tear.
B. a lateral collateral ligament tear.
C. an anterior cruciate ligament tear.
D. a meniscal tear.

Radiologic Findings:

7-8. Figure 7–26 is an axial image. There is a high-signal intensity line through the triangular anterior glenoid labrum representing an anterior glenoid labral tear (C). (*C* is the correct answer to Question 7-8.) In Fig. 7–26, A is the posterior labrum, B is the biceps tendon, and D is the belly of the subscapularis muscle.

7-9. Figure 7–27 is a lateral radiograph of the knee obtained with a horizontal x-ray beam. There is a joint effusion with a fat-fluid level (*arrowheads*). This fat-fluid level is called a *lipohemarthrosis*. It is important to perform horizontal cross table lateral films in the acute trauma setting in order to demonstrate this. Frequently,

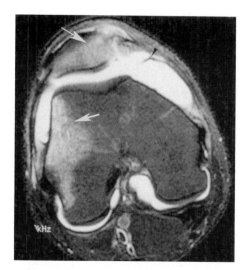

Fig. 7–28.

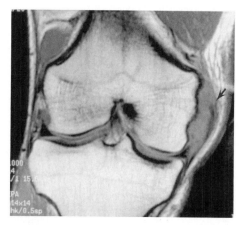

Fig. 7–29.

there is a fracture to account for the presence of fat within the joint because the fat has entered from the bone marrow cavity. (*B* is the correct answer to Question 7-9.) Fat-fluid levels may also be seen in patients who have acute tears of ligaments, especially the ACL.

7-10. Figures 7–28, the axial image on the little girl injured by tripping over the electrical cord, shows a large joint effusion and high-signal-intensity areas on the medial aspect of the patella and the lateral aspect of the lateral femoral condyle (*arrows*). These are also in essence a type of "kissing contusion." However, in this instance, the contusions result from impingement of the medial aspect of the patella onto the lateral femoral condyle as the patella dislocates laterally. For this to happen, there has to be a stretch or tear of the medial retinaculum (*arrowhead*). (*C* is the correct answer to Question 7-10.) This constellation of findings is typical of transient patellar dislocation-relocation.

7-11. Figure 7–29, a coronal image of the football player injured during a game, shows a complete tear of the medial collateral ligament (MCL) (*arrow*). (*A* is the correct answer to Question 7-11.) Injuries to the medial side of the knee occur from lateral trauma (valgus stress). The clinician in this instance noticed the medial joint laxity and suspected an MCL tear.

Discussion

INSTABILITY DISORDERS

Instability disorders are functional joint disorders generally manifested by pain, a feeling of insecurity around the joint, or a sensation of the joint giving way and abnormal motion around the joint. There may be no radiographic evidence of joint abnormality because often only soft-tissue injuries, such as ligamentous or fibrocartilaginous tears, are present. These abnormalities can often only be demonstrated by stress views or MR examinations of the joint in question.

SHOULDER INSTABILITY

The glenohumeral joint is the most inherently unstable ball-in-socket joint in the body. The major stability of the shoulder joint is provided by the joint capsule, the rotator cuff muscles, and the ligaments and tendons that surround it. The glenoid labrum, a fibrocartilaginous structure, contributes to shoulder joint stability by deepening the socket (glenoid labral complex) for this ball (humeral head).

A variety of soft-tissue injuries are associated with the anterior instability syndrome. The most common injuries from anterior glenohumeral dislocation are anteroinferior glenoid labral tears (the Bankart lesion), capsular stripping, Hill-Sachs deformity (compression fracture of the posterolateral aspect of the humeral head), and glenoid labral tears associated with osseous fracture (Figs. 7–30 and 7–31). Tears of the posterior aspect of the glenoid labrum are seen following posterior dislocation (Fig. 7–32). As we discussed in the last section, ruptures or tears of the rotator cuff tendons (SITS) are common causes of shoulder joint dysfunction and instability. The supraspinatus is the most commonly torn tendon in the shoulder. When the subscapularis tendon tears, an

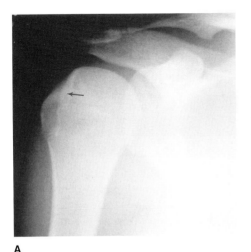

A

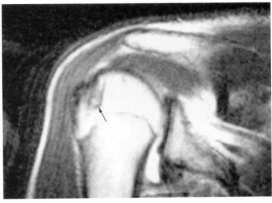

B

Fig. 7–30. **A** Frontal postreduction radiograph of a patient who had an anterior dislocation shows the compression fracture of the posterolateral aspect of the humeral head (*arrow*). This abnormality is called the Hill-Sachs lesion. **B** Oblique coronal MR image of same patient also shows the Hill-Sachs deformity (*arrow*).

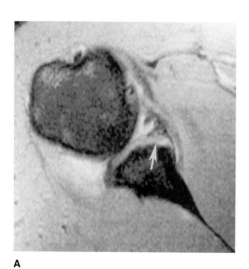

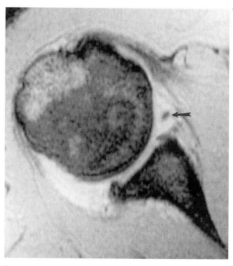

A   **B**

Fig. 7–31. A Axial MR image of a patient who had an anterior dislocation showing a fracture of the anterior and inferior aspect of the glenoid (*arrow*). This is also called the "bony" Bankart lesion. **B** Higher axial MR image in the same patient showing the associated anterior labral tear (*arrow*).

associated dislocation of the biceps tendon usually occurs. This results from a tear of the transverse ligament, a fascial extension across the intertubercular sulcus that holds the biceps tendon in place (Fig. 7–33).

The shoulder joint is best evaluated with MR imaging if there is a suspicion of a tendon abnormality. Shoulder arthrography and CT arthrography may also be requested by the orthopedic surgeon and used as alternative investigational tools in patients who have undergone rotator cuff repairs or who have had recent surgery to vital structures with residual ferromagnetic metallic clips. These tests are also used in patients who have aneurysm clips or metallic substances in the body (especially those located in or close to the eyes).

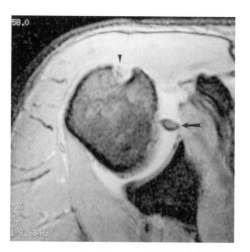

Fig. 7–33. Axial MR image of a patient who had a subscapularis tendon tear showing dislocation of the biceps tendon medially (*arrow*). Notice the empty intertubercular sulcus (*arrowhead*).

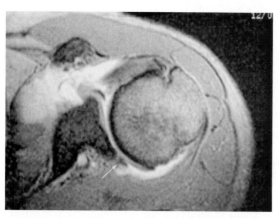

Fig. 7–32. Axial MR image of patient who had a posterior dislocation showing a posterior labral tear (*arrow*).

KNEE JOINT INSTABILITY

Stability of the knee, which is a hinge joint, is provided by the muscles and the ligamentous complexes. The most important of these are the anterior and posterior cruciate ligaments and the lateral and medial collateral ligament complexes. The major knee muscles and tendons that cross the joint include the quadriceps muscle and tendon and the patella ligament anteriorly; the biceps femoris tendon, tensor fascia lata, and popliteus muscles laterally; the pes anserinus tendons (sartorius, gracilis, and semitendinosus muscles—"Say grace before tea" is a phrase to help us remember these!) medially; and the gastrocnemius and plantaris muscles posteriorly. Rupture of any of the tendons, ligaments, or muscles compromises stability of the knee joint. All of these structures can be exquisitely demonstrated with MR imaging, which is the best imaging test to evaluate instability in this joint.

EXERCISE 7-4: ARTHRITIDES

Clinical Histories:

Case 7-12. A 75-year-old man presented with bilateral hip pain of several years' duration. Figure 7–34 is a frontal view of his pelvis.

Case 7-13. A 45-year-old woman with generalized body "aches and pains" presented to her rheumatologist. Her erythrocyte sedimentation rate (ESR) was elevated at 70 mm. Figure 7–35 is a frontal view of both of her hands.

Case 7-14. A 59-year-old woman with renal failure and a long history of hemodialysis was seen in the emergency room having experienced 2 days of intense right hip pain and fever. She had a fall 8 days ago. She has substantial limitation of motion in the right hip on physical examination. Figure 7–36 is the frontal view of her right hip.

Case 7-15. A 60-year old man presented to the emergency room with intense foot pain. He was a known ethanol abuser. An oblique view of his right foot is shown in Fig. 7–37.

Case 7-16. A 39-year-old man with a long history of back pain presented with limitation of movement in his neck. His HLA-B27 antigen was elevated. Figure 7–38 is a lateral view of his cervical spine.

Case 7-17. A 58-year-old man with a "rash" on his elbows presented to his rheumatologist with hand pain. Figure 7–39A is a frontal view of his hands and Figure 7–39B is a coned down view of the distal phalanges of his left hand.

Questions:

7-12. The frontal pelvis view in Fig. 7–34 shows all of the following features except
- **A.** loss of articular space.
- **B.** geode formation.
- **C.** juxta-articular osteopenia.
- **D.** bony sclerosis.

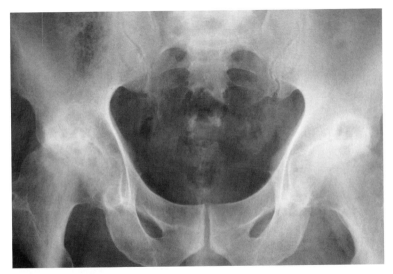

Fig. 7–34.

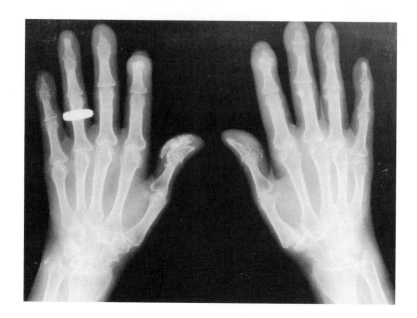

Fig. 7–35.

7-13. The hands of the 45-year-old woman in Fig. 7–35 show soft tissue calcifications that are most consistent with a diagnosis of
    A. osteoarthritis.
    B. scleroderma.
    C. systemic lupus erythematosus (SLE).
    D. psoriasis.

7-14. The radiograph of the right hip in Fig. 7–36 is most compatible with
    A. osteoarthritis.
    B. gout.

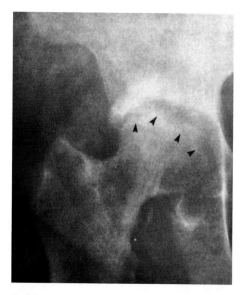

Fig. 7–36.

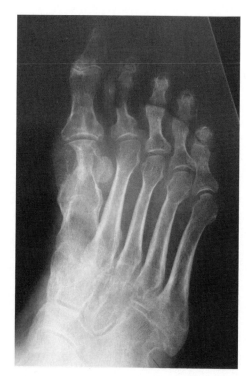

Fig. 7–37.

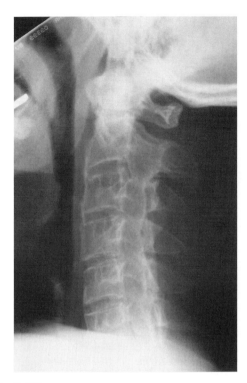

Fig. 7–38.

C. septic arthritis.
D. scleroderma.

7-15. The imaging findings at the first metatarsal phalangeal joint in Fig. 7–37 are most likely due to

A. scleroderma.
B. ankylosing spondylitis.
C. gout.
D. osteoarthritis.

7-16. The linear ossifications connecting the cervical vertebral bodies in Fig. 7–38 are called
A. osteophytes.
B. erosions.
C. soft-tissue swelling.
D. syndesmophytes.

7-17. The "pencil-in-cup" deformity of the distal interphalangeal joints in Fig. 7–39 is most compatible with a diagnosis of
A. psoriasis.
B. gout.
C. ankylosing spondylitis.
D. SLE.

Radiologic Findings:

7-12. The frontal radiograph of both hips in this case (Fig. 7–34) shows articular space narrowing, sclerosis, and subchondral cyst formation (also called *geodes*) bilaterally. There is no significant juxta-articular osteopenia. Therefore, the correct answer to Question 7-12 is *C* and the findings are most compatible with bilateral osteoarthritis (OA) of the hips.

7-13. In this case (Fig. 7–35), the most prominent feature of this lady's hand is soft-tissue calcification and acroosteolysis of the distal tuft. The features are most compatible with a diagnosis of scleroderma. (*B* is the correct answer to Question 7-13).

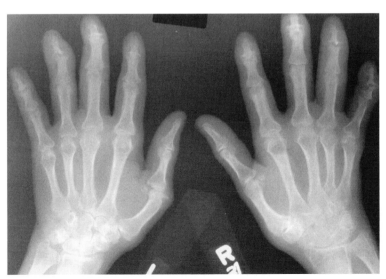

A

Fig. 7–39.

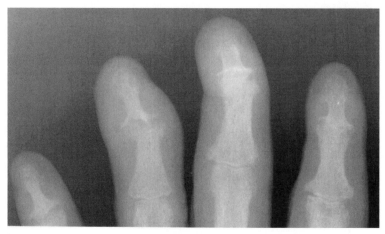

Fig. 7–39. *Cont.*   **B**

7-14. In this case (Fig. 7–36), the radiograph of the right hip shows articular space narrowing, bony erosion in the acetabulum and femoral head (*arrowheads*), and irregular bony sclerosis. The findings are most compatible with septic arthritis. (*C* is the correct answer for Question 7-14.)

7-15. Figure 7–37 shows marked soft-tissue swelling and erosion of the distal aspect of the first metatarsal as well as erosions involving the proximal aspect of the proximal phalanx. These erosions have "overhanging margins." This radiographic appearance and the location of these changes at the first metatarsal phalangeal joint are characteristic of "podagra" associated with the initial attack of gout. (*C* is the correct answer to Question 7-15.)

7-16. The lateral view of the cervical spine in Fig. 7–38 shows prominent thin vertically oriented connections between the anterior aspects of the vertebral bodies and fusion of the posterior elements of the spine. The thin vertically oriented ossifications are located anatomically in the outer layers of the annulus fibrosis and represent syndesmophytes that are associated with ankylosing spondylitis. (*D* is the correct answer to Question 7-16.)

7-17. Figure 7–39 shows soft-tissue swelling at the PIP and DIP joints and "pencil-in-cup" erosions of the distal interphalangeal joint of the second through fifth digits bilaterally. (Fig. 7–39*B* is a magnified view of Fig. 7–39*A.*) There is associated periosteal reaction. These findings are most compatible with a diagnosis of psoriasis. (*A* is the correct answer to Question 7-17.)

Discussion:

Osteoarthrosis (osteoarthritis): The frontal view of the pelvis of Case 7-12 (Fig. 7–34) shows the classic findings

of osteoarthritis. These include cartilage loss with resultant articular space narrowing, subchondral cysts, and osteophyte formation. The findings of osteoarthritis are similar regardless of the joint in which they occur. In the knee, the articular space narrowing initially involves the medial compartment (Fig. 7–40), but may progress to involve the lateral and patellofemoral compartments. In the hands, the articular space narrowing typically

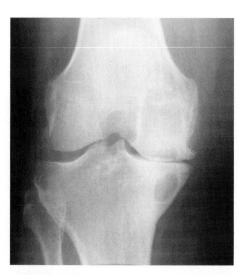

Fig. 7–40. Frontal view of a 65-year-old man shows the classic features of osteoarthritis of the knee with medial articular space narrowing, subchondral cyst formation, sclerosis, and osteophyte formation. Osteoarthritis of the knee initially involves the medial compartment but may, over time, progress to involve the lateral and patellofemoral compartments.

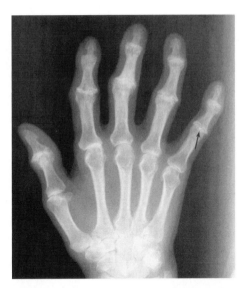

Fig. 7–41. Frontal radiograph of the right hand in a 56-year-old woman shows the classic changes of erosive oeteoarthritis. Note the "gull-wing" appearance (*arrow*) of the PIP joint of the fifth digit.

involves the distal interphalangeal joints. Another classic "target area" of osteoarthritis in the hand is the first carpal metacarpal joint (trapezio-first metacarpal joint). There is a variant of osteoarthritis, *erosive osteoarthritis,* which can present with a cyclical clinical phase of involvement that mimics rheumatoid arthritis. Patients with erosive osteoarthritis develop central erosions within the joints of the hand in a classic "gull wing" appearance as shown at the proximal interphalangeal joint of the fifth digit in the patient's hand in Fig. 7–41.

CONNECTIVE-TISSUE DISEASES AND SERONEGATIVE SPONDYLOARTHROPATHIES

Generally, a history of polyarticular stiffness suggests a polyarthritis and the initial imaging investigation is a radiographic survey of the affected joint or joints. These images target the most common regions of involvement and usually include films of the hands, wrists, pelvis, knee, feet, and ankles. The findings on these films, coupled with the ESR value, should indicate whether a connective-tissue disorder is the cause of the arthropathy. Often patients will be tested for rheumatoid factor (discussed in the next paragraph). If this test is negative and the patient has symptoms involving the peripheral joints and spine, then a *seronegative spondyloarthropathy* is considered.

Perhaps the most common and characteristic connective-tissue disease producing arthritis is rheumatoid arthritis (RA). Females (especially middle-aged

women) are more commonly affected by this disease than men. RA is thought to be a malfunction of the immune system, and patients with this disorder usually produce a measurable immune complex called rheumatoid factor (RF). They also characteristically have an elevated ESR. The disease often progresses in a symmetrical fashion. The major initial pathologic process in RA is a synovitis, which produces periarticular osteopenia because of the associated hyperemia. Later in the disease, synovial proliferation with pannus formation may then cause erosions in the juxta-articular regions (the so-called "bare areas"). These erosions occur at the cortex where the synovium contacts it and it is not protected by articular cartilage. Subsequently, the disease may progress to secondary degenerative changes and eventually to fibrous or bony ankylosis of the joint. In the wrist, the carpal bones will show osteopenia, carpal crowding, or subluxations. In fact, the ulnar styloid is often one of the first sites of erosions and "pencilling." Juxta-articular osteopenia is seen in the bones of the hands and wrists. Symmetric swelling at the proximal interphalangeal joints of the hand is present, and bone ends show erosions, especially at the metacarpophalangeal and proximal interphalangeal joints (Fig. 7–42).

Systemic lupus erythermatosus is a connective-tissue disorder that can be seen in conjunction with other connective tissue diseases (the so-called "overlap syndrome"). Patients with SLE may show profound osteopenia, including resorption of the tufts, but it does not characteristically result in erosions. The typical appearance is joint instability with multiple subluxations at the wrists and metacarpophalangeal joints. In fact, SLE is the most common cause of a nonerosive subluxing arthropathy (Fig. 7–43). Subluxations also occur in RA, but the subluxations in RA are associated with the "bare area" erosions.

Scleroderma (progressive systemic sclerosis, or PSS) is a disorder characterized by fibrosis and skin thickening. Soft-tissue calcification is a prominent feature of this disorder. The major effects of this disease are not on the joints per se, but are secondary to the diffuse sclerosis with resultant joint stiffness for which the patient may seek treatment initially. About 10% of patients with PSS have synovitis that is indistinguishable from RA at presentation, and many of these patients eventually develop Raynaud's phenomenon. The typical imaging findings are periarticular calcification and resorption of the terminal phalangeal tufts (acroosteolysis) (Fig. 7–35). Scleroderma may also be associated with other connective disorders such as rheumatoid arthritis and SLE in the same individual.

Psoriasis, Reiter's disease, ankylosing spondylitis, and inflammatory bowel disease comprise the major seronegative spondyloarthropathies. Psoriasis is a

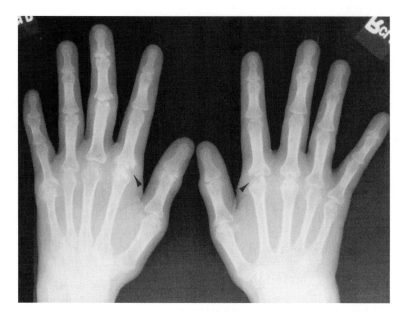

Fig. 7–42. Frontal view of both hands in a patient with long-standing rheumatoid arthritis showing marked carpal destruction and radiocarpal joint narrowing with substantial erosive change as well as the characteristic "bare area" erosions best exhibited at the second metacarpophalangeal joint (*arrowheads*). Also note the soft-tissue swelling at multiple joints.

connective-tissue disorder that primarily affects the skin. However, about 15% of patients with psoriasis develop bone and joint changes and these findings may be the initial manifestations of the disease. Radiographic findings of psoriasis include periosteal reaction (periostitis) and/or focal cortical thickening in the digits. The earliest manifestation of the disease is juxta-articular osteopenia that is less profound than in RA. The disease may then progress to show erosions at the bone ends (marginal erosions). The distribution of these findings in psoriasis is mainly the distal interphalangeal joints, unlike the findings in patients with RA, which are predominately in the proximal interphalangeal joints and carpus. The "pencil-in-cup" erosions seen in Fig. 7–39 are typical of psoriasis. Patients with psoriasis and other seronegative spondyloarthropathies also develop abnormalities of the spine and sacroiliac joints (hence the term *spondyloarthropathy*).

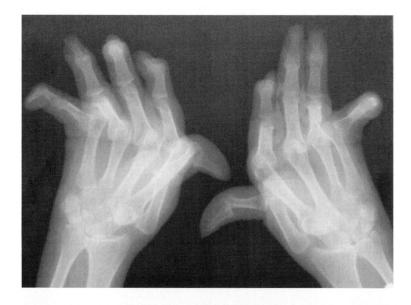

Fig. 7–43. Frontal view of both hands in a patient with long-standing SLE shows marked ulna deviation at the metacarpophalangeal joint as well as subluxation of the thumb. Note the absence of erosions. These findings are classic for this disease.

Reiter's disease is a postinfective disorder of the immune system that is characterized by the triad of nongonococcal urethritis, conjunctivitis/iritis, and arthritis. Seen most frequently in male patients, Reiter's disease was originally thought to be caused by *Chlamydia,* but other organisms, including *E. coli* and *Salmonella* organisms, have also been implicated. The imaging findings of Reiter's disease are often indistinguishable from those of psoriatic arthritis except that Reiter's disease most commonly affects the feet and psoriasis most commonly involves the hands. Both diseases show periostitis, erosions, and enthesopathic changes. An *enthesis* is an area of attachment of a ligament or tendon to bone by the perforating fibers of Sharpey. An *enthesopathy* is, therefore, an abnormality at this site and is seen on the radiograph as bony excrescences in these areas. A typical example of enthesopathy in Reiter's disease is the bony excrescence on the inferior aspect of the calcaneus, which develops at the site of attachment of the plantar fascia and the short flexors in the foot (Fig. 7–44).

Ankylosing spondylitis (AS) is a rheumatic disease causing arthritis of the spine and sacroiliac joints and can cause inflammation of the eyes, lungs, and heart valve. The typical clinical scenario is intermittent back pain that occurs throughout life. The pain may progress to severe chronic disease attacking the spine, peripheral joints, and other organs resulting in marked loss of motion and deformity over time. The cause of AS is not known, but most of the spondyloarthropathies share a common genetic marker called the HLA-B27 antigen. The disease usually presents in the adolescent and young adult and is most common in Native Americans.

Figure 7–38 shows the typical features of ankylosing spondylitis (AS) in the cervical spine. The thin vertically oriented ossifications connecting the vertebral bodies, syndesmophytes, are anatomically located in the outer layers of the anulus fibrosus. Also typical in this case is the fusion of the posterior elements. In fact, the classic appearance of AS is the "bamboo spine" (Fig. 7–45). This appearance is caused by fusion of all the synovial joints of the spine and predisposes the patient to the development of fractures (insufficiency-type fractures). This insufficiency fracture (also called a *pseudoarthrosis*) is a well-documented complication of ankylosing spondylitis.

The mainstay of treatment for AS is nonsteroidal anti-inflammatory medication to control pain. However, some patients with severe disease may be given methotrexate.

SEPTIC ARTHRITIS

Septic arthritis is usually bloodborne (hematogenous) and is most commonly monoarticular (involving only one joint at any time). A common cause of septic arthritis in the adult is *Staphylococcus aureus*, although other infective agents including streptococcus, gonococcus, and other gram-negative organisms may also be encountered. Streptococcus and gram-negative organisms are particularly important in the pediatric age group.

The radiographic examination of the patient in Case 7-14 (Fig. 7–36) provides general anatomic information,

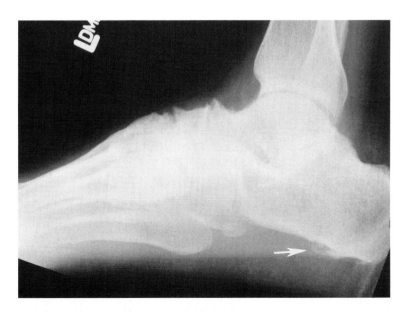

Fig. 7–44. Lateral foot radiograph in a patient with long-standing Reiter's disease shows marked narrowing of the hindfoot and midfoot, proliferative changes, and sclerosis. Note the prominent calcaneal spur representing enthesopathic change (*arrow*). Reiter's and psoriasis look identical except that Reiter's more commonly involves the foot.

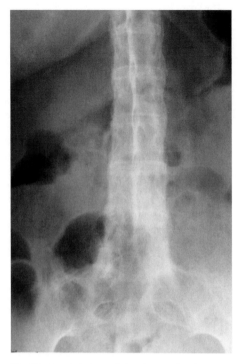

Fig. 7–45. Frontal view of the thoracolumbar spine showing the classic "bamboo" appearance of the spine in ankylosing spondylitis. This appearance results from fusion of the vertebral bodies and posterior elements.

helps to determine whether further imaging is necessary, and aids in deciding whether further intervention is appropriate. Her physicians were very worried about septic arthritis in this clinical setting of previous renal transplant (i.e., relatively immunocompromised) and a hip aspiration was requested. Twenty milliliters of bloodstained turbid fluid was aspirated and sent to the microbiology laboratory for Gram stain, culture, and sensitivity studies. The cultures grew *Staphylococcus aureus*, a common pathogen in septic arthritis.

Figure 7–36 shows the classic radiographic findings of septic arthritis and osteomyelitis. These include articular space narrowing, erosion of bone on both sides of the joint, and sclerosis. An effusion will always be present and can be identified by ultrasound or MR imaging. Septic joints will also be "hot" on bone scan because of the marked hyperemia and bony proliferation.

CRYSTAL DEPOSITION DISEASES

Gout, a disorder most common in middle-aged men, is an inflammatory arthritis caused by abnormal deposition of urates (called *tophi*) in the soft tissues and carti-

lage. These deposits cause episodic joint inflammation and are associated with pain and disability. In the earlier stages of the disease, radiographs of the bone and joints may be normal except for soft-tissue swelling and in some instances soft-tissue calcification. The classic initial presentation of gout is *podagra*, an acute inflammation of the joint, usually the first metatarso–phalangeal joint (Fig. 7–37). At presentation the patient will have severe joint pain and the overlying soft tissues will be swollen and red. With repeated attacks over years (usually at least 15–20 years), bony erosions with "overhanging edges" (or overhanging margins) may develop adjacent to the joint but not within the joint. When the patient is severely incapacitated by pain and not moving the joint, "disuse" osteopenia can be seen at radiography. Occasionally, osteopenia may be due to intraosseous deposition of tophaceous material. The typical areas to screen for gout are the first metatarsophalangeal joint, the heel, the back of the elbow joint (olecranon fossa), and the hands and wrists. Screening for elevated serum levels of uric acid and joint aspiration are probably the best ways to confirm the clinical suspicion of gout. The joint aspirate will show birefringent uric acid crystals in the synovial fluid on polarized light microscopy.

Calcium pyrophosphate dehydrate crystal deposition (CPPD) disease is another common crystal deposition joint disorder. In CPPD disease there is calcification in the fibrocartilage and hyaline articular cartilage (so-called "chondrocalcinosis"). The most common association with chondrocalcinosis is aging although it may also be seen in pseudogout (CPPD disease), gout, ochronosis, hemochromatosis, and hyperparathyroidism. The presence of calcification alone is not diagnostic of CPPD, however. The clinical syndrome of pain from the presence of abnormal cartilage calcification is referred to as the CPPD syndrome, and symptoms may be provoked by various stresses (e.g., surgical procedures). Aspiration of the joint thought to be involved by CPPD and discovery of the typical calcium pyrophosphate crystals confirm the diagnosis.

EXERCISE 7-5: MISCELLANEOUS JOINT DISORDERS

Clinical Histories:

Case 7-18. A 24-year-old male medical student, an avid tennis player, had intermittent joint swelling and minimal knee pain. Lately the pain had worsened and was interfering with his tennis game. Nonsteroidal anti-inflammatory agents were not working well and an orthopedic resident requested

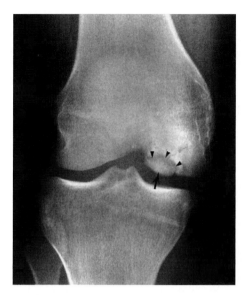

Fig. 7–46.

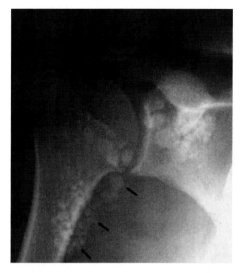

Fig. 7–47.

that he get a knee x-ray (Fig. 7–46). After looking at the radiograph, the resident scheduled an appointment for the student with an attending surgeon.

Case 7-19. A 20-year-old man complained of a feeling of fullness and gritty sensations in his right shoulder. He has never had a shoulder dislocation, although on several occasions he has been unable to raise the shoulder and has felt a painful "catch" at times. A radiograph of his right shoulder was obtained (Fig. 7–47).

Case 7-20. A 10-year-old boy was referred to an orthopedic surgeon for investigation of a limp. There was no reliable history of trauma. A frontal radiograph of the pelvis is shown and is abnormal (Fig. 7–48).

Case 7-21. A 35-year-old man with episodic right hip pain that began 4 to 6 months ago presented with a dull aching pain now in both hips. A frontal radiograph of both hips was obtained (Fig. 7–49).

Questions:

7-18. The most likely diagnosis in Fig. 7–46 is
    A. synovial osteochondromatosis.
    B. pigmented villonodular synovitis.
    C. avascular necrosis of the femoral condyle.
    D. osteochondritis dissecans (OCD) of the femoral condyle.

7-19. The most likely diagnosis in Fig. 7–47 is
    A. hemochromatosis.
    B. synovial osteochondromatosis (SOC).
    C. pigmented villonodular synovitis.
    D. calcified Heberden's nodes.

7-20. The most likely diagnosis in Fig. 7–48 is
    A. chronic changes of transient synovitis of the right hip.
    B. chronic changes of slipped capital femoral epiphysis (epiphysiolysis).
    C. chronic changes of Legg-Calvé-Perthes disease of the right hip.
    D. none of the above.

7-21. Concerning Fig. 7–49, the observations include all of the following except
    A. osteophytes in both femoral heads.
    B. irregularity and loss of sphericity of the right femoral head.
    C. depression/subchondral fracture of right femoral head.
    D. bilateral acetabular sclerosis.

Radiologic Findings:

7-18. The AP view of the right knee (Fig. 7–46) shows an ovoid bony fragment on the inner aspect of the medial femoral condyle (*arrow*) separated from the femur by a lucency (*arrowheads*). This appearance is diagnostic of OCD of the knee. (*D* is the correct answer to Question 7-18.)

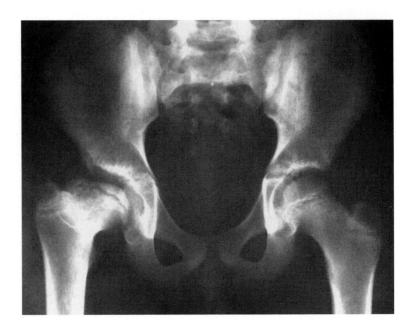

Fig. 7–48.

7-19. The radiograph of the right shoulder in Fig. 7–47 shows multiple rounded calcific bodies overlying the proximal humerus and glenoid process of the scapula. The distribution of these is within the joint and axillary recess (*arrows*). This appearance is classic for SOC. (*B* is the correct answer to Question 7-19.)

7-20. The radiograph of the pelvis in Fig. 7–48 shows collapse of the right capital femoral epiphysis, which is broad and short, and forms an acute angle with the shaft of the femur. The femoral head is displaced laterally and is not completely covered by the mildly deformed acetabulum. The left hip is normal. The findings are characteristic of the late changes in Legg-Calvé-Perthes disease. (*C* is the correct answer to Question 7-20.)

7-21. The radiograph of both hips in Fig. 7–49 demonstrates that the right femoral head is no longer smooth and spherical (loss of spherocity), and this is due to the presence of subchondral collapse in the superio-lateral aspect (*arrow*). The left femoral head is still

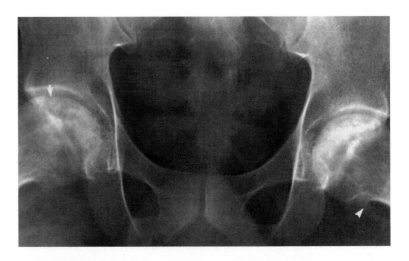

Fig. 7–49.

spherical but shows sclerosis. Also note the marginal osteophytes arising from the inferior and medial aspect of the left femoral head (*arrowhead*). The acetabuli are normal and these radiographic features are typical of avascular necrosis (osteonecrosis) of the femoral head. (*D* is the correct answer to Question 7-21.)

Discussion:

Osteochondritis dissecans (OCD) is a bone disorder that produces joint symptoms because of the intra-articular location of the abnormality. OCD, as classically demonstrated in Fig. 7–46, is seen on the radiograph as a semicircular focus of bone and overlying cartilage separated from the convex articular surface of the native bone by a lucency. The etiology is uncertain but current opinion favors repetitive microtrauma and vascular insult to the subchondral bone. Almost any joint may be affected, but the knee (distal femur), ankle (dome of the talus), and elbow (capitellum) joints are the most commonly involved sites. The disease is slightly more common in active young men but is increasingly being encountered in young women because they are more actively involved in athletics today. In the knee, OCD most commonly involves the non-weight-bearing aspect of the medial femoral condyle (i.e., the inner aspect and area shown in Fig. 7–46) and the lateral femoral condyle. MR imaging is the most appropriate modality to stage the lesion, predict whether the fragment may become separated entirely, and plan definitive treatment. CT or CT arthrography is an alternate test to use in patients who cannot undergo MR imaging.

Synovial osteochondromatosis (SOC) is a joint abnormality characterized by the presence of cartilaginous and osseous loose bodies within the synovial cavity in the joint. The exact cause is not known, but "primary" SOC is thought to be caused by synovial metaplasia and "secondary" OCD is assumed to be due to fractures of osteophytes or articular cartilage that shed into the joint cavity. Radiography may show only a joint effusion if the intrasynovial fragments are not ossified. These intra-articular bodies can be seen if they are calcified (Fig. 7–47, *arrows*). MR imaging is the best modality to use to show both ossified and nonossified intra-articular fragments and to evaluate the other soft-tissue structures around the joint.

Pigmented villonodular synovitis is a condition of unknown etiology characterized by hyperplasia or excessive villous proliferation of the synovium. This condition may occur in a single joint (localized form) or involve multiple joints (diffuse form). Thought to be caused by hemorrhage, PVNS shows hemosiderin-laden macrophages within the synovium best appreciated by gross examination. Radiographs often show a joint effusion with preservation of the articular space and normal bone mineral density. The later stages of the disease result in erosions on both sides of the joint. Joint aspiration yields dark brown fluid ("chocolate" effusion) due to the presence of the hemosiderin-laden macrophages. MR imaging is an excellent preoperative test to evaluate PVNS because the pigmented material (hemosiderin) shows low signal intensity on both the short TE (T_1-weighted) and the long TE (T_2-weighted) MR sequences. In fact, this finding is a very specific appearance for this disease. Heberden's node is a disfigurement of the interphalangeal joints as a result of severe osteoarthritis. Initially, it is due to soft-tissue inflammatory changes and is subsequently due to bony changes at the distal interphalangeal joints. It is more commonly seen in female patients.

Osteonecrosis can occur in any bone and is associated with a variety of disorders, including sickle cell hemoglobinopathy, Gaucher's disease, SLE, pancreatitis, alcoholism, steroid treatment, and barotrauma. When the process occurs at a bone end, it is known as *avascular necrosis*; when it occurs in the metaphysis of the bone, it is commonly referred to as a *bone infarct*. Eponyms have been used to designate osteonecrosis in certain sites. For example, *Perthes' disease* (Legg-Calvé-Perthes disease) is the eponym used to refer to idiopathic osteonecrosis of the femoral head occurring in a child as shown in Case 7-20 (Fig. 7–48). Other common eponyms include *Freiberg's infraction* (avascular necrosis of the head of the second or third metatarsal), *Köhler's disease* (tarsal navicular), *Panner's disease* (capitellum of the humerus), and *Kienböck's disease* (carpal lunate). The exact mechanism of the development of osteonecrosis is unknown, although bone-marrow edema after thrombosis and occlusion of the osseous capillaries and end arterioles are believed to be primarily responsible.

Radiography is a rather insensitive diagnostic tool for evaluating the early manifestations of osteonecrosis. Osteonecrosis does cause zones of increased sclerosis and osteolysis in the affected bone that can be appreciated on radiographs. However, these changes are late and early treatment cannot be performed at this stage (Fig. 7–49). If the disease is not diagnosed and treated early, the affected bone may go through a phase of subchondral collapse and become deformed. Subsequently, secondary osteoarthrosis will develop in the affected joint as a complication of neglected or poorly treated disease. Traditionally, nuclear medicine bone scanning has been used in this setting, but today MR imaging is the most sensitive available modality for the early diagnosis of this disease (Fig. 7–50).

Hemochromatosis is a rare disorder of iron metabolism, in which iron is deposited in the skin, parenchymal

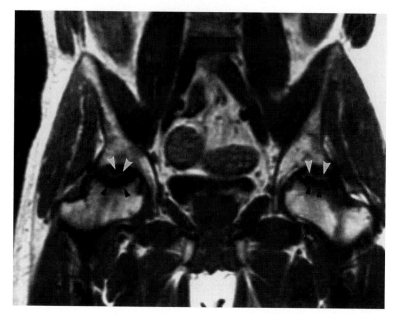

Fig. 7–50. A coronal T$_1$-weighted image of the pelvis of a patient with osteonecrosis of both hips shows focal areas of abnormally low signal intensity in both femoral heads superiorly (*arrowheads*). The low-signal (*dark*) areas are separated from the normal bone by linear high-signal (bright) areas.

organs, and articular cartilage. This predisposes the joint to degenerative disease. Arthritis due to hemochromatosis is characterized by loss of joint space and formation of peculiar hooked osteophytes especially at metacarpal heads.

BIBLIOGRAPHY

1. Berquist TH. *MRI of the Musculoskeletal System.* 4th ed. Philadelphia: Lippincott Williams & Wilkins; 2001.
2. Chew FS, Bui-Mansfield LT, Kline MJ. *Musculokeletal Imaging.* Philadelphia: Lippincott William & Wilkins; 2003.
3. Kaplan P. *Musculoskeletal MRI.* Philadelphia: Saunders; 2001.
4. Resnick D. *Diagnosis of Bone and Joint Disorders.* 4th ed. Philadelphia: Saunders; 2002.
5. Rogers LF. *Radiology of Skeletal Trauma.* 3rd ed. Philadelphia: Churchill Livingstone; 2002.
6. Stoller DW. *Magnetic Resonance Imaging in Orthopedics & Sports Medicine.* 2nd ed. Philadelphia: Lippincott-Raven; 1997.
7. Yochum TR, Rowe LJ. *Essentials of Skeletal Radiology.* 2nd ed. Baltimore: Williams & Wilkins; 1996.

PART 4

Abdomen

Plain Film of the Abdomen

8

Michael Y. M. Chen

In recent years, new techniques such as ultrasonography, computerized tomography (CT), and MR imaging have been used widely and have altered the use of plain films of the abdomen in the evaluation of abdominal diseases. Plain films of the abdomen are still used primarily to assess calcifications and intestinal perforation or obstruction. The plain radiograph is commonly used as a preliminary radiograph before other studies such as CT and barium enema. Plain abdominal radiography is routinely employed before intravenous urography (IVU) because stones in the urinary tract can be obscured by iodinated contrast material but may be shown on plain abdominal radiographs. The yield of plain radiographs is higher in patients with moderate or severe abdominal symptoms and signs than in those with minor symptoms.

TECHNIQUE AND NORMAL IMAGING

Technique

The most common plain radiograph of the abdomen is an anteroposterior (AP) view with the patient in the supine position. The AP view of the abdomen is also called a KUB film because it includes the kidneys, ureters, and bladder. When acute abdominal disease is suspected clinically, an erect film of the abdomen and a posteroanterior (PA) view of the chest are also required. Digital imaging is becoming more common, and abdominal images may be viewed on computer monitor rather than on films.

Normal Imaging

SOFT TISSUE

The abdomen is composed primarily of soft tissue. The density of soft tissue is similar to the density of water, and the difference in density between solid and liquid is not distinguishable on a plain radiograph. The liver is a homogeneous structure located in the right upper quadrant; the hepatic angle delineates the lower margin of the posterior portion of the liver (Fig. 8–1). In the left upper quadrant a similar angular structure, the splenic angle, can be identified by the fat shadow around the spleen (see Fig. 8–1).

Organ enlargement can be recognized by the effect of displacement on nearby bowel loops or by obliteration of the adjacent normal fat or gas pattern. Hepatomegaly may compress the proximal transverse colon below the right kidney. Splenomegaly may push the splenic flexure of the colon downward. A large fused renal shadow across the psoas muscle and lumbar spine suggests a horseshoe kidney.

FAT SHADOW

Fat density, which is between that of soft tissue and that of gas, outlines the contour of solid organs or muscles. In obese patients, fat may not be distinguishable from ascitic fluid on plain abdominal film. The flank stripe, also called the *properitoneal fat stripe,* is a line of fat next to the muscle of the lateral abdominal wall (see Fig. 8–1). The flank stripes are symmetrically concave or slightly convex in obese people located along the side of the abdominal wall. The normal properitoneal fat stripe is in proximity to the gas pattern seen in the ascending or descending colon. Widening of the distance between the properitoneal fat stripe and the ascending or descending colon suggests fluid, such as abscess, ascitic fluid, or blood within the paracolic gutter.

Fat is present in the retroperitoneal space adjacent to the psoas muscle (see Fig. 8–1). The psoas muscle shadow may be absent unilaterally or bilaterally as a normal variant or as a result of inflammation, hemorrhage, or neoplasms of the retroperitoneum. Unilateral convexity of the psoas muscle contour suggests an intramuscular mass or abscess. The quadratus lumborum muscles may be delineated by fat located lateral to the psoas shadow (see Fig. 8–1). In the pelvis, the fatty envelope of the obturator internus muscle is seen on the inner aspect of the pelvic inlet (see Fig. 8–1). The dome of the urinary bladder may be delineated by fat.

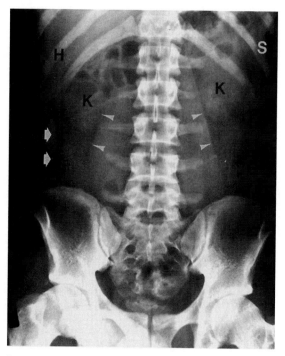

A

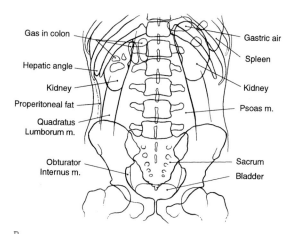

B

Fig. 8–1. **A** Normal plain film of the abdomen. The lower margins of the posterior portion of the liver, the hepatic angle (H), and the lower part of the spleen (S) are delineated by a fat shadow. Both kidneys (K) and the psoas muscle shadows (*arrowheads*) are outlined by a fat shadow. The properitoneal fat stripe is also shown bilaterally (*arrows*). **B** Diagram of normal abdominal plain film.

GAS PATTERN

Gas has the lowest density (radiolucency) in the abdomen. It is seen in the stomach and colon, but it is rarely seen in the normal small bowel because the air rapidly traverses the organ. The presence of more than a minimal amount of gas in the small bowel should be considered abnormal and is indicative of a functional ileus or mechanical obstruction. Identification of the differences between the gas shadows of the jejunum, ileum, or colon helps to assess the location of bowel obstruction (Fig. 8–2). A gas pattern in distended intestinal loops is usually limited above the point of mechanical obstruction, but functional ileus has a more diffuse distribution in both the small intestine and the colon. If the gas shadow in the intestine is displaced to an unusual location, a soft-tissue mass, either inflammatory or neoplastic, may be suspected. The presence of air-fluid levels in a distended small intestine on upright films suggests either functional ileus or mechanical obstruction. Fluid levels within the stomach or colon are ordinarily of no pathologic importance, because fluid may be introduced by oral agents or by cleansing enemas. The presence of solid material with a mottled appearance and small bubbles of gas surrounded by the colonic contour suggests feces in the colon.

A large amount of gas seen in the peritoneal cavity indicates postoperative status or bowel perforation. Air bubbles in the peritoneal cavity indicate a perforated viscus, abscess, or necrotic tumor. In the right upper quadrant, air that is seen in the biliary tree or around the gallbladder suggests cholecystoenteric fistula or emphysematous cholecystitis. A finely arborizing gas pattern over the right upper quadrant that extends peripherally to the edge of the liver is characteristic of hepatic portal vein gas. In the bowel wall, multiple air bubbles may indicate pneumatosis cystoides intestinalis. Extraluminal gas also may appear within the retroperitoneal structures, including the lesser omental bursa, a subhepatic site, the paraduodenal fossa, and the pericecal or periappendiceal areas. A gas pattern seen below the bony pelvis indicates an inguinal or femoral hernia.

BONY STRUCTURE OR CALCIFICATION

Bony structures or calcifications have the highest density (radiopacity) that is seen on plain films. Bony structures comprise the ribs superiorly, the lumbar spine, and the pelvis. Calcifications in the abdomen include calcified arteries, calculi in the urinary or biliary tract, prostatic calculi, pancreatic calcifications (which are usually indicative of chronic pancreatitis, with or without carcinoma), appendicolith, or ectopic gallstone in the small bowel associated with mechanical obstruction from

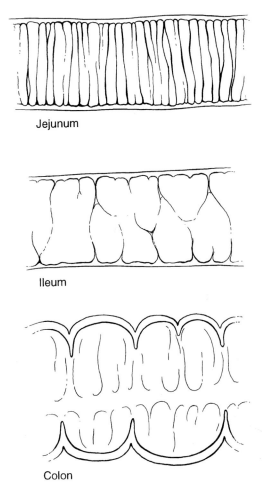

Fig. 8–2. Schematic illustration of portions of bowel. The jejunum shows numerous mucosal folds, whereas the ileum has fewer folds. Both serosa of the jejunum and the ileum are smooth. The colon has serosa indented by haustra, and mucosal folds do not cross the lumen.

gallstone ileus. Some foreign bodies, including ingested foreign bodies, bullets, or surgical clips, may be seen in the abdomen. Other rare structures, such as parasitic, metastatic, or heterotopic bone formations, also may be seen in the abdomen.

Suspicion of urinary calculi is a common indication for abdominal radiography. About one-half of calculi in the urinary tract that are visible via unenhanced helical CT can be detected on plain abdominal films. On the other hand, about 15% of gallstones are radiopaque and are seen on abdominal plain radiographs. Ultrasonography is the better choice for evaluating gallstones. Oral cholecystography (OCG) is occasionally used to demonstrate radiolucent gallstones.

TECHNIQUE SELECTION

The routine abdominal films consist of supine and upright views. If the patient cannot stand for an erect abdominal film and a PA view of the chest, the cross-table lateral projection with the right side elevated may be used to assess pneumoperitoneum and air-fluid levels. As little as 1 to 2 mL of free air in the peritoneal space may be identified if the films are appropriately obtained. The PA view of the chest is usually obtained as part of an acute abdominal series because an abnormality in the chest may have symptoms referred to the abdomen.

Oblique views and conventional tomography of the abdomen are obtained, especially in examination of the urinary tract, when full delineation of the ureters and depiction of the renal collecting system are desirable. Likewise, oblique studies of the ureter and urinary bladder are helpful in delineating abnormalities of that organ.

Plain abdominal radiography is less sensitive in evaluating solid organs or metastases. In recent years, increased use of cross-sectional techniques, such as ultrasonography and CT, has shown them to be more sensitive in assessing disorders of the abdominal solid organs and metastatic diseases. Acute cholecystitis is better assessed by ultrasonography or nuclear medicine studies.

EXERCISES

EXERCISE 8-1: UPPER ABDOMINAL CALCIFICATIONS

Clinical Histories:

Case 8-1. A 44-year-old woman presents with right upper quadrant pain (Fig. 8–3).

Case 8-2. A 36-year-old woman presents with flank pain (Fig. 8–4).

Case 8-3. A 48-year-old man who is an alcoholic presents with epigastric pain (Fig. 8–5).

Case 8-4. A 59-year-old woman is seen who underwent colectomy surgery for colon cancer 10 years ago (Fig. 8–6).

Questions:

8-1. What is the most likely diagnosis in Case 8-1 (Fig. 8–3)?
- **A.** Adrenal calcification
- **B.** Calcified gallstones
- **C.** Kidney stones
- **D.** Milk-of-calcium bile in the gallbladder

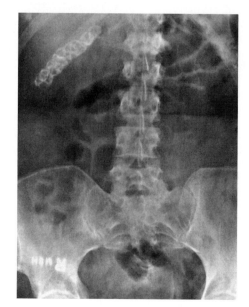

Fig. 8–3.

8-2. What is the most likely diagnosis in Case 8-2 (Fig. 8–4)?
- **A.** Adrenal calcification
- **B.** Calcified gallstones
- **C.** Kidney stones
- **D.** Medullary nephrocalcinosis

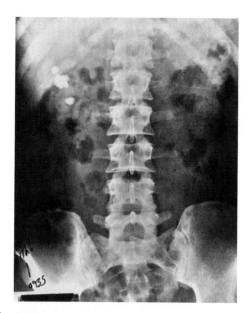

Fig. 8–4.

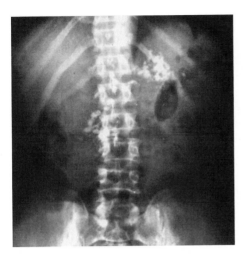

Fig. 8–5.

8-3. What is the most likely diagnosis in Case 8-3 (Fig. 8–5)?
A. Adrenal calcification
B. Calcified hepatic metastases
C. Pancreatic calcification
D. Primary calcified mucoproducing adenocarcinoma in the colon

8-4. What is the most likely diagnosis in Case 8-4 (Fig. 8–6)?
A. Adrenal calcification
B. Calcified hepatic metastases

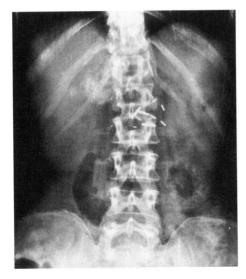

Fig. 8–6.

C. Pancreatic calcification
D. Primary calcified mucoproducing adenocarcinoma in the colon

Radiologic Findings:

8-1. Figure 8–3 demonstrates multiple faceted calcifications in the right upper quadrant, which are characteristic for gallstones. (*B* is the correct answer to Question 8-1.)

8-2. Figure 8–4 shows three separate deposits of calcified density confined to the right renal shadow. The largest one measures 2 cm in greatest diameter. (*C* is the correct answer to Question 8-2.)

8-3. Figure 8–5 shows multiple stippled calcifications in the upper abdomen adjacent to the lumbar spine. In a patient with a history of alcoholism, pancreatic calcification from chronic pancreatitis would be the most likely diagnosis. (*C* is the correct answer to Question 8-3.)

8-4. Figure 8–6 shows stippled and discrete calcifications overlying the right 12th rib, just above the renal outline. When calcification in the lung base, skin, retroperitoneum, pancreas, kidney, and adrenal glands is excluded, hepatic calcification should be considered in a patient with a history of colon cancer. (*B* is the correct answer to Question 8-4.)

Discussion:

About 15% to 20% of gallstones are calcified sufficiently to be seen on a plain abdominal film. Most gallstones comprise mixed components, including cholesterol, bile salts, and biliary pigments. Pure cholesterol and pure pigment stones are uncommon. Calcified gallstones vary in size and shape. Most gallstones have thin, marginal calcification with central lucency and are laminated, faceted, or irregular in shape. Some gallstones contain gas in their fissures whether calcified or noncalcified, called the *Mercedes Benz sign.* Milk of calcium or "limy" bile occurs in patients with longstanding cystic duct obstruction. The bile contains a high concentration of calcium carbonate and is densely radiopaque on plain radiograph (Fig. 8–7). Calcification of the gallbladder wall (porcelain gallbladder) develops in patients with chronic cholecystitis, cholelithiasis, and cystic duct obstruction. Porcelain gallbladder is characterized by curvilinear calcification in the muscular layer of the gallbladder mimicking a calcified cyst (Fig. 8–8).

Nephrolithiasis is the most common cause of calcification within the kidneys. Most renal calculi (85%) contain calcium complexed with oxalate and phosphate salts. Any process that creates urinary tract stasis may cause the development of urinary calculi. Renal calculi

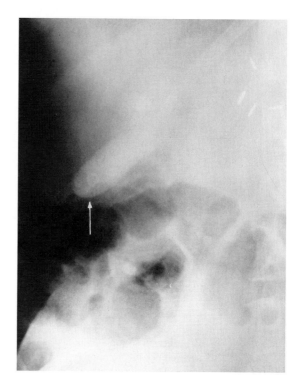

Fig. 8–7. Milk-of-calcium bile. Plain radiograph shows homogeneous density of the gallbladder. A small gallstone is also seen within the gallbladder (*arrow*). (From Chen MY et al. Abnormal calcification on plain radiographs of the abdomen. *The Radiologist.* 1999; 7:65–83; used with permission.)

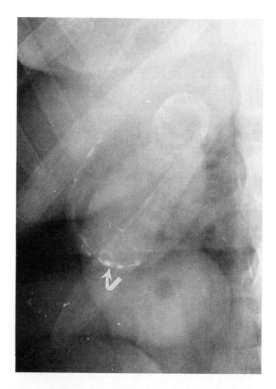

Fig. 8–8. Porcelain gallbladder. Plain radiograph shows curvilinear discontinuous calcification in the gallbladder wall (*arrow*). (From Chen MY et al. Abnormal calcification on plain radiographs of the abdomen. *The Radiologist.* 1999;7:65–83; used with permission.)

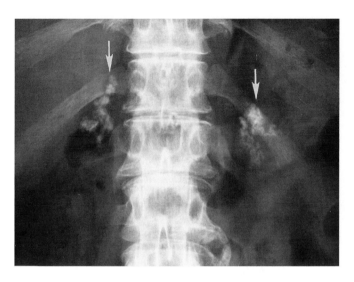

Fig. 8–9. Solid adrenal calcifications. Bilateral discrete, stippled adrenal calcifications (*arrows*) in the normal-sized glands in an asymptomatic patient with a history of complicated childbirth. (From Chen MY et al. Abnormal calcification on plain radiographs of the abdomen. *The Radiologist.* 1999;7:65–83; used with permission.)

are usually small and lie within the pelvicalyceal system or in a calyceal diverticulum. They may remain and increase in size, or they may pass distally. When calcifications are seen projecting over the renal shadows on routine films of the abdomen, an oblique view or conventional tomography is often needed to localize the densities in relation to the kidneys. A staghorn calculus contains calcium mixed with magnesium, ammonium, and phosphate and forms in the environment of recurrent urinary tract infection with alkaline urine. In general, CT is more sensitive than plain radiography in evaluating urinary calculi.

The adrenal gland is located at the superomedial part of the adjacent kidney. The right gland is lower than the left. Normally the adrenal gland measures less than 2.5 × 3 cm. Stippled, mottled, discrete, or homogeneous calcifications may appear as a portion of the adrenal gland or may occupy the entire organ, forming a triangular clump in the adrenal glands (Fig. 8–9). Most adrenal calcifications are incidental findings in normal-sized glands. They are caused by neonatal adrenal hemorrhage, prolonged hypoxia, severe neonatal infection, or birth trauma. Less than one-fourth of patients with Addison's disease have adrenal calcifications.

In the United States, 85% to 90% of patients with pancreatic lithiasis are alcoholics. Conversely, less than half of patients with chronic pancreatitis ever develop pancreatic calcifications visible on plain radiograph. Although gallstones passing through the biliary tract can cause acute pancreatitis, chronic pancreatitis or pancreatic calcification is rarely caused by cholelithiasis.

Hepatic calcifications are caused primarily by neoplasms, infections, or parasitic infestations. Primary hepatic tumors, both benign and malignant, may have calcifications. Colonic carcinoma and papillary serous cystadenocarcinoma of the ovary are the most frequent primary tumors causing calcified metastases in the liver. Other primary neoplasms in the thyroid gland, lung, pancreas, adrenal gland, stomach, kidney, and breast may cause calcified hepatic metastases. Inflammatory calcified granulomas related to tuberculosis or histoplasmosis are common in miliary calcifications. Calcified cystic lesions, such as *echinococcus* disease in the liver, are commonly seen in areas of the world where the causative organism is endemic.

EXERCISE 8-2: PELVIC CALCIFICATIONS

Clinical Histories:

Case 8-5. A 15-year-old boy presents with right lower quadrant pain and fever (Fig. 8–10).

Case 8-6. A 64-year-old man presents with hematuria (Fig. 8–11).

Case 8-7. A 48-year-old woman presents with lower abdominal fullness (Fig. 8–12).

Case 8-8. A 14-year-old girl presents with lower abdominal pain and a palpable mass in the pelvis (Fig. 8–13).

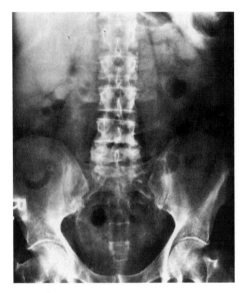

Fig. 8–10.

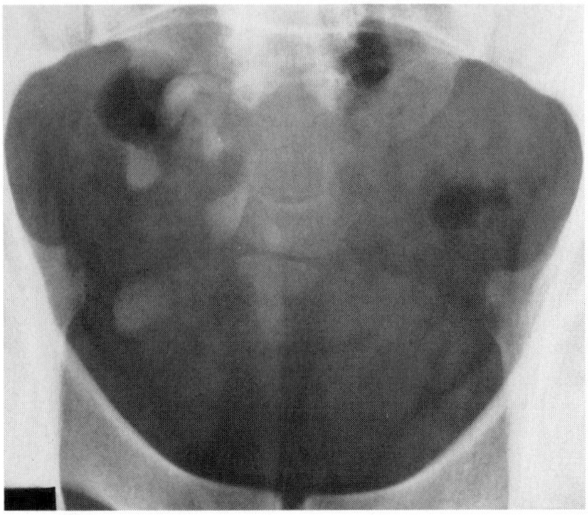

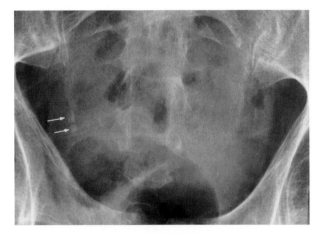

Fig. 8–13.

Fig. 8–11.

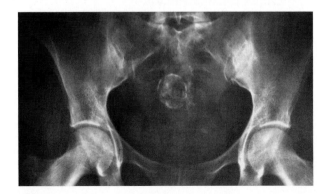

Fig. 8–12.

Questions:

8-5. What is the most likely diagnosis in Case 8-5 (Fig. 8–10)?
  A. Appendicolith
  B. Ectopic gallstone
  C. Pelvic phlebolith
  D. Right ureteral calculus

8-6. What is the most likely diagnosis in Case 8-6 (Fig. 8–11)?
  A. Appendicolith
  B. Multiple phleboliths
  C. Multiple ureteral calculi
  D. Prostatic calculi

8-7. What is the most likely diagnosis in Case 8-7 (Fig. 8–12)?
  A. Bladder calculus
  B. Chondrosarcoma of the sacrum
  C. Cystadenoma of the ovary
  D. Uterine fibroid calcifications

8-8. What is the most likely diagnosis in Case 8-8 (Fig. 8–13)?
  A. Bladder calculi
  B. Calcified vas deferens
  C. Ovarian dermoid cyst
  D. Uterine fibroid calcification

Radiologic Findings:

8-5. This case (Fig. 8–10) is that of a boy with acute appendicitis. (*A* is the correct answer to Question 8-5.) An oval calcification measuring 0.8 cm in diameter projects over the iliac bone and laterally to the right sacroiliac joint with a distended appendiceal lumen filled with gas. At surgery, gangrenous appendicitis with perforation and an obstructing appendicolith were found.

8-6. This case (Fig. 8–11) demonstrates a 5- × 5-m and a 4- × 4-mm calcified density (*arrows*) along the expected course of the right distal ureter. These densities were formerly identified in the right kidney and have migrated inferiorly to their current positions, indicating right ureteral calculi. With the history of hematuria, the most likely choice would be right ureteral calculi. (*C* is the correct answer to Question 8-6.)

8-7. Figure 8–12 shows a large, 2-cm-diameter mottled calcification and curvilinear calcifications in the midpelvis. These calcifications overlie the sacrum and are consistent with calcification in uterine fibroids. (*D* is the correct answer to Question 8-7.)

8-8. Figure 8–13 shows several "teeth-like" calcifications in the right side of the pelvis. With a palpable pelvic mass, the most likely diagnosis is ovarian dermoid cyst. (*C* is the correct answer to Question 8-8.)

Discussion:

Calcified appendiceal stones are present in only about 10% of patients with appendicitis; however, in a symptomatic child, an appendicolith indicates at least a 90% chance of acute appendicitis. Prophylactic appendectomy has been recommended in the child with an incidentally discovered appendicolith because of a high incidence of gangrene and perforation.

Ureteral calculi are always a consideration in patients with hematuria. About 50% of urinary calculi are radiographically opaque and shown on the plain abdominal radiograph. Close scrutiny of the abdominal film is crucial because ureteral calculi may be elusive when they project over the lumbar transverse processes or the sacroiliac region. To confirm a ureteral calculus, CT or intravenous urography is often needed to localize the density to the ureter. CT is more sensitive in evaluating ureteral calculi. Phleboliths are thrombi within the pelvic veins, and this location accounts for their circular shape. Calcification within these thrombi starts peripherally with a typical radiolucent center that is seen radiographically. Phleboliths have little clinical significance except that they can be confused with other pelvic densities, particularly distal ureteral calculi. In general, ureteral stones lie above and medially to the ischial spines, and they lack a radiolucent center.

Most uterine leiomyoma calcifications appear as multiple mottled or speckled calcifications or as dense, smooth, curvilinear calcifications around the mass. The real soft-tissue mass is often larger than the area of calcification. Other calcifications in the pelvis include calcified ovarian tumors (Fig. 8–14), foreign material, lymph nodes, or prostate.

Ovarian dermoid cysts account for about 10% of ovarian neoplasms. Ovarian dermoid cysts range from 6 to 15 cm in diameter and contain teeth, abortive bone, and curvilinear capsular calcification, which may be seen on plain radiographs. A dermoid cyst may contain sebaceous material simulating low-density fat compared to surrounding soft tissue.

Bladder stone is often seen in association with bladder outlet obstruction. Bladder calculi are composed of mixed calcium oxalate and phosphate salts that are radiopaque. Other calcifications in the bladder include foreign body, transitional cell carcinoma,

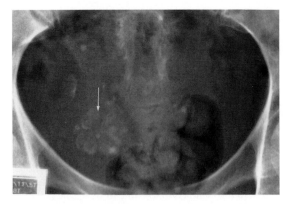

Fig. 8–14. Calcifications in ovarian tumor. Multiple sporadic calcifications (*arrow*) in the central pelvis from an ovarian cystadenocarcinoma. (From Chen MY et al. Abnormal calcification on plain radiographs of the abdomen. *The Radiologist.* 1999;7:65–83; used with permission.)

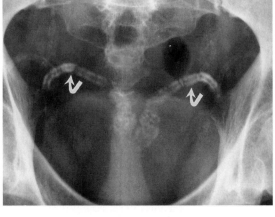

Fig. 8–16. Calcifications of vas deferens. Calcifications (*arrows*) in the tortuous ampullary segment of the vas deferens. (From Chen MY et al. Abnormal calcification on plain radiographs of the abdomen. *The Radiologist.* 1999;7:65–83; used with permission.)

urachal carcinoma, schistosoma infestation, tuberculosis, or alkaline encrusting cystitis. Calcifications in the same area include prostatic calculi (Fig. 8–15) and calcified vas deferens (Fig. 8–16). The prostate gland may be calcified. If enlarged, it may protrude into the bladder.

EXERCISE 8-3: INCREASED ABDOMINAL DENSITY OR MASSES

Clinical Histories:

Case 8-9. A 57-year-old man presents with history of hepatitis (Fig. 8–17).

Case 8-10. A 35-year-old woman presents with fever and anemia (Fig. 8–18).

Case 8-11. A 40-year-old man presents with back pain (Fig. 8–19).

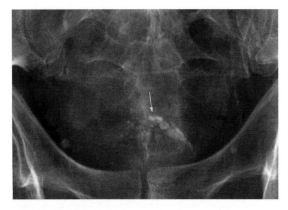

Fig. 8–15. Prostate calculi. Diffuse and symmetric coarse calcifications (*arrow*) in an enlarged prostate. (From Chen MY et al. Abnormal calcification on plain radiographs of the abdomen. *The Radiologist.* 1999;7:65–83; used with permission.)

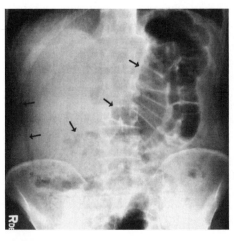

Fig. 8–17.

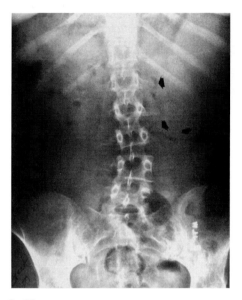

Fig. 8–18.

Case 8-12. A 45-year-old woman presents with lower abdominal fullness (Fig. 8–20).

Questions:

8-9. What is the most likely diagnosis of the soft-tissue mass (*arrows*) in Fig. 8–17?
A. Ascites
B. Cirrhosis

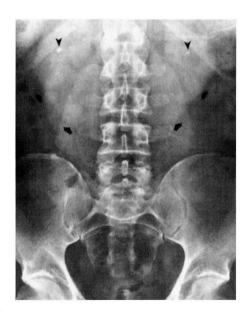

Fig. 8–19.

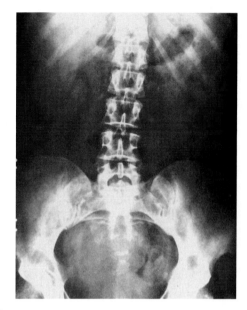

Fig. 8–20.

C. Hepatomegaly
D. Nephromegaly

8-10. What is the most likely diagnosis of the soft-tissue mass (*arrows*) in Fig. 8–18?
A. Adrenal carcinoma
B. Gastric outlet obstruction
C. Renal cell carcinoma
D. Splenomegaly

8-11. What is the most likely diagnosis of the soft-tissue mass (*arrows*) in Fig. 8–19?
A. A pseudotumor sign of small bowel obstruction
B. Gastric outlet obstruction
C. Hepatomegaly
D. Horseshoe kidney

8-12. What is the most likely diagnosis in Case 8-12 (Fig. 8–20)?
A. Ovarian cyst
B. Pelvic abscess
C. Pelvic hematoma
D. Pelvic kidney

Radiologic Findings:

8-9. In this case (Fig. 8–17), the right side of the abdomen shows increased density and is relatively free of gas. Displacement of the gas pattern in the duodenum and jejunum to the left side is indicative of hepatomegaly. (*C* is the correct answer to Question 8-9.) A radionuclide liver scan showed hepatic metastases from lung cancer.

8-10. In this case (Fig. 8–18), a soft-tissue mass in the left upper quadrant displaces the gas in the splenic flexure of the colon downward. Left adrenal or renal cell carcinoma rarely presents as a large mass to the left of the midline. The most likely diagnosis is splenomegaly. (*D* is the correct answer to Question 8-10.)

8-11. In this case (Fig. 8–19), a mass in the midabdomen delineates the lower poles of both kidneys, which are fused at the midline, consistent with horseshoe kidney. (*D* is the correct answer to Question 8-11.) Small renal calculi (*arrowheads*) are present bilaterally.

8-12. Figure 8–20 shows a soft-tissue mass in the pelvis. In a middle-aged woman, an ovarian or uterine mass would be the most likely considerations. Ultrasonography of the pelvis showed a large, fluid-filled mass, confirmed surgically as an ovarian cyst. (*A* is the correct answer to Question 8-12.)

Discussion:

Although abdominal plain radiographs are useful in detecting hepatomegaly or splenomegaly, they are of little use in diagnosing hepatic disease, particularly if hepatomegaly is not present. Other imaging modalities, such as ultrasonography, CT, MR imaging, and radionuclide liver scans, are more sensitive and accurate for evaluating hepatic primary diseases or metastases. In addition, barium studies of the gastrointestinal tract and intravenous urograms may be helpful in excluding gastric outlet obstruction, carcinoma, or renal cell carcinoma.

Fusion of the kidneys may occur in the embryologic stage during the second month of gestation. Most (95%) of these fusions occur at the lower poles of the kidneys. Intravenous urography shows the kidney to be vertical or even in the reverse oblique direction and its position to be lower than normal. Horseshoe kidney may be associated with other congenital anomalies, as well as a high incidence of urinary tract obstruction, infection, or stone formation. A horseshoe kidney may also deviate the upper ureters laterally.

When a plain film suggests the presence of a pelvic mass, a specific diagnosis is often not possible. Intravenous urography and barium enema are useful in excluding a mass arising from the lower urinary tract or colon and in showing extrinsic involvement of these structures. On the other hand, pelvic ultrasonography, CT, or MR imaging better demonstrates the pelvic organs and their interrelationship and will differentiate between solid or fluid content in the mass.

EXERCISE 8-4: INTESTINAL DISTENTION

Clinical Histories:

Case 8-13. A 66-year-old man presents with fever, chills, and abdominal pain (Fig. 8–21).

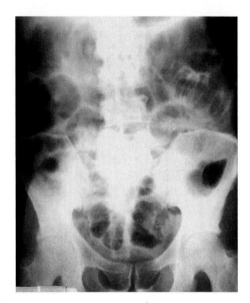

Fig. 8–21.

Case 8-14. A 65-year-old woman presents with abdominal distention and a history of abdominal surgery (Fig. 8–22).

Case 8-15. A 70-year-old man presents with abdominal distention (Fig. 8–23).

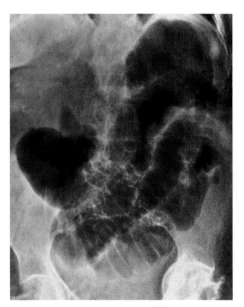

Fig. 8–22.

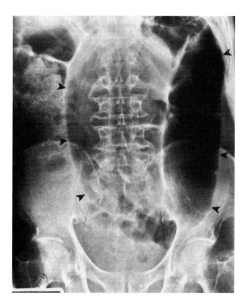

Fig. 8–23.

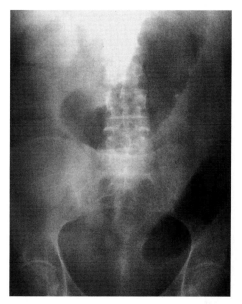

Fig. 8–24.

Case 8-16. A 66-year-old woman presents with abdominal distention and constipation for 3 days (Fig. 8–24).

Questions:

8-13. What is the most likely diagnosis in Case 8-13 (Fig. 8–21)?
- **A.** Functional ileus of the bowel
- **B.** Mechanical obstruction of the colon
- **C.** Mechanical obstruction of the small bowel
- **D.** Pneumoperitoneum

8-14. What is the most likely diagnosis in Case 8-14 (Fig. 8–22)?
- **A.** Functional ileus of the bowel
- **B.** Gastric outlet obstruction
- **C.** Mechanical obstruction of the small intestine
- **D.** Pneumoperitoneum

8-15. What is the most likely cause of the distended bowel loop (*arrowheads*) in Fig. 8–23?
- **A.** Cecal volvulus
- **B.** Functional ileus of the bowel
- **C.** Pneumoperitoneum
- **D.** Sigmoid volvulus

8-16. What is the most likely diagnosis in Case 8-16 (Fig. 8–24)?
- **A.** Ascites
- **B.** Functional ileus of the bowel
- **C.** Mechanical obstruction at the colon
- **D.** Mechanical obstruction at the small bowel

Radiologic Findings:

8-13. In this case (Fig. 8–21), a diffuse abnormal gas pattern with distention of the small bowel, colon, and rectum suggests functional ileus. Two days later the patient underwent laparotomy, and small bowel ischemia was found (Fig. 8–25). (*A* is the correct answer to Question 8-13.)

8-14. Figure 8–22 shows gaseous distention of the stomach, duodenum, and jejunum on the supine film, but no gas is seen in the colon, suggesting mechanical small bowel obstruction. Gastric outlet or duodenal obstruction is unlikely because many jejunal loops are dilated. At surgery, an obstructing jejunal adhesion was found. (*C* is the correct answer to Question 8-14.)

8-15. The patient in Fig. 8–23 has a huge distended and folded colonic loop in the midabdomen and pelvis (the "coffee bean" sign). The most likely consideration is a sigmoid volvulus. (*D* is the correct answer to Question 8-15.)

8-16. Figure 8–24 shows a distended transverse colon and descending colon and no gas in the sigmoid colon and rectum. The small bowel is not distended. Mechanical obstruction of the colon distal to the level of descending colon is likely. (*C* is the correct answer to Question 8-16.) Barium enema (Fig. 8–26) shows an irregular narrowing at the rectosigmoid region, indicative of sigmoid carcinoma.

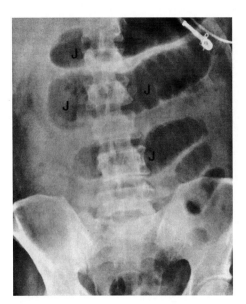

Fig. 8–25. Two days later, a follow-up abdominal plain film in the same patient shown in Fig. 8-21 shows a gas pattern in several separated loops of the jejunum (J) at midabdomen, which is indicative of enteric ischemia.

Discussion:

Generalized or diffuse distribution of gas, both in the small bowel and in the colon, is more indicative of a functional ileus. The most common causes of functional ileus are postoperative status, neuromuscular diseases, ischemia, and intrinsic or extrinsic inflammations. Air-fluid levels

may be seen in patients with functional ileus when plain films are obtained with the patient in an upright position.

Limited distribution of abnormal gas in the intestine favors a mechanical obstruction. Air-fluids levels may also be seen in patients with mechanical obstruction when an upright abdominal radiograph is obtained. The most common causes of mechanical obstruction in the small bowel are adhesions, internal or external hernias, neoplasms, or intussusceptions. Ileocolic intussusception is common in children.

When the small bowel is filled with a large amount of fluid, a row of small gas bubbles may be trapped between the valvulae conniventes. The row of gas bubbles is called the *string of beads* or *string of pearls sign* and is seen on the decubitus or upright view of the abdomen (Fig. 8–27). A fluid-filled, closed-loop small-bowel obstruction may appear as an oval mass in the abdomen and is known as the *pseudotumor sign* (Fig. 8–28). These signs suggest a mechanical obstruction and possible strangulation.

Sigmoid volvulus may twist along the mesenteric axis and the long axis of the bowel. The twisted and overdistended sigmoid colon may appear as an inverted U shape or a coffee bean shape, without haustra or septa, at the upper pelvis and abdomen crossing the transverse colon. The colon above the sigmoid may be distended; however, the small bowel is rarely distended in a patient

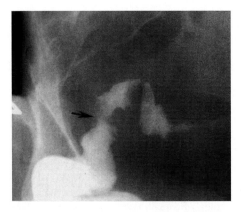

Fig. 8-26. Barium enema shows a narrowing (*arrow*) with an irregular contour at the rectosigmoid region, suggesting sigmoid carcinoma as the cause of colonic obstruction.

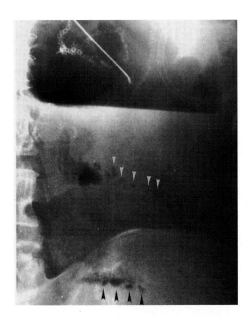

Fig. 8–27. Small-bowel obstruction. Two rows of air bubbles (*arrowheads*) with fluid levels in the left midabdomen are indicative of mechanical obstruction in the small intestine.

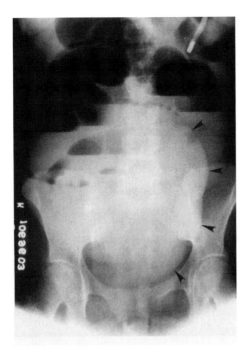

Fig. 8–28. Small-bowel obstruction shows a huge mass (*arrowheads, pseudotumor sign*) in the midabdomen with several adjacent fluid levels. (From Chen MYM, Zagoria RJ, Ott DJ, Gelfand DW. *Radiology of the Small Bowel.* New York: Igaku-Shoin; 1992; used with permission.)

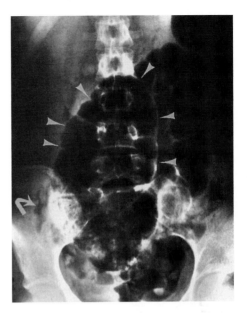

Fig. 8–29. A distended cecum and right colon (*arrowheads*) are seen at midabdomen. The terminal ileum (*curved arrow*) is located laterally to the cecal volvulus. Barium enema may delineate the twisted point in the ascending colon.

with sigmoid volvulus. Barium enema may show a beaking sign adjacent to the twisted point. Vascular insufficiency may occur if volvulus cannot be corrected.

A small-bowel volvulus may be caused by internal hernia or adhesion similar to that of sigmoid volvulus. Small-bowel volvulus may be located outside the pelvis with no proximal colonic dilatation. Cecal volvulus is the cause of 1% to 2% of intestinal obstructions. Most often a cecal volvulus is twisted and relocated in the midabdomen or left upper quadrant (Fig. 8–29).

Mechanical obstruction of the colon is commonly caused by colonic neoplasm, volvulus, or inflammatory mass caused by diverticulitis of the left colon. All colonic segments proximal to the mechanical obstruction are distended with gas or a combination of gas and feces. When intestinal secretions and fecal matter fill the distended bowel loop, solid and liquid contents produce a mottled appearance. Whether the small bowel becomes distended from a colonic obstruction depends on its duration and severity, and also on the competency of the ileocecal valve.

EXERCISE 8-5: INCREASED OR DECREASED DENSITY IN THE ABDOMEN

Clinical Histories:

Case 8-17. A 35-year-old man is seen who underwent laparotomy 2 days earlier (Fig. 8–30).

Case 8-18. A 49-year-old woman presents with acute abdominal pain (Fig. 8–31).

Case 8-19. A 40-year-old woman presents with abdominal distention (Fig. 8–32).

Case 8-20. A 45-year-old woman is seen who had a motor vehicle accident (Fig. 8–33).

Questions:

8-17. What is the most likely diagnosis in Case 8-17 (Fig. 8–30)?
    A. Bullous emphysema
    B. Colon interposition
    C. Pneumoperitoneum
    D. Tension pneumothorax

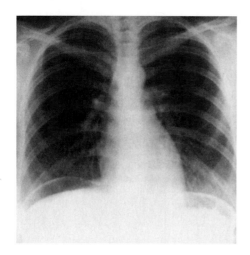

Fig. 8–30.

8-18. What is the most likely diagnosis in Case 8-18 (Fig. 8–31)?
　　A. Functional ileus of the bowel
　　B. Mechanical obstruction of the colon
　　C. Mechanical obstruction of the small bowel
　　D. Pneumoperitoneum

8-19. What is the most likely diagnosis in Case 8-19 (Fig. 8–32)?
　　A. Ascites
　　B. Functional ileus

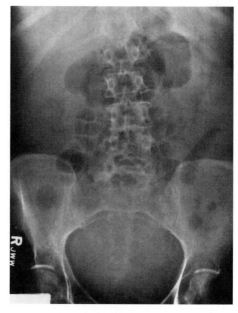

Fig. 8–32.

　　C. Gallstone ileus
　　D. Mechanical obstruction in the small bowel

8-20. What is the most likely diagnosis in Case 8-20 (Fig. 8–33)?

　　A. Ascites
　　B. Hemoperitoneum
　　C. Pelvic teratoma
　　D. Uterine fibroma

Radiologic Findings:

8-17. Figure 8–30 shows crescent-shaped lucencies beneath both hemidiaphragms outlining the liver on the

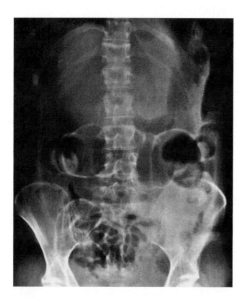

Fig. 8–31.

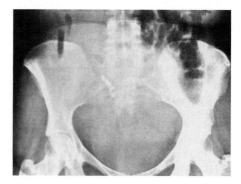

Fig. 8–33.

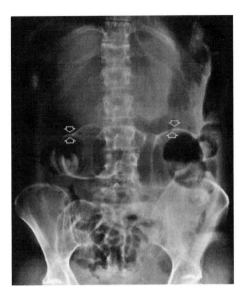

Fig. 8–34. In a patient with pneumoperitoneum, the double-wall sign shows inner and outer walls of the transverse colon (*arrows*) delineated by air in the colon and in the peritoneal cavity.

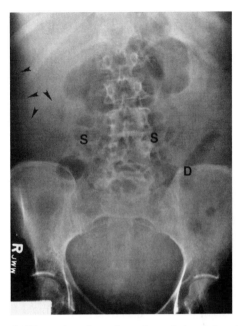

Fig. 8–35. Ascites shows hepatic angle (*arrowheads*, Hellmer's sign) and descending colon (D) displacing medially, small-bowel loops (S) located centrally, and increased density in the pelvis.

right and the spleen on the left in the PA chest film, suggesting pneumoperitoneum. (*C* is the correct answer to Question 8-17.)

8-18. Figure 8–34 shows both the inner and outer walls of the transverse colon (*arrows*). This double-wall sign is seen on the supine film of the abdomen because there is air within the intestinal lumen and in the peritoneal cavity, caused by rupture of a viscus. (*D* is the correct answer to Question 8-18.)

8-19. In Fig. 8–35, the hepatic angle (*arrowheads*) and the descending colon (D) are displaced medially, the small bowel (S) is located centrally in the abdomen, and there is increased density in the pelvis, suggesting ascites. (*A* is the correct answer to Question 8-19.)

8-20. In this case (Fig. 8–33), the soft-tissue density with no gas pattern in the pelvis is consistent with hemoperitoneum in this motor vehicle accident victim. CT better evaluates hemoperitoneum (Fig. 8–36). (*B* is the correct answer to Question 8-20.)

Discussion:

In adults, the most common causes of pneumoperitoneum are postoperative status, ruptured abdominal viscus, and peritoneal dialysis. Residual air in the abdomen after surgery may persist for 1 to 2 weeks. Serial abdominal films, however, should show a gradual reduction in the amount of free peritoneal air. A persistent or

increasing amount of air on postoperative serial films suggests a perforated viscus or ruptured surgical anastomosis. Spontaneous pneumoperitoneum is commonly caused by the perforation of a duodenal ulcer. Less common causes include pneumomediastinum, pulmonary emphysema, pneumatosis intestinalis, and entrance of air per vagina.

Pneumoperitoneum is most readily detected on the upright film of the chest, even if only a small amount of air is present. The left lateral decubitus view is useful and may show a small amount of free air accumulating between the right lateral margin of the liver and the peritoneal surface. Normally, the interface between the air and inner intestinal wall is visible, but the serosal surface is not appreciated because its density is similar to that of the adjacent peritoneal contents. When gas is present in the peritoneal cavity, however, both inner and outer walls will be delineated; this is called the *double-wall sign* or *Rigler's sign.* A visible serosal margin of bowel can also be simulated by normal adjacent omental fat or adjacent contiguous loops of small or large bowel (Fig. 8–37). If in doubt, the upright or left lateral decubitus film may confirm pneumoperitoneum. CT is more sensitive than plain radiograph in assessing pneumoperitoneum. Colon interposition occurs on the right between the liver and hemidiaphragm, and haustrations

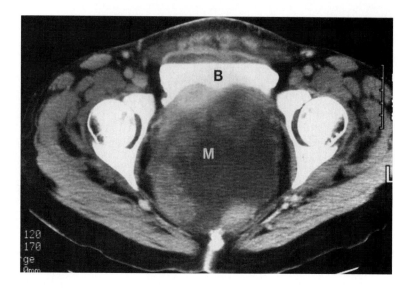

Fig. 8–36. CT shows a large soft-tissue mass (M) shadow with different attenuation in the pelvis, pushing the bladder (B) anteriorly. Hemoperitoneum was the diagnosis in this patient with a history of trauma.

are usually recognized that aid differentiation from pneumoperitoneum.

Although plain film of the abdomen is not sensitive in assessing small amounts of intraperitoneal fluid, the plain film can demonstrate moderate and large amounts of fluid collections. In ascites, the hepatic angle may be obscured or displaced medially (Hellmer's sign). The ascending or descending colon may be displaced medially by fluid in the paracolic gutter. A large amount of fluid may accumulate in the pelvis, causing increased density and symmetrical bulges (*dog ears sign*). Other signs, such as separation of the small bowel loops and overall higher density in the abdomen, are also seen, but not often. CT and ultrasonography more accurately assess intraperitoneal fluid and coexistent masses.

Blood and pus have a similar density to that of ascitic fluid in the peritoneal cavity; therefore, hemoperitoneum may produce signs similar to those found in ascites. High density in the pelvis is a sign of hemoperitoneum in patients with a history of trauma. CT better evaluates hemoperitoneum.

EXERCISE 8-6: EXTRALUMINAL GAS PATTERN

Clinical Histories:

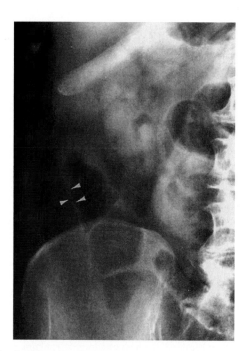

Fig. 8–37. False double-wall sign. Both inner and outer walls of the ascending colon (*arrowheads*) are outlined by air inside the colon and fat shadow outside. (*Courtesy of Stanley Bohrer, M.D., Winston-Salem, NC.*)

Case 8-21. A 42-year-old man presents with mild abdominal pain (Fig. 8–38).

Case 8-22. A 66-year-old woman is admitted with vague abdominal pain and vomiting (Fig. 8–39).

Case 8-23. A 77-year-old woman presents with fever and a 1-week history of abdominal pain (Fig. 8–40).

Case 8-24. A 64-year-old man presents with fever, abdominal pain, and distention (Fig. 8–41).

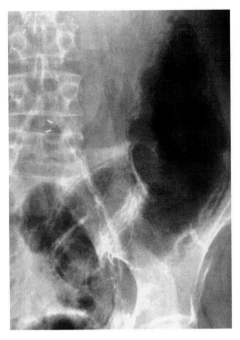

Fig. 8–38.

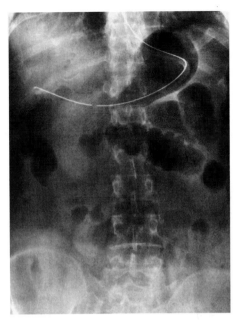

Fig. 8–39.

Questions:

8-21. What is the most likely diagnosis in Case 8-21 (Fig. 8–38)?
A. Colonic diverticulitis
B. Mechanical obstruction of the colon
C. Pneumatosis cystoides intestinalis
D. Pneumoperitoneum

8-22. What is the most likely diagnosis in Case 8-22 (Fig. 8–39)?
A. Abscess
B. Functional ileus
C. Gallstone ileus with gas in the biliary tree
D. Hepatic portal vein gas

8-23. What is the most likely diagnosis in Case 8-23 (Fig. 8–40)?
A. Gallstone ileus with gas in the biliary tree
B. Hepatic portal venous gas
C. Pneumoperitoneum
D. Right subdiaphragmatic abscess

8-24. What is the most likely diagnosis in Case 8-24 (Fig. 8–41)?
A. Gallstone ileus with gas in the biliary tree
B. Hepatic portal venous gas
C. Pneumoperitoneum
D. Subdiaphragmatic abscess

Radiologic Findings:

8-21. Figure 8–38 shows linear air streaks along the descending and sigmoid colon in a patient with mild abdominal pain. These streaks indicate pneumotosis cystoides intestinalis. (*C* is the correct answer to Question 8-21.)

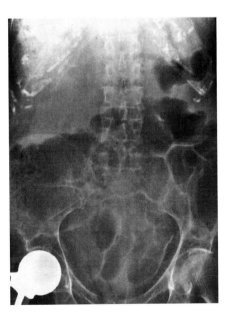

Fig. 8–40.

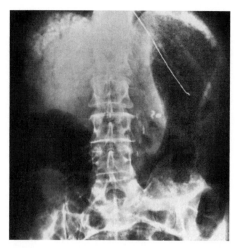

Fig. 8–41.

8-22. Figure 8–39 shows a distended proximal jejunum and a few air bubbles in the right upper quadrant, indicating gallstone ileus with mechanical obstruction and air in the biliary tree (Fig. 8–42A). An upper gastrointestinal study demonstrates a distended proximal small bowel, a fistula (Fig. 8–42B) between the

biliary tree and the duodenum, and three gallstones in the small bowel (Fig. 8–42C). CT shows air in the biliary tree (Fig. 8–42D). (C is the correct answer to Question 8-22.)

8-23. In this case (Fig. 8–40), multiple air bubbles in the right upper quadrant in a patient with fever are consistent with a subdiaphragmatic abscess (Fig. 8–43). Bilateral linear rib calcifications and right hip replacement are also seen. (D is the correct answer to Question 8-23.)

8-24. Figure 8–41 shows a fine arborizing linear gas pattern in the right upper quadrant that extends to the periphery of the liver, indicating portal venous gas. (B is the correct answer to Question 8-24.)

Discussion:

Pneumatosis cystoides intestinalis appears as linear streaks of gas or intramural cystic collections of gas in the small bowel or colon. The cysts range in size from 0.5 to 3 cm and may extend into the adjacent mesentery. Pneumatosis intestinalis is an incidental finding in most patients, usually with a self-limited benign course; simple bowel obstruction, volvulus, and air from the mediastinum or retroperitoneum are commonly associated. Pneumatosis intestinalis may be caused by ischemic and necrotizing enterocolitis in patients with leukemia or

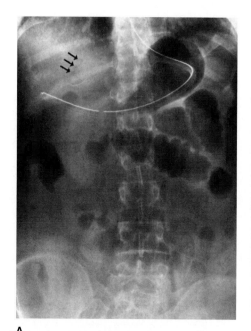

A

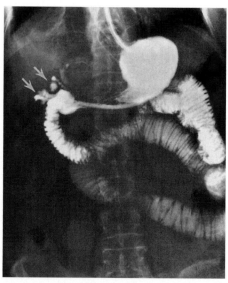

B

Fig. 8–42. **A** Gallstone ileus in the same patient shown in Fig. 8–39 is seen as distended small-bowel loops and air bubbles at the right upper quadrant (*arrows*). **B** Upper gastrointestinal series shows reflux of barium suspension into the biliary tree through a cholecystoduodenal fistula (*arrows*).

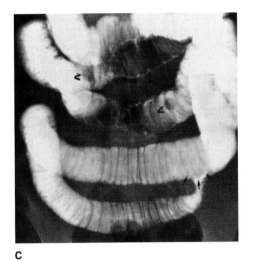

C

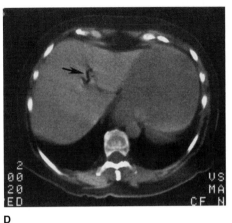

D

Fig. 8–42. **C** Small- bowel examination shows three gallstones in the small bowel (*arrows*), with the distal stone (*straight arrows*) causing obstruction. **D** CT study demonstrates air (*arrow*) in the biliary tree in the same patient. (A–D from Chen MYM, Dyer RD, Zagoria RJ, et al. CT of gallstone ileus. *Appl Radiol.* 1991;20:37–38; used with permission.)

non-Hodgkin lymphoma and in those who have had bone marrow transplantation.

Gallstone ileus, the mechanical obstruction of the small bowel by an impacted gallstone, is commonly

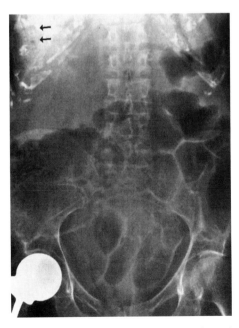

Fig. 8–43. Multiple air bubbles (*arrows*) in the right upper quadrant indicate a subdiaphragmatic abscess.

seen in elderly women. Clinical presentation in gallstone ileus is nonspecific, and the mortality rate is high (15%). A gallstone enters the intestinal lumen via a cholecystoenteric fistula. Major radiographic signs include small-bowel obstruction, air in the biliary tree, and an ectopic gallstone seen on plain abdominal film, upper gastrointestinal series, or CT study.

Abscess in the subphrenic and subhepatic spaces is a serious problem, with a mortality rate of 30%. Subphrenic abscess may arise spontaneously or as a complication of abdominal surgery, pancreatitis, diverticulitis, or appendicitis. A cluster of gas may be seen on plain film in 70% of abscesses. Left-sided abscess is difficult to discern because gas in the splenic flexure, stomach, or jejunum may mimic gas within the abscess. Other radiographic findings include elevation of the adjacent hemidiaphgram, pleural effusion, and basilar atelectasis.

In the right upper quadrant, when multiple tubular lucencies are seen reaching the lateral hepatic margins, portal venous gas is a likely consideration. Biliary tree gas is located in the central hepatic zone near the porta hepatis. Benign portal venous gas has been noted in sigmoid diverticulosis, nonobstructed splenic flexure carcinoma, ulcerative colitis, and bronchopneumonia. Mesenteric vascular insufficiency and necrotizing intestinal infection are common causes of hepatic portal venous gas. In children, necrotizing enterocolitis produces intramural gas within mesenteric veins to the liver; the mortality rate in patients with the sign of hepatic portal venous gas is higher than in those without portal venous gas.

BIBLIOGRAPHY

Baker SR, Cho KC. *The Abdominal Plain Film with Correlative Imaging.* 2nd ed. Stamford, Conn: Appleton & Lange; 1999.

Chen MYM, Bechtold RE, Bohrer SP, Zagoria RJ, Dyer RB. Abnormal calcification on plain radiographs of the abdomen. *Crit Rev Diagn Imaging.* 1999;40:63–202.

Gore RM, Levine MS. *Textbook of Gastrointestinal Radiology.* 2nd ed. Philadelphia: WB Saunders; 2000.

Meyers MA. *Dynamic Radiology of the Abdomen: Normal and Pathologic Anatomy.* 5th ed. New York: Springer-Verlag; 2000.

Radiology of the Urinary Tract

9

Judson R. Gash & D. Matthew Bowen

Radiology imaging has advanced dramatically since the first edition of this text. Technological advances and other innovations have greatly modified imaging of the urinary tract, with the dominant change being an increasing emphasis on cross-sectional modalities, especially CT. The result has been improved accuracy and earlier diagnoses of urinary tract disorders.

This chapter introduces the basic concepts in imaging of the urinary tract. The available imaging modalities and principles of their interpretation are discussed, especially in terms of its anatomy and its variants. The importance of choosing the most appropriate study for a given clinical scenario cannot be overemphasized and the next section of the chapter reviews technique selection. Clinical exercises and case examples are used to demonstrate important imaging concepts and diseases of the urinary tract. Finally, a bibliography of suggested readings is provided at the end of the chapter.

TECHNIQUES AND NORMAL ANATOMY

This section introduces the common radiologic techniques used in evaluation of the urinary tract. Emphasis is on a detailed description of each technique as it applies to the urinary tract. Also, a discussion of normal anatomy and some important fundamental concepts of interpretation is included. A basic knowledge of the gross anatomy is assumed with emphasis placed on the radiographic anatomic considerations.

Abdominal Radiography

Conventional radiographs (plain films) can occasionally provide important clues to diseases of the urinary tract. Radiographs of the abdomen when used to evaluate the urinary tract are often referred to as KUBs (kidney, ureter, and bladder). KUBs may serve a role as preliminary films (scouts) prior to an examination such as an intravenous urography, or they may be used as a general evaluation of the abdomen or the urinary tract. As stated, abnormalities of the urinary tract may be suggested on conventional radiographs and, among other things, the bones and soft tissues should be evaluated and abnormal densities, especially calcifications, should be sought. "Gas, mass, bones, stones" can be used as a reminder of main areas to examine on the KUB (Fig. 9–1). Soft tissue masses can occasionally be detected and suggest renal or pelvic lesions. Sclerotic bony lesions can suggest metastatic prostate cancer and lytic bony lesions can be seen with disseminated renal cell carcinoma. Additionally, the bony changes of renal osteodystrophy (diffuse bony sclerosis) may be identified on plain radiographs. Vertebral anomalies are associated with congenital malformations of the urinary tract.

In the setting of trauma, fractures of the lumbar transverse processes suggest possible renal injuries and pelvic fractures raise concern for coexistent bladder or urethral trauma. Air and calcifications should be specifically sought over the urinary tract. Emphysematous pyelonephritis, a urologic emergency with high mortality, is the result of a renal infection by gas-producing

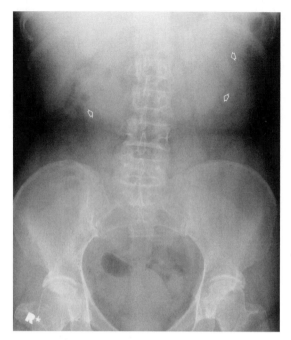

Fig. 9–1. Normal KUB. Note that portions of the normal renal contours (*arrows*) are visible and should be evaluated. No abnormal calcifications, soft tissue densities, or bony lesions are evident.

organisms and may be diagnosed on plain films by mottled or linear collections of air within the renal parenchyma. If emphysematous pyelonephritis is suspected, emergency computed tomography (CT) should be performed to delineate the extent of involvement and immediate urologic consultation obtained.

Finally, radiographs are useful for detecting and evaluating urinary tract calculi. It has been reported that 90% of calculi are radiopaque and can be identified on conventional radiographs. However, recent studies suggest that no more than 40% to 60% of urinary tract stones are detected and accurately diagnosed on plain radiographs. The sensitivity for detection of stones is limited when the calculi are small, of lower density composition, or when overlapping stool, bony structures, or air is obscuring the stones. Additionally, the specificity of conventional radiography is somewhat limited because a multitude of other calcifications occur in the abdomen, including arterial vascular calcifications, pancreatic calcifications, gallstones, leiomyomas, and many more. (More than 200 causes of calcification in the abdomen have been described.) Phleboliths, which are calcified venous thromboses, are especially problematic because they frequently overlap the urinary tract and are difficult to differentiate from

distal ureteral stones. Lucent centers are a hallmark of phleboliths, whereas renal calculi are often most dense centrally. Additionally, oblique films and tomograms may be useful to differentiate true renal calculi from densities within the tissues anterior or posterior to the kidney.

Intravenous Urography

Intravenous urography (IVU), also known as *intravenous pyelography* (or more commonly, the IVP), has dominated imaging of the urinary tract for more than 50 years. Although recent advances in other techniques have substantially reduced its role, IVU remains an important study for some urinary tract disease processes. More importantly, however, decades of use of the IVU have established the fundamentals of imaging evaluation of the urinary tract. An understanding of these principles forms a foundation for radiologic interpretation of the urinary tract with the IVU or other more "advanced" imaging modalities. Thus, the IVU technique is explained with interspersed discussion of anatomy, normal variants, and, most importantly, some fundamentals of interpretation.

Although an urgent examination should not be delayed to prepare a patient for an IVU, overlying stool can obscure important detail on an intravenous urogram and therefore a mild bowel preparation of clear liquids and laxatives before an elective study is recommended. The study should always begin with a scout KUB. This has several purposes including detection of calcifications (which may be obscured after contrast material is injected), assurance of proper technique (patient positioning, exposure parameters) prior to contrast administration, and exclusion of contraindications to the study (retained barium, etc.). The scout film should encompass the area from the adrenals to the symphysis pubis, and sometimes more than one film may be required.

Intravenously injected iodinated contrast is excreted primarily by glomerular filtration in the kidney, opacifying the urinary tract as it progresses from the kidney through the ureter and to the bladder. Capturing this sequential "opacification" on radiographs is the fundamental basis of the IVU. There are many variations in the filming sequence for the urogram that are acceptable as long as it optimizes visualization of specific anatomy of the urinary tract during maximum contrast opacification.

Optimal visualization of the kidney is accomplished very early in the examination. Within 1 to 3 minutes after injection, the contrast bolus is filtered by the glomeruli and fills the nephron, resulting in intense opacification of the renal parenchyma; this phase of contrast opacification is called the *nephrogram*. Evaluation of the

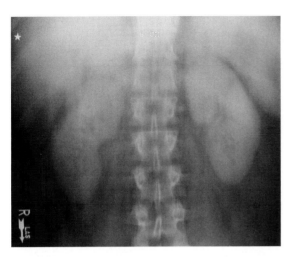

Fig. 9–2. Normal nephrotomogram. Note the position of the kidneys within the abdomen, with the right kidney slightly lower than the left; the size of the kidneys, between three and four lumbar vertebra lengths; the symmetry of the nephrograms; and the renal contour, which is smooth.

kidneys during the nephrographic phase is often enhanced with *tomograms* (nephrotomograms) (Fig. 9–2). The kidneys should be evaluated for their position, orientation, size, contour, and radiographic density. The kidneys are typically located at the level of the upper lumbar spine with the right kidney slightly lower than the left. They generally lie with their axes along the psoas muscles with the upper pole slightly more medial than the lower. Alterations in position and orientation of the kidneys may be related to congenital anomalies such as pelvic kidneys or may be secondary to mass effect from an adjacent lesion.

The size of the kidneys is somewhat variable depending on age and sex of the patient, but on the intravenous urogram the kidneys normally range from 11 to 14 cm. The right kidney is typically slightly smaller than the left. Measurement of renal size is also dependent on the examination. For example, on the IVU the kidneys appear artificially larger due to magnification. To account for this as well as other parameters such as overall body size, a generalization is that the kidneys should measure between three and four lumbar vertebra lengths. Additionally, the kidneys should be symmetric in size with a discrepancy greater than 2 cm requiring an explanation. There are a number of causes of abnormal renal size, ranging from incidental anomalies such as congenital renal hypoplasia to significant conditions such as renal artery stenosis (small kidney) or infiltrating renal neoplasm (large kidney).

The kidneys should have a reniform shape and a smooth contour. Embryologically, the kidney is composed of lobes that smoothly fuse to create the kidney; however, not uncommonly, small residual clefts remain where the lobes fail to completely fuse, a condition referred to as *persistent fetal lobation*. This must be distinguished from true renal scarring, which most often results from chronic vesicoureteral reflux/chronic bacterial pyelonephritis or from renal infarcts. The clefts of fetal lobation occur between lobules, i.e., the cortex between calyces, whereas scarring typically occurs in the cortex over the calyx. Additionally, the calyces are generally distorted and rounded with chronic reflux disease. Bulges to the renal contour are of more concern because they raise suspicion for a mass. A key concept in evaluation of a possible mass is parenchymal thickness as measured from calyces to edge of the kidney. A fairly common normal variant is the *dromedary hump*, which is a bulge created along the lateral mid aspect of the left kidney related to splenic impression on the kidney. This bulge is differentiated from a mass by a typical calyx that extends out toward the bulge, keeping the parenchymal thickness similar to the rest of the kidney. A true mass results in increased parenchymal thickness or even mass effect on the adjacent calyces, which are displaced away from the bulge. The radiographic density of the kidneys following contrast injection is related to arterial supply, renal function and excretion, and venous outflow. Alterations in any of these parameters may result in abnormalities of one or both of the nephrograms. For example, ureteral obstruction results in a delayed and increasingly dense nephrogram.

Soon after the nephrographic phase, contrast begins filling the intrarenal collecting system including the calyces and renal pelvis. This portion of the study is termed the *pyelographic phase* (Fig. 9–3). Several films are used to evaluate the collecting system (intrarenal collecting system and ureter) beginning at our institution with a KUB obtained 5 minutes after contrast injection. Evaluation of the intrarenal collecting system is improved by placing a compression device over the lower abdomen, thereby compressing the ureters on the sacrum, resulting in increased distention and improved visualization of the proximal ureters and renal collecting system. Compression is contraindicated in several settings, including ureteral obstruction, abdominal aortic aneurysm, and recent abdominal surgery. Typically, compression is applied after the 5-minute KUB has been obtained and evaluated by the radiologist. A film of the kidneys is performed after 10 minutes, allowing for the compression of the ureter to result in proximal distention. The intrarenal collecting system consists of calyces, infundibula, and the renal pelvis. Normally, each kidney consists of 7 to 14 evenly distributed

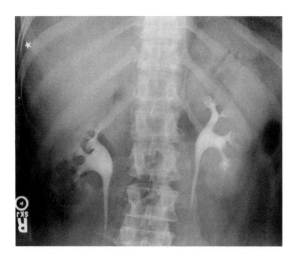

Fig. 9–3. Normal pyelogram. Note the delicate cup-shaped appearance of the calyces and the relative symmetry of the renal pelvis with no evidence of dilation or mass effect.

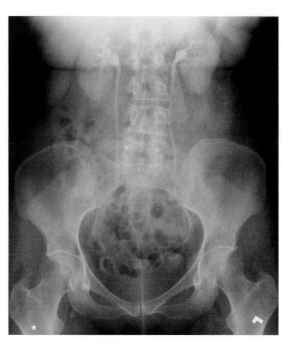

Fig. 9–4. Normal KUB showing contrast opacified ureters. Note the course of the ureters lateral to the lumbar spine overlying the psoas muscles proximally, crossing over the sacrum, and curving laterally in the pelvis before turning medially to insert in the urinary bladder. Due to peristalsis, the ureter may not be visible in its entirety.

calyces. The individual renal calyx, from the Latin for "chalice," is a delicate appearing cup-shaped structure. Not uncommonly, partial fusion of the calyces occurs, especially in the renal poles, creating the compound calyx. Other calyceal variants occur, including variants of number (polycalycosis, unicalyx kidney) and size (megacalycosis, microcalyx) and must be differentiated from true pathology. The calyces may not be visualized if compressed or may be deviated by masses. The normal delicate, cup-like appearance can be distorted or irregular in conditions such as papillary necrosis, tuberculosis, or transitional cell carcinoma. Subtle rounding or ballooning of the calyces is one of the earliest signs of urinary tract obstruction. Diverticula may arise from the calyces, creating a haven for stone formation, recurrent infection, or even transitional cell malignancy. The renal pelvis is also quite variable in appearance. A common variation is the so-called "extrarenal" pelvis, where the pelvis lies outside the renal sinus. In this setting the pelvis tends to be more prominent and rounded, mimicking hydronephrosis. This can be differentiated from true obstruction by normal appearing calyces. The renal pelvis should be evaluated for filling defects and mass effect.

Release of compression results in a bolus of contrast material entering the ureters, which is evaluated with a KUB, and often with oblique films, obtained immediately after release of the device at 15 minutes (Fig. 9–4). Occasionally, fluoroscopy may be utilized to visualize suspicious areas of the ureter not seen on the conventional films. The ureter extends from the ureteral pelvic junction to the ureteral vesicle junction. Proximally, the ureter passes over the psoas muscle and should generally lay just lateral to the lumbar spine. The midportions of the ureters course over the lateral sacrum with the distal portion gently curving laterally in the pelvis before entering the bladder. The ureter is an actively peristalsing structure that is not normally seen in total on the IVU. In fact, complete visualization of the ureter may suggest distal obstruction. The ureter should be inspected for filling defects, which can be caused by stones or tumor, and should be symmetric in size. Evaluation of the ureteral course is important. Typically, the ureter should be no more lateral than the tips of the lumbar transverse processes and no more medial than the lumbar pedicles. Deviations of the normal ureter generally suggest extrinsic diseases, such as mass lesions. However, in patients with large psoas muscles the ureters may be displaced laterally as an incidental result.

Finally, the bladder is opacified last on the study beginning around 5 minutes after injection. Early filling films, later distended films, and postvoiding images

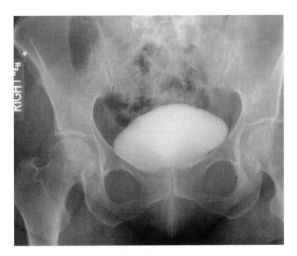

Fig. 9–5. Normal bladder. Note the location of the bladder just above the pubic symphysis, as well as its smooth contour. No filling defects should be seen.

complete the evaluation of the bladder (Fig. 9–5). The bladder is an oval to rounded structure that normally lies just above the pubic symphysis on the IVU. Not uncommonly, especially on early filling films, some extrinsic compression of the bladder can be seen due to the sigmoid colon. In women, the dome of the bladder may normally be indented by the uterus. These normal findings must be differentiated from abnormal extrinsic mass effects. Bladder wall thickness can sometimes be visualized and assessed, especially if thickened. Additionally, the bladder mucosa should be scrutinized for irregularity or filling defects that may suggest a mass.

Films in addition to the typical IVU sequence may be used, taking advantage of the greater density of contrast material than that of urine, and include prone and upright films as well as delayed films as needed. Regardless of the filming routine, the best IVU is the one monitored by the radiologist and tailored for the patient based on the study indication.

Retrograde Pyelography/ Cystography/ Urethrography

Direct injection of water-soluble iodinated contrast material is a useful method of examining various regions of the urinary tract. The advantage of this method of evaluation is the direct control over the contrast injection rather than reliance on secondary excretion from the kidney. Retrograde pyelography, often carried out in conjunction with cystoscopy, is performed by placing a small catheter into the distal ureter. Contrast material is

then injected through this catheter into one or both ureters. Fluoroscopy and conventional radiographs should then be obtained. This study usually results in excellent evaluation of the ureter and intrarenal collecting system. The ureter is typically seen in its entirety, which rarely occurs with other imaging studies. Interpretation is similar to that of the IVU with the caveat that the contrast within the collecting system is under greater pressure than physiologic conditions and mild ballooning of the calyces as well as occasional extravasation can occur normally.

Imaging of the bladder is performed with a cystogram, for which a catheter is placed into the bladder and contrast material is then injected. The contrast material is optimally injected under fluoroscopic observation but occasionally is performed with only static conventional radiographs, such as in the trauma setting. Anatomic considerations and evaluation are similar to the IVU with a few caveats. One advantage to cystography is that vesicoureteral reflux can be evaluated during the conventional cystogram unlike during IVU. Recently, CT cystography, in which after contrast instillation CT imaging is utilized instead of conventional films, has been used, especially in the setting of trauma to evaluate for bladder injury.

The urethra may be evaluated with contrast material via two methods. In one, the urethra is evaluated during voiding, often following a cystogram (voiding cystourethrogram or VCUG). Alternatively, a retrograde study may be performed (retrograde urethrogram). The urethra in the male consists of four portions, including the prostatic, membranous, bulbous, and penile portions. During voiding, the urethra is fairly uniformly distended and tubular in appearance (Fig. 9–6). On a retrograde study, the more posterior urethra (prostatic and membranous) is often contracted and seen as a thin wisp of contrast. The female urethra appears as a short, slightly funnel-shaped tubular structure during voiding (Fig. 9–7) (Note that a special catheter is required for evaluation of the female urethra in a retrograde fashion.) The urethra in males is generally evaluated for injuries but may also be examined for filling defects, masses, strictures, and fistula. The female urethra is most commonly examined for diverticula.

Ultrasonography

Ultrasonography is a useful technique for evaluation of the urinary tract, made especially attractive by its ease of use and lack of complications (no contrast material or ionizing radiation). The kidneys are generally well seen in all but the largest of patients (Fig. 9–8). The renal medulla is hypoechoic (darker) relative to renal cortex and can be identified in most normal adults as cone-shaped central structures. (Occasionally, this corticomedullary

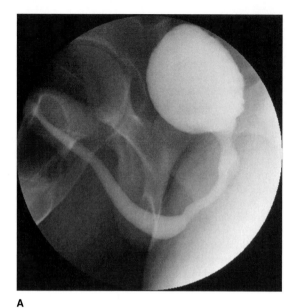

A

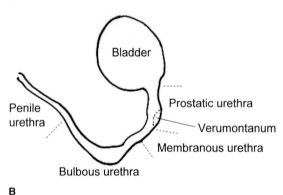

B

Fig. 9–6. Normal antegrade urethrogram and drawing. The mild areas of narrowing and dilation are normal. On an antegrade study, unlike a retrograde examination, the proximal urethral is distended and readily assessed. No evidence of stricture or extravasation is seen.

are often nonspecific, ultrasonography allows a more detailed evaluation including the ability to confidently diagnose the most common renal mass—the simple cyst. Solid masses, however, remain nonspecific and generally require further evaluation. Like the IVU, there are normal variants that can mimic mass lesions including dromedary humps and persistent collections of normal renal tissue within the substance of the renal parenchyma referred to as *persistent columns of Bertin.* Additionally, the parenchyma near the renal hila may appear prominent as well, occasionally mimicking a mass. Each of these lesions may be distinguished by their echogenicity being equal to surrounding tissue, lack of mass effect, and characteristic location. Occasionally, additional imaging may be required in equivocal cases.

The renal sinus is the area engulfed by the kidney medially, harboring the renal pelvis, arteries, veins, nerves, and lymphatics that enter and exit the kidney, all contained within a variable amount of fat. Fat is typically brightly echogenic on ultrasound, and fat within

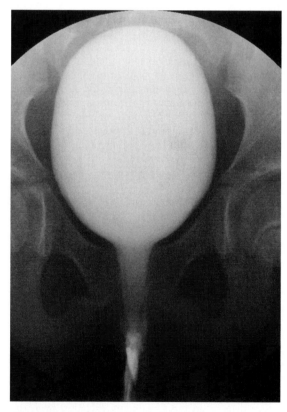

Fig. 9–7. Normal female VCUG. Note the smooth contour of the urinary bladder and the short, conical appearing urethra.

distinction is not visible.) The renal cortex is isoechoic or slightly hypoechoic compared with the echogenicity of the adjacent liver. Renal echogenicity exceeding that of the liver is abnormal and requires explanation. Most commonly hyperechoic kidneys are seen in the setting of medical renal disease, such as end-stage hypertensive glomerulosclerosis.

In addition to echogenicity, the kidneys should be assessed for size, location, and symmetry. Scarring and masses can be evaluated. Unlike the IVU, where masses

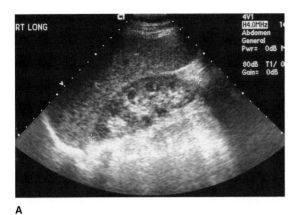

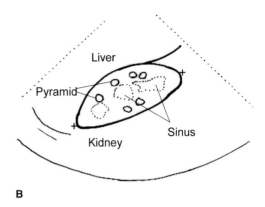

A **B**

Fig. 9–8. Normal renal ultrasound: long axis view and drawing. Note the smooth contour of the kidney. The rounded to cone-shaped medullary pyramids are hypoechoic to the cortex and should not be mistaken for a mass or dilated collecting system. The renal cortex should be similar to or slightly hypoechoic compared with liver. In addition, notice the hyperechoic fat of the renal sinus—the central echo complex.

the renal sinus dominates the ultrasonographic appearance, creating what is known as the *central echo complex.* The size of the central echo complex is variable, often more prominent in the elderly and minimal in the child. Absence of the central echo complex may suggest a mass such as a transitional cell carcinoma replacing the normal fat. Alternatively, the complex may be very prominent in the benign condition of renal sinus lipomatosis. Calcifications are characteristic on ultrasound, being brightly echogenic and resulting in shadowing posteriorly as the sound waves are attenuated. Renal stones or calcifications may be detected within the renal parenchyma or in the intrarenal collecting system. The echogenicity of the normal renal sinus, however, creates difficulty because sometimes it obscures or mimicks small stones.

Ultrasonography is also excellent for detecting hydronephrosis with the distended collecting system being easily recognized within the central echo complex. The ureters are not normally seen on ultrasound due to obscuring overlying tissue and their small size. Evidence of their patency may be verified by Doppler detection of urine rapidly entering the bladder from the distal ureters, i.e., distal ureteral jets (Fig. 9–9). The bladder is seen as a rounded or oval anechoic (fluid) structure in the pelvis. The bladder may demonstrate mass lesions, such as transitional cell carcinoma, or stones. The urethra is not typically seen on an ultrasound image although urethral diverticula may occasionally be demonstrated.

Computed Tomography

CT is now the dominant radiologic imaging modality for evaluation of the urinary tract. The advent of multidetector spiral CT has further propelled CT to the forefront of

urologic imaging. Several factors make CT effective in assessing the urinary tract. The high contrast resolution and spatial resolution afforded by CT allow detection and evaluation of subtle differences in very small structures. Mathematical calculations of the attenuation of the CT x-ray beam allow quantitative evaluation of the relative density of structures (i.e., their Hounsfield units), and it is through these "CT numbers" that much unique diagnostic information of the urinary tract is gained. Examinations can be performed amazingly fast because thin-slice CT scans of the entire urinary tract are now obtainable in just a few seconds. Finally, the wide availability and relative safety of CT furthers its appeal.

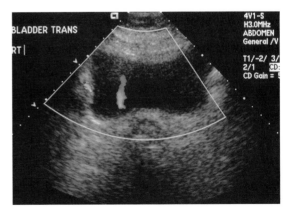

Fig. 9–9. Normal ultrasound image of a ureteral jet. Doppler image shows the stream of urine entering the urinary bladder through the ureteral orifice, consistent with an unobstructed normal ureter.

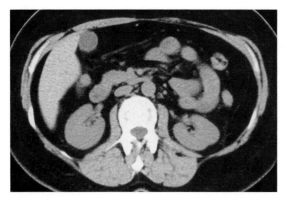

Fig. 9–10. Normal noncontrast CT image of the kidneys. Note the smooth contour and relative symmetry of the kidneys and their sharp interface with the perirenal fat.

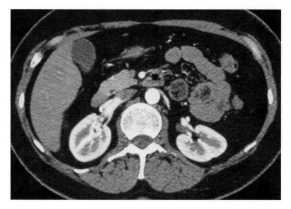

Fig. 9–11. Normal CT of the corticomedullary phase of renal opacification. In this early phase, the cortex enhances more than the medulla because the cortex initially receives the majority of the arterial blood flow. The cortex and medulla are easily distinguished by CT.

CT scans of the urinary tract may be performed with and/or without intravenous iodinated contrast material depending on the indications. Noncontrast studies may be performed to evaluate stone disease and other calcifications. Additionally, noncontrast views of the kidneys serve as a baseline to evaluate for lesion enhancement after contrast administration, a critical factor in mass evaluation. On noncontrast examinations the kidneys are homogeneous and have a density similar to most soft tissue (Fig. 9–10). In all but the thinnest adults, fat is seen surrounding the kidneys and extending into the renal sinus. Contrast-enhanced studies of the kidneys are best performed with a mechanical power injector.

With rapid scanning and contrast bolus timing, several sequential phases of opacification within the kidney can be delineated by CT including corticomedullary, nephrographic, and excretory phases. The corticomedullary phase can be seen if scanning is performed during the first 20 to 90 seconds after contrast administration and represents the early preferential blood flow to the renal cortex (Fig. 9–11); however, small masses could be missed during this phase, being obscured within the unenhanced renal medulla. Subsequently, contrast begins to pass into the distal collecting tubules within the renal medulla, resulting in a more homogeneous opacification of the renal parenchyma, termed the *CT nephrographic phase*. This generally occurs around 2 to 4 minutes after contrast medium injection. Finally, the excretory phase is seen when contrast opacifies the collecting system (Fig. 9–12). Each different phase of opacification may better demonstrate different disease processes and thus various scanning protocols are used to evaluate the kidneys depending on the indication.

One of the major recent advances in imaging has been the ability to noninvasively evaluate the vascular system, and thin-section early CT images accurately

demonstrate the main arterial and venous structures of the kidney (Fig. 9–13). Just as with IVU or any modality, the kidneys should be evaluated for position, orientation, size, and radiographic density. Unlike IVU, however, CT provides much greater specificity regarding renal disease, including mass lesions. The ubiquitous simple cyst is generally easily diagnosed and differentiated from the more concerning solid mass. Fat within a solid mass generally allows the diagnosis of the benign

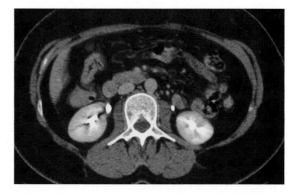

Fig. 9–12. Normal CT of the nephrographic/pyelographic phase of renal enhancement. In this later phase of enhancement, the renal parenchyma becomes homogeneous as contrast passes into the collecting ducts of the renal medulla—the nephrographic phase. Also shown in this example is contrast within the intrarenal collecting system—the pyelographic or excretory phase.

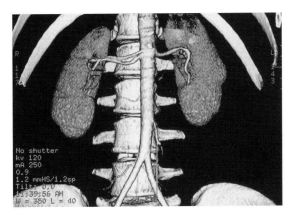

Fig. 9–13. Normal CT angiogram of the renal arteries, 3-D reconstruction. Note that this image clearly demonstrates that there are two right renal arteries. This is a normal variant. In this case, the renal arteries are patent without evidence of significant stenosis.

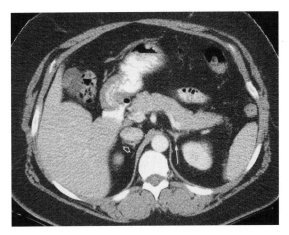

Fig. 9–14. Normal CT of the adrenals. The left adrenal has the characteristic inverted Y shape (*arrow*), whereas the right, located immediately behind the inferior vena cava, is somewhat more linear in appearance (*open arrow*) in this case.

angiomyolipoma. The solid, non-fat-containing mass in the adult should be considered a renal cell carcinoma until proven otherwise. CT is sensitive in detecting renal masses and, although not always supplying a specific diagnosis, typically provides important information allowing for appropriate patient management.

CT is also useful in staging renal neoplasms. Non-neoplastic renal disease, such as trauma and complicated infections, is accurately demonstrated on CT images, which provide specific information regarding the extent and severity of the process. Unlike conventional radiographs, IVU, or even ultrasound, CT provides a thorough evaluation of the adrenal glands, which appear as small inverted Y-shaped structures above the kidneys (Fig. 9–14). Additionally, the remainder of the retroperitoneum, containing fat, the normal occupants of the retroperitoneum (kidneys, adrenals, pancreas, duodenum, and parts of the colon), and vascular structures, is well seen by CT, and diseases such as inflammation, infection, and tumor are easily demonstrated.

Until recently, the ureters and their disorders were the domain of the IVU or retrograde pyelogram. However, since the mid-1990s, spiral CT has become the study of choice for evaluating suspected ureteral stones. Two factors were key in this transition. First, the invention of spiral CT technique allowed for continuous coverage of the entire ureter without skip areas. Second, virtually all stones are dense and conspicuous on CT. There are many other advantages to using CT to evaluate suspected ureteral stones including speed of the examination, identification of alternative explanations

for the pain (appendicitis, divertculitis, aneurysm, etc.), and elimination of intravenous contrast complications (because the study is performed without contrast). Scans no thicker than 5 mm are performed from the top of the kidneys to the symphysis pubis. The ureter can be visualized and followed from the renal pelvis to the bladder in most cases and appears as a tubular 2- to 3-mm fluid structure surrounded by retroperitoneal fat (Fig. 9–15).

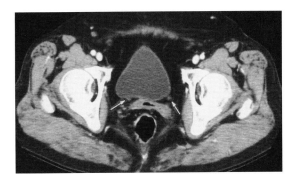

Fig. 9–15. Normal CT image of the distal ureters and urinary bladder. Although contrast has been administered, it has not yet reached the bladder. Note that despite their small size and lack of contrast, the ureters can be identified (*arrows*) within the retroperitoneal fat. The right ureter is seen near its point of entrance to the bladder. The bladder contains water density urine and a thin, smooth wall can be delineated.

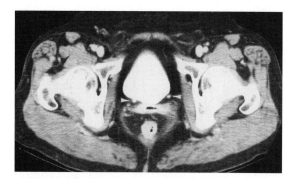

Fig. 9–16. Normal CT showing the distal ureters and urinary bladder opacified with IV contrast. After a 5-minute delay, the distal ureters (*arrowheads*) and bladder are easily identified. Delayed images may be necessary to evaluate the ureter or bladder in certain circumstances.

Stones can be diagnosed by their high density and location within the ureter. Secondary signs of obstruction have been described, including dilation of the proximal ureter, hydronephrosis, renal enlargement and stranding in the fat surrounding the kidney. As on the IVU, phleboliths can prove troubling due to their frequent close approximation with the distal ureter; however, their central lucency, lack of surrounding inflamed ureteral wall, and lack of secondary signs of obstruction usually allow their distinction.

When contrast material has been administered, the ureters appear as dense, rounded structures in the retroperitoneum (Fig. 9–16). On CT, the bladder appears as a rounded water or contrast density structure in the pelvis. One pitfall is that the first few images of contrast beginning to enter the bladder may mimic a bladder mass. The bladder wall should be evaluated for thickening and irregularity, which may suggest hypertrophy, inflammation, or carcinoma. Stones may be detected within the bladder. The urethra is not normally seen on CT.

Magnetic Resonance Imaging

Just like CT, technical advances in magnetic resonance (MR) imaging have led to increasing use in urinary imaging. Fast-scanning techniques that allow breath-hold imaging, combined with the spectacular tissue contrast of MR imaging and the ability to directly image in any plane, make this an attractive modality for evaluating the urinary tract. Lack of ionizing radiation adds to its appeal, but cost, availability, claustrophobia, and the contraindication of certain materials including pacemakers remain major drawbacks. Finally, MR imag-

ing of the kidney is performed with gadolinium as the contrast agent, not iodinated contrast material. In renal imaging one of the main advantages of gadolinium versus iodine is the virtual lack of nephrotoxicity at clinical doses. On MR imaging, the kidneys appear to be of variable signal intensity, depending on the imaging factors and, like CT, contrast-enhanced phases of imaging (arterial, corticomedullary, nephrographic, and excretory) are all visible (Fig. 9–17).

Specific imaging sequences are designed to manipulate imaging factors to allow for optimum evaluation of the particular clinical concern. The ability to image in any plane creates a unique advantage for MR imaging (Fig. 9–18). The kidneys should be evaluated in a fashion similar to that of other modalities. Recently, two techniques have been developed to allow the ureters to be evaluated. In one method, the high signal intensity of water (urine) is utilized to make the ureters conspicuous compared to other tissues. In the other technique, the MR imaging contrast agent gadolinium is given and the ureters opacify similar to IVU or contrast-enhanced CT. The bladder is well visualized, similar to CT. Finally, the adrenal glands are well seen, as in CT, and the normal shape is the same as that described for CT and the signal intensity depending on particular imaging parameters. The ureters, bladder, and adrenals are evaluated in a fashion similar to that used for CT.

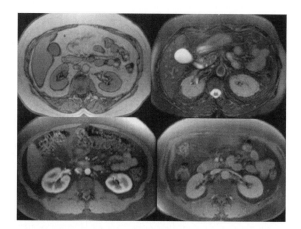

Fig. 9–17. Normal MRI of the kidneys. The appearance of the kidneys is variable on MR imaging depending on imaging factors. The top left image is a T_1-weighted sequence and the top right is T_2 weighted. The bottom images were obtained after gadolinium injection and demonstrate the corticomedullary and nephrographic phases.

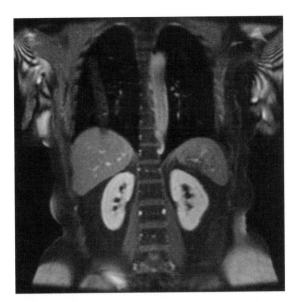

Fig. 9–18. Normal MR imaging of the kidneys. This image was obtained in the coronal plane and after gadolinium injection.

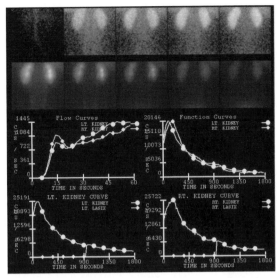

Fig. 9–19. Normal ^{99m}Tc-MAG$_3$ renogram. Images are shown in the upper portion of the figure demonstrating the radioisotope progressing through the urinary tract. In the bottom portion of the figure, quantitative data are expressed in renogram curves.

Nuclear Medicine

The basic technique of a nuclear medicine study is discussed in Chapter 1; here, we briefly examine the more specific role in evaluation of the urinary tract. In general, the value of nuclear imaging in the urinary tract is several-fold: Functional information related to quantifiable collected data is obtained, the radiation dose is lower than that for traditional radiographic techniques, and the incidence of complications is very low.

Renal evaluation is typically performed by intravenous bolus injection of renal-specific agents such as technetium-labeled mercaptoacetyltriglycine (^{99m}Tc-MAG$_3$). Images are acquired every few seconds that demonstrate renal blood flow, with additional images obtained over several minutes that show renal uptake and excretion. Recall that the recorded data can be used to produce images, but are also quantifiable and employed to generate time–activity curves (Fig. 9–19).

Information about renal perfusion, morphology, relative function of each kidney, and excretion can be extremely useful in evaluation of conditions such as renovascular hypertension, obstruction, and renal transplant examination. Although anatomically oriented data can be obtained with other radioisotopes that aggregate more in the renal parenchyma, in general, nuclear medicine renal studies suffer from fairly low spatial resolution and, therefore, are often used in conjunction with other imaging studies.

Radionuclide cystography is another useful test used to diagnose and monitor vesicoureteral reflux. Here, technetium pertechnetate is mixed with saline and infused into the bladder with subsequent images obtained over the urinary tract. This study is quite sensitive for the detection of significant reflux but at a considerably lower radiation dose than conventional cystography. Another important study is the radioactive iodine labeled metaiodobenzylguanidine (MIBG) examination. MIBG collects in adrenal medullary tissue and is useful in diagnosis and evaluation of pheochromocytoma. Additional radioisotopes are available for urinary tract imaging, usually in fairly specific roles.

Angiography

The role of angiography as a diagnostic tool continues to diminish with the increasing accuracy of noninvasive techniques to evaluate the vascular system. The renal arteriogram is performed after puncture of a more peripheral vessel such as the common femoral artery, with advancement of a catheter into the renal artery origin. Contrast material is injected via the catheter and rapid, typically digital, conventional radiographic images are obtained. The renal arterial vessels are well demonstrated, along with nephrographic images of the kidney and views of the venous drainage (Fig. 9–20). Delayed images may be obtained to demonstrate the renal collecting

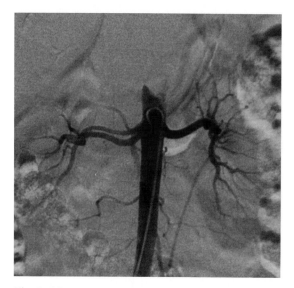

Fig. 9–20. Normal renal arteriogram. The renal arterial system is visualized in detail with spatial resolution superior to that of other techniques. Delayed images can be obtained to show the venous phase and/or the collecting system filling with contrast material.

system. The still superior spatial resolution of angiography permits detailed evaluation of the renal arterial supply and has a small but important diagnostic role in evaluating the small vessels of the kidney for such diseases as vasculitis and fibromuscular dysplasia. The angiogram plays little role in diagnostic evaluation of the renal parenchyma, having been supplanted by cross-sectional imaging techniques. The main role for angiography today, as discussed later, is aiding and guiding interventional techniques.

TECHNIQUE SELECTION

No one ideal technique is yet available for the comprehensive evaluation of the urinary tract. Each technique has strengths and weaknesses that affect their thoroughness and accuracy in evaluating urinary tract diseases and also patient complaints. Importantly, imaging techniques are not necessarily exclusive and in some circumstances are complementary—taken alone they may not provide enough information but together allow a correct clinical diagnosis. A knowledge of which tests are most appropriate for a given clinical question is paramount for physicians involved with the treatment of urinary tract disease. Issues of cost, complications, and time are consequences of an injudicious study choice. However, most importantly, the diagnosis of a patient's condition may not be made unless the appropriate test has been used to evaluate the condition.

The plain radiograph (KUB) has fairly limited use for evaluating the GU tract. Although abnormal "stones, bones, gases and masses" may be demonstrated by the KUB, the utility of the study is limited by its lack of sensitivity and specificity. The KUB can be used effectively to follow radiographically visible stone disease such as assessing stone burden or ureteral stone passage; it is also used to assess stent position, especially ureteral stents. The KUB is also essential as a screening image prior to an IVU or other studies.

Several factors have made the IVU central to evaluating the urinary tract for many decades. The IVU is able to assess both function and morphology, to evaluate the entire urinary tract, and has high spatial resolution allowing for subtle lesion detection, especially of the collecting system. Its lack of sensitivity and specificity for many disorders, however, has always been a shortcoming. For example, less than 50% of renal masses less than 3 cm will be detected on an IVU. Moreover, even mass lesions detected are nonspecific and require further evaluation with additional modalities. However, due to the strengths of the study as discussed earlier, the IVU is still a useful test in certain circumstances. The IVU can be used to evaluate the urinary tract for congenital anomalies, to assess obstruction, and to evaluate for mucosal lesions such as transitional cell carcinoma of the upper tracts or papillary necrosis. As technology has advanced, the IVU has been supplanted in many indications by more modern modalities. The IVU is no longer generally indicated for assessing renal masses, urinary tract infection, trauma, ureteral colic, and vascular diseases, such as renovascular hypertension.

The conventional radiographic techniques that utilize direct contrast injection (retrograde pyelogram, cystogram, and urethrogram) maintain specific roles. For example, the voiding cystogram for evaluating ureteral reflux and the retrograde male urethrogram in suspected urethral injuries remain studies of choice.

Nuclear medicine sustains its role in functional evaluation of the urinary tract, especially the kidney. Renal scintigraphy is an important tool in the assessment of renal function and can be useful in evaluating obstruction, renovascular hypertension, renal transplants or an occasional problematic pseudomass. The ability to quantitatively assess relative renal function is frequently an important issue for the surgeon, determining whether nephrectomy or attempted renal sparing surgery is most appropriate. The nuclear medicine cystogram, due to its high sensitivity and lower radiation dose, remains a key tool in evaluating and following ureteral reflux. The MIBG study plays a unique role regarding the pheochromocytoma. The diagnosis of pheochromocytoma is generally made with a classic clinical history combined with confirmatory biochemical evidence, with MIBG providing a confirmatory diagnosis. More important is the role for MIBG in detecting metastatic or recurrent disease or in locating extra-adrenal lesions. Molecular imaging promises to revolutionize radiology and may play a future role in the urinary tract, especially in oncologic imaging.

The safety and ease of ultrasound solidify the utility of this modality, especially in pediatric imaging. Ultrasound is useful in evaluating the kidney for masses, scarring, and hydronephrosis, especially in children. For example, it is used to exclude postobstructive (hydronephrosis) etiologies of acute renal failure, to evaluate for sequelae (scarring) of vesicoureteral reflux in children, and to diagnose simple renal cysts. Ultrasound is generally the study of choice in evaluating the renal transplant as well. However, the relatively small and sometimes technically limited (in large patients) field of view, lack of visualization of the ureters, and lack of functional assessment limit the use of ultrasound in some circumstances. For instance, in the setting of obstruction ultrasound may demonstrate hydronephrosis, but often the etiology of the obstruction, such as ureteral stone or mass, is not identified. Additionally, solid renal masses are nonspecific on ultrasound and require further imaging, usually with CT. Finally, the ultrasound has only moderate sensitivity for detecting renal stone disease.

As stated in the discussion of techniques, the diagnostic role of conventional angiography continues to diminish as noninvasive CT and MR angiography develop. Patient comfort, speed of examination, diminished complications, and reduced cost all favor noninvasive vascular imaging. However, two main factors allow for a persistent important role for the angiogram. Compared to CT and MR, conventional angiography still has superior resolution for small-vessel evaluation. Thus, diagnostic angiography may play a role in diagnosis of small-vessel renal disease such as polyarteritis nodosa. More importantly, unlike CT and MR, catheter angiography allows for the ability to simultaneously treat abnormalities diagnosed at the time of angiography. For example, although many modalities are used to evaluate for renovascular hypertension, angiography alone allows for treatment at the time of diagnosis as in the patient with fibromuscular dysplasia whose hypertension may be cured with transluminal angioplasty at the time of arteriography. The angiogram is similarly used in acute renal hemorrhage, acute arterial obstruction, and occasional renal mass management. The important and wide-ranging role of the interventional radiologist in the management of urinary tract disease is beyond the scope of this chapter.

MR imaging continues to grow in utility for evaluating the urinary tract and is the study of choice in certain instances. Like CT, MR imaging has excellent spatial and contrast resolution and can evaluate the renal vasculature and renal and adrenal anatomy, characterize lesions, and evaluate the bladder and prostate. Fluid/contrast-enhancing techniques are beginning to allow evaluation of the ureters and the remainder of the collecting system. MR imaging is thus an excellent choice to screen for renovascular hypertension, to stage renal cell carcinoma, to problem solve difficult renal masses, and to evaluate the adrenal mass, and it is gaining favor in evaluation of certain ureteral and bladder conditions. Finally, unlike CT, MR imaging does not use iodinated contrast material and is especially useful in the setting of chronic renal insufficiency when an iodinated contrast agent is contraindicated. However, high cost, limited availability, and contraindications such as pacemakers and claustrophobia limit the widespread use of MR imaging.

Finally, CT is now the examination of choice for urinary tract imaging. From the adrenal glands to the prostate, the CT scan is the preferred study for many GU conditions including trauma, complicated infections, renal and adrenal masses, neoplastic conditions, retroperitoneal disease, renovascular hypertension, and ureteral colic. CT may be the sole study needed or may serve as an adjunct to other studies. With the advent of thinner slices and faster scans, the ability of CT to evaluate the urinary tract mucosa will emerge, and the CT urogram will almost certainly completely replace one of the last indications for the IVU. As discussed previously, CT benefits from wide availability, speed, high contrast and spatial resolution, and patient ease. CT is limited when iodinated contrast is contraindicated or radiation exposure is of special concern such as in pregnancy.

In summary, there is as yet no one comprehensive best imaging examination for the urinary tract; each has its advantages and disadvantages and their value depends on indications of the study. The 25-year-old pregnant woman with hematuria is quite different from the 75-year-old man with the same symptom, and the issue of which imaging modality is best will vary with these considerations. The physician must combine evidence-based knowledge of the accuracy and utility of various studies with the art of medicine, combining science with finesse to ultimately result in the best possible evaluation and care of the individual patient. Finally, although the requesting physician should be well informed about the utility, accuracy, strengths, and weaknesses of available tests, the best care, especially in the fast changing field of imaging, is provided by close consultation between the physician and radiologist.

EXERCISES

EXERCISE 9-1: ADRENAL MASSES

Clinical Histories:

Case 9-1. A 52-year-old male patient presents with vague right abdominal pain. A CT scan of the upper abdomen is shown in Fig. 9–21.

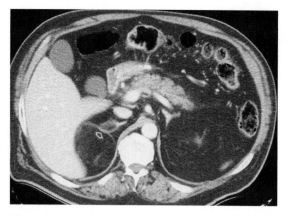

Fig. 9–21.

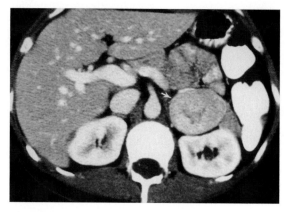

Fig. 9–23.

Case 9-2. A 47-year-old patient with newly diagnosed lung cancer presents to the emergency room for right flank pain. A CT scan without contrast of the upper abdomen is shown in Fig. 9–22.

Case 9-3. A 39-year-old male patient presents with refractory hypertension and episodes of headaches and palpitations. A CT scan with contrast of the abdomen was performed (Fig. 9–23).

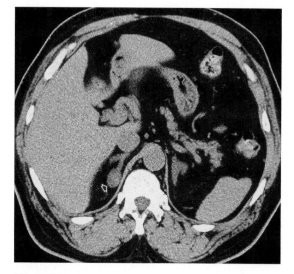

Fig. 9–22.

Questions:

9-1. In Case 9-1, the most likely diagnosis is
  A. adrenal metastasis.
  B. renal angiomyolipoma.
  C. adrenal myelolipoma.
  D. retroperitoneal liposarcoma.

9-2. Regarding Case 9-2, in a patient with a primary neoplasm elsewhere, the most common adrenal mass is
  A. metastasis.
  B. adenoma.
  C. adrenal carcinoma.
  D. acute adrenal hemorrhage.

9-3. In Case 9-3, the most likely diagnosis is
  A. pheochromocytoma.
  B. metastasis.
  C. adrenal cyst.
  D. adrenal lymphoma.

Radiologic Findings:

9-1. In Fig. 9–21, a predominantly fat-containing 5-cm mass (*arrow*) is seen within the right upper abdomen. The mass lies just medial to the right lobe of the liver and is seen to arise from the posterior aspect of the adrenal gland. (*B* is incorrect.) Although subtle, the thin rim of tissue surrounding the lesion demarcates the mass and differentiates it from normal adjacent retroperitoneal fat. The fatty nature of the lesion is confirmed by the low-density tissue within the mass, similar to that of adjacent normal retroperitoneal and subcutaneous fat. Fat is rare within adrenal metastasis. (*A* is incorrect.) Although the retroperitoneal sarcoma is a consideration for a retroperitoneal fatty mass, the adrenal origin of the lesion as well as the fatty nature make adrenal myelolipoma the most likely diagnosis. (*C* is the correct answer to Question 9-1.)

9-2. In this case, the diagnosis or exclusion of metastatic disease is one of the most important issues facing the radiologist in daily practice. The diagnosis of metastatic disease allows appropriate therapy for the patient including the possible prevention of unnecessary surgery. Perhaps more importantly, misdiagnosing a benign lesion as metastatic disease may mistakenly prevent potentially curative therapies such as surgery. In Fig. 9–22, there is a small 2-cm homogeneous mass (*arrow*) arising from the medial limb of the right adrenal gland. Recall that the density of a lesion can be quantitated on CT with Hounsfield unit measurements (although not shown, the Hounsfield unit measurements of the mass was 8 HU). Acute adrenal hematomas are high-density masses on noncontrast CT scan measuring between 50 to 90 HU. (*D* is incorrect.) Adrenal carcinomas are typically large heterogeneous lesions and are quite rare. (*C* is incorrect.) The distinction between adrenal metastasis and adenoma is a critical one. Although there can be overlap in their appearances, certain imaging characteristics of adrenal adenomas allow a confident diagnosis in the vast majority of cases as we will see. Even with a known primary malignancy, however, statistically the most likely etiology of a small adrenal mass is benign adrenal adenoma. (*B* is the correct diagnosis to Question 9-2.)

9-3. In this case, the CT scan of Fig. 9–23 demonstrates a 4-cm solid mass (*arrow*) appearing just anterior to the left kidney. Note the fat plane that clearly shows the mass to not be arising from the kidney. No specific characteristics are seen such as fat. The lesion is denser than surrounding muscle, making a cyst unlikely. (*C* is incorrect.) Adrenal lymphoma is typically bilateral and usually shows diffuse enlargement of the adrenal glands and is typically accompanied by retroperitoneal adenopathy. (*D* is incorrect.) Although metastatic disease can have variable appearances and cannot be radiographically excluded, the lesion is also typical for a pheochromocytoma and, given the clinical history, is the most likely diagnosis. (*A* is the correct answer to Question 9-3.)

Discussion:

The adrenal mass is a common problem for the radiologist and is being incidentally diagnosed more often with the increased use of cross-sectional imaging, especially CT and MR imaging. In fact, the term *adrenal incidentaloma* has been coined for the small adrenal mass identified on imaging studies obtained for other reasons. Although there are many causes of adrenal masses, the most common include benign adenomas, metastatic disease, adrenal carcinoma, and myelolipomas.

The most common adrenal mass is the adrenal adenoma. Although they can be hyperfunctioning and result in clinical syndromes, the majority of adrenal adenomas are not functioning and are diagnosed incidentally. Distinguishing these incidentalomas from more significant pathology is critical. Fortunately, most adenomas have specific characteristics that allow a confident diagnosis. Adenomas are similar to normal adrenal cortical tissue in that they contain a high proportion of cellular lipid material. This results in a low-density appearance and Hounsfield measurements on unenhanced CT. MR imaging can be used to demonstrate the same characteristic by using special imaging sequences that reveal intracellular lipid. This feature along with other characteristics of adenomas, including small size and uniform appearance, allow a confident imaging diagnosis in most patients. The adrenal gland is a common site of metastatic disease, with breast and lung carcinoma being most common sources. The imaging characteristics of metastatic disease are quite variable. Lesions may be unilateral or bilateral, homogeneous or heterogeneous in appearance (Fig. 9–24). The larger the metastatic lesion, generally, the more necrosis and hemorrhage and the more heterogeneous the lesion appears. Smaller lesions tend to be more uniform. Fortunately, metastatic disease does not contain high intracellular lipid-like adenomas and thus do not show the lipid-type imaging changes that characterize adenomas. However, metastatic disease can be indistinguishable from other adrenal pathology, and histologic confirmation with biopsy may be necessary. Pheochromocytomas are an unusual catecholamine-producing tumor that most commonly arises

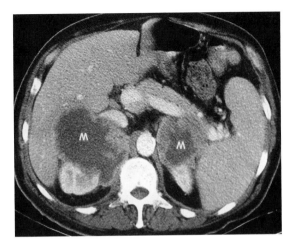

Fig. 9–24. CT scan with contrast shows large bilateral adrenal masses (M) with extensive central necrosis typical of advanced adrenal metastatic disease.

in the adrenal medulla, although in 10% of cases they may arise in an extra-adrenal location. Most tumors arise sporadically although a small percentage occur in certain syndromes. Most pheochromocytomas produce a constellation of symptoms referable to their catecholamine production including hypertension and episodic headaches and palpitations. Most pheochromocytomas appear as a nonspecific adrenal mass on CT. Many of these lesions are fairly homogeneous solid masses. However, necrosis, calcification and cystic formation all occur. On MR imaging, the diagnosis may be suggested by the fairly specific finding of a very bright adrenal mass on T_2-weighted images. Finally, MIBG, which collects in adrenal medullary-type tissue, can provide important information about these tumors. Although they may be used to confirm the diagnosis of a suspected adrenal pheochromocytoma, a more important role for MIBG imaging is in the evaluation of metastatic disease or recurrent tumor or for the localization of extra-adrenal lesions. The MIBG scan typically shows a brightly intense area of activity at the site of the lesion (Fig. 9–25).

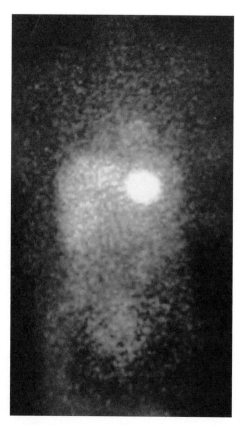

Fig. 9–25. MIBG scan showing an intense area of increased activity within this proven left adrenal pheochromocytoma.

EXERCISE 9-2: RENAL MASS

Clinical Histories:

Case 9-4. A 35-year-old woman with recurrent urinary tract infections underwent an IVU. A single view of the kidneys obtained during this study (Fig. 9–26) reveals another finding.

Case 9-5. A 45-year-old woman presents for a right upper quadrant ultrasound to evaluate for gallbladder disease. An image of her right kidney obtained during this study is displayed in Fig. 9–27 A. A subsequent CT scan of the lesion is shown in Fig. 9–27 B.

Case 9-6. A 55-year-old man presents with a history of right flank pain and hematuria. A CT with contrast of the abdomen is obtained (Fig. 9–28).

Case 9-7. A 60-year-old man presents with left flank pain and hematuria. A CT scan of the abdomen is shown in Fig. 9–29.

Questions:

9-4. In Case 9-4, the most likely diagnosis is a
  A. dromedary hump.
  B. malignant primary renal neoplasm.
  C. simple renal cyst.
  D. metastatic lesion from a distant primary malignancy.

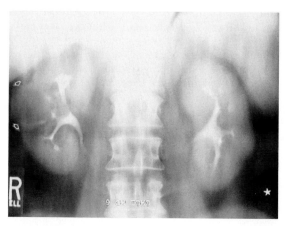

Fig. 9–26.

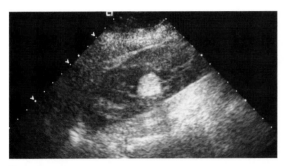

A

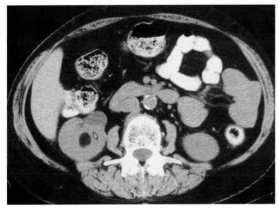

B

Fig. 9–27.

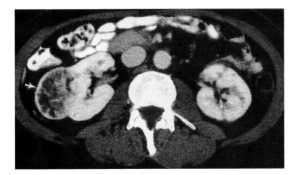

Fig. 9–28.

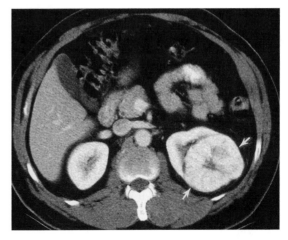

Fig. 9–29.

9-5. Which is *NOT* true of the lesion shown in Fig. 9–27?
A. This lesion contains fat.
B. CT is the key to definitive diagnosis.
C. The ultrasound finding is nonspecific.
D. The lesion shown is the most common malignant renal neoplasm.

9-6. Which of the following is *NOT* true of the lesion seen in Fig. 9–28?
A. This is the most common primary renal malignancy.
B. This lesion is classically associated with the clinical triad of flank pain, hematuria, and a palpable mass.
C. This type of lesion often contains fat.
D. This lesion does enhance with IV contrast.

9-7. How can one differentiate the lesion in Fig. 9–29 from that seen in Fig. 9–28?
A. By CT densitometry.
B. By ultrasonographic characteristics.
C. These lesions cannot be distinguished by imaging.
D. By MR signal characteristics.

Radiologic Findings:

9-4. In this case, the nephrotomogram (Fig. 9–26) shows a well-defined, rounded lesion (*arrows*) that arises from the midportion of the right kidney and causes slight smooth distortion of the renal calyceal morphology. This lesion has no distinguishable wall and has a distinct interface with the adjacent renal parenchyma. The lesion appears lucent compared with normal enhancing renal parenchyma suggesting it may be water density. Therefore, *C* is the correct answer to Question 9-4.

9-5. In this case, the ultrasound image (Fig. 9–27*A*) reveals a hyperechoic lesion with echogenicity similar to that of adjacent perirenal fat. However, this appearance on ultrasound is nonspecific and requires further evaluation and a CT should generally be obtained. The CT

(Fig. 9–27 *B*) shows that this lesion (*arrow*) does indeed contain fat. The presence of definitive fat within a renal mass is virtually pathognomonic for the diagnosis of angiomyolipoma, which is a benign lesion containing fat, blood vessels, and smooth muscle. Therefore, *D* is the correct answer to Question 9-5.

9-6. In this case, the lesion seen in Fig. 9–28 is an inhomogeneous soft tissue mass (*arrow*) arising from the right kidney, which proved to be a renal cell carcinoma. It displays many of the common CT characteristics of renal cell carcinoma including a somewhat rounded shape with irregular margins, enhancement with IV contrast, and inhomogeneity (which can be due to hemorrhage, proteinaceous debris, and even calcifications). Renal cell carcinomas almost never contain fat, making *C* the correct choice.

9-7. In this case, the lesion has imaging and clinical characteristics indistinguishable from renal cell carcinoma. However, the lesion (Fig. 9–29, *arrows*) is an oncocytoma, a benign tumor arising from the distal tubule or collecting ducts. Classically, oncocytoma is often associated with a characteristic central stellate scar. However, scarring can be seen in a renal cell carcinoma as well and these lesions cannot be reliably distinguished by imaging alone, making *C* the correct answer for Question 9-7.

Discussion:

These cases demonstrate examples of the most common renal masses, both benign and malignant. In general, all of these renal masses expand and displace normal renal parenchyma and normal collecting system structures. They are distinguished from infiltrating processes (such as infiltrating neoplasms, infections, and infarctions), which tend to preserve normal renal morphology. Expansile or exophytic renal masses may be seen by plain film, IVU, and cross-sectional imaging (ultrasonography, CT, and MR imaging). In many, but not all cases, the characteristics revealed by various imaging modalities can provide accurate diagnoses and/or determine the need for further follow-up imaging and/or tissue diagnosis.

The simple cyst is the most common renal mass, present in up to 50% of the population older than age 50. They are almost always asymptomatic and discovered incidentally. Although they occasionally may become infected, hemorrhage, or cause pain, their main importance lies in differentiating the lesions from renal tumors. Cysts can be single or multiple, unilateral or bilateral, and vary greatly in size. Pathologically they are thought to be acquired lesions arising from blocked collecting ducts or tubules. They have thin fibrous capsules lined with epithelial cells and contain clear serous fluid. Only the largest of renal cysts may be evident on plain radiographs. On the IVU a renal cyst classically is well defined, lucent, and with imperceptible walls. Although

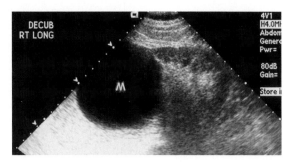

Fig. 9–30. Ultrasonography shows an anechoic mass (M) with no distinguishable wall and enhanced through-transmission of sound.

these findings suggest a cyst, even the most characteristic of lesions are still nonspecific and require further evaluation with additional studies. On cross-sectional imaging modalities, cysts are sharply demarcated from adjacent parenchyma, homogeneous in appearance, rounded with imperceptible walls, and do not enhance with the administration of contrast material. By ultrasonography, a clearly anechoic lesion with no distinguishable wall, a sharp interface with adjacent parenchyma, and enhanced through-transmission of sound can be diagnosed as a simple cyst (Fig. 9–30). By CT, cysts measure near water density and show no enhancement or associated solid components. Lesions meeting the criteria for simple cysts do not require follow-up. Cystic appearing lesions that do not meet the above criteria, such as those with thick enhancing walls, those containing internal debris, or those with calcifications, can represent cystic neoplasms and must be evaluated further by serial imaging and/or by histological diagnosis.

Solid renal masses are of even greater concern. One such lesion, the angiomyolipoma, or AML, is most easily distinguished from other renal masses by the presence of internal fat. These lesions are hamartomous tumors of mesenchymal origin that are usually well differentiated and benign. In addition to fat, they contain sheets of smooth muscle and thick-walled blood vessels. They most commonly occur in middle-aged females. Although these are usually asymptomatic, they are predisposed to spontaneous hemorrhage, especially when large. They can occur as sporadic solitary lesions or in association with tuberous sclerosis, in which case multiple angiomyolipomas are often present. As stated, the demonstration of fat in a renal mass by CT is essentially diagnostic of angiomyolipoma. Although these lesions are benign, they are often removed when greater than 4 to 5 cm due to the increased risk of hemorrhage, and for this reason smaller angiomyolipomas require follow-up to monitor the lesion for growth.

Another benign renal neoplasm that deserves comment is the oncocytoma, which originates from the epithelium of the distal tubules or collecting ducts. A characteristic, although nonspecific, pathologic feature of these lesions is a central stellate scar. They are typically asymptomatic and discovered incidentally, although they may occasionally be associated with a flank mass, pain, or hematuria. On IVU, they present as a solid renal mass, requiring further evaluation. On cross-sectional imaging studies, an oncocytoma appears as a well-defined renal mass. The diagnosis of oncocytoma may be suggested by a central stellate scar. However, even when classic, the imaging characteristics described above cannot be used to reliably differentiate them from malignant renal cell carcinoma and excision is generally indicated. Note that biopsy is generally not recommended because the cytologic appearance of oncocytoma and renal cell carcinoma (RCC) may be indistinguishable.

RCC is the most common primary renal malignancy, originating from the epithelium of the proximal tubule, having a male predominance, and a peak incidence in adults in their 50s. Any renal mass lesion that cannot be definitively identified as one of the benign entities mentioned above must be assumed to be renal cell carcinoma until proven otherwise, most often by tissue diagnosis. Classically, RCC is associated with the clinical triad mentioned above of flank pain, a flank mass, and hematuria, although all three are present in less than 10% of cases. More commonly, these lesions are being discovered incidentally before symptoms have developed. They have the IVU characteristics of a solid renal mass and may demonstrate calcifications in up to 30% of cases. On ultrasound, a nonspecific renal mass is seen. Note that these lesions may be hyperechoic and mimic angiomyolipomas or have central necrosis mimicking the central scar of oncocytomas. By CT, they tend to be rounded, soft-tissue masses, enhancing after the administration of intravenous contrast agent. When small, they are often homogeneous, although when larger they are more heterogeneous frequently with necrosis and often with calcifications. One important role for imaging beyond detecting renal cell carcinoma is evaluating the extent of tumor spread. Renal cell carcinoma can extend locally and invade adjacent soft tissues, especially when large and extensive. In addition, RCC has a propensity to spread into the renal veins and beyond and the extent of this must be delineated prior to surgery. Evidence of enlarged lymph nodes and spread to liver, lung, bones, and other areas, suggesting metastatic disease, should be sought. Surgical excision is the treatment of choice for resectable lesions, making accurate staging to determine surgical candidacy all the more important.

EXERCISE 9-3: STONE DISEASE

Clinical Histories:

Case 9-8. A 36-year-old female presents with acute right flank pain. A CT scan without intravenous contrast is obtained (Fig. 9–31).

Case 9-9. A 41-year-old female presents with a history of vague flank pain and recurrent urinary tract infections. An ultrasound of the right kidney is shown in Fig. 9–32.

Questions:

9-8. In Case 9-8, what is the most likely diagnosis?
- **A.** Acute appendicitis
- **B.** Right ureteral calculus
- **C.** Ruptured aortic aneurysm
- **D.** Pelvic phlebolith

9-9. In Case 9-9, what is the most likely diagnosis?
- **A.** Medullary nephrocalcinosis
- **B.** Cortical nephrocalcinosis
- **C.** Renal tuberculosis
- **D.** Emphysematous pyelonephritis

Radiographic Findings:

9-8. In this case, a CT scan (Fig. 9–31) of the abdomen was obtained without intravenous contrast. Stranding in the fat planes can be seen on the right in the retroperitoneum. Stranding within the fat planes on a CT is a nonspecific finding resulting from many conditions. In

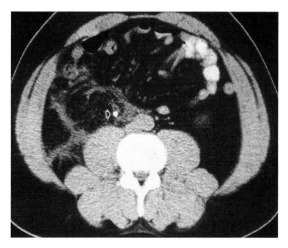

Fig. 9–31.

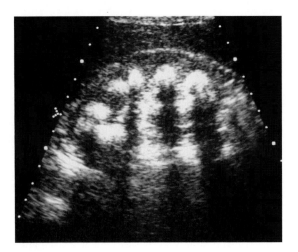

Fig. 9–32.

general, the stranding can be related to inflammation such as recent surgery, infection, or abnormal fluid collections such as blood or urine. Thus, the stranding seen in this case could result from any of the first three listed possible answers. However, within the right ureter is a high-density rounded structure consistent with a ureteral calculus (*arrow*). (*B* is the correct answer to Question 9-8.) Two main parameters that should be noted are the size and location of a stone, because these two factors are directly related to the likelihood of stone passage. Additionally, once the diagnosis of a ureteral stone is made, the radiologist must continue to evaluate the remainder of the scan because additional abnormalities may also exist.

9-9. In this case, a renal ultrasound (Fig. 9–32) demonstrates rounded highly echogenic areas throughout the central parenchyma of the kidney. Several important additional observations include strong uniform shadowing posteriorly from the echogenic areas consistent with sound attenuation and suggesting calcification. Although attenuation of the ultrasound beam occurs with air, such as might occur with emphysematous pyelonephritis, the shadowing in those cases is often "dirty" in appearance, being somewhat inhomogeneous. (*D* is incorrect.) Also, the calcifications are located in the medullary area of the kidney, unlike the cortical location of cortical nephrocalcinosis. (*A* is the correct answer to Question 9-9.)

Discussion:

Suspected stone disease is a common indication for urinary tract imaging. Calcifications occurring in the kidney can be dystrophic, related to abnormal tissue such as within tumors, cysts, or infection. This type of calcification is to be distinguished from nephrocalcinosis

and nephrolithiasis. Nephrocalcinosis refers to the development of calcification within the renal parenchymal, generally unrelated to an underlying renal pathology. Furthermore, nephrocalcinosis should be distinguished from nephrolithiasis, which are stones within the collecting system. Note that nephrocalcinosis and nephrolithiasis may coexist.

Nephrocalcinosis is additionally subdivided into two categories depending on location. That which occurs in the renal cortex is termed *cortical nephrocalcinosis* and that within the medulla is called *medullary nephrocalcinosis.* Cortical nephrocalcinosis is less common and occurs most frequently in the setting of chronic glomerulonephritis or acute cortical necrosis, the latter condition being seen as a result of toxic ingestions such as ethylene glycol or related to acute hypotensive events. Cortical nephrocalcinosis may be detected on plain radiographs or cross-sectional imaging modalities such as CT or ultrasonography. The diagnosis is usually made by demonstrating thin linear bands of calcification at the extreme periphery of the kidney that may extend into the columns of Bertin but should not involve the renal medulla. Medullary nephrocalcinosis is more frequently observed than cortical disease and is most often due to hypercalcemic states such as hyperparathyroidism, renal tubular acidosis, or medullary sponge kidney. On plain films and CT studies, medullary nephrocalcinosis appears as speckled or dense calcifications within the renal medulla, sparring the cortex. In medullary sponge kidney, an anatomic condition of abnormally dilated collecting tubules, the condition may be unilateral or even focal, although medullary nephrocalcinosis from other causes is typically bilateral and diffuse. On ultrasound examination, shadowing echogenic foci are noted within the renal medulla.

Nephrolithiasis (better known to the public as kidney stones) is much more common than nephrocalcinosis. In fact, urinary tract calculi occur in as many as 12% of the population of the United States. Although there are clearly definable causes in some cases (hereditary conditions, metabolic diseases such as gout, certain urinary tract infections, and predisposing anatomic conditions), the vast majority of cases are labeled idiopathic. Many small stones that are located within the intrarenal collecting system are asymptomatic; however, stones that pass into the ureter (ureterolithiasis) may obstruct the urinary tract and result in excruciating pain. Additionally, stones may cause hematuria or be a nidus for recurrent infection. Conventional radiographs have long been used to evaluate stone disease; in fact, the first description of urinary calculi was in April 1896, only a few months after the discovery of the x-rays by Roentgen.

Stones appear as calcific densities on plain radiograph overlying the urinary tract (Fig. 9–33). Urinary tract calculi are variably opaque and visible depending on their

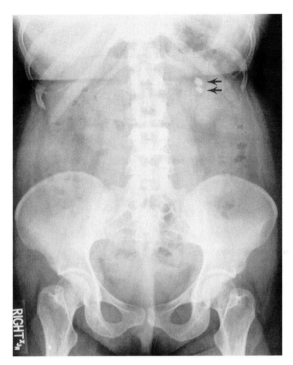

Fig. 9–33. KUB shows two dense 1-cm calcifications (*arrows*) projecting over the mid-portion of the left kidney consistent with nephrolithiasis.

size, composition, and location. The accuracy of conventional radiographs for detecting stones has long been overestimated. Perhaps only 50% of stones are identified prospectively and one can never be certain that an individual calcification on an isolated plain radiograph is within the urinary tract or simply overlies it. Confusing calcifications are many, including phleboliths, arterial calcifications, calcified lymph nodes, and other calcified masses.

The IVU has also long been used to evaluate stone disease. The IVU is used to confirm the location of a calcification in the urinary tract, to identify underlying predisposing issues (diverticula, anomalies), and finally to assess obstruction by stones in the ureter. Stones on ultrasound appear as brightly echogenic structures and often with posterior shadowing. However, not all stones shadow, and because there are many small noncalcific echogenic foci (vessels, fat) normally within the kidney, the accuracy for detecting renal calculi is only moderate with ultrasound. Additionally, ultrasound suffers from its inability to visualize only the most proximal and distal ureters and must rely on nonspecific indirect signs such as hydronephrosis and absent ureteral jets to suggest ureteral stones and obstruction. CT has now moved to

the forefront in the imaging evaluation of stone disease. Virtually all urinary tract stones are dense on CT and show up as bright foci. Even stones as small as 1 mm are usually visible with current CT scanners. Additionally, the entire urinary tract can be visualized on CT without overlapping or obscuring structures. In patients who present acutely with flank pain and are suspected of having ureteral stones, CT has become the study of choice. The diagnosis is confirmed by directly identifying a stone within the ureter. Secondary findings of obstruction may also be identified on CT, helping to confirm the diagnosis. Renal enlargement, perinephric stranding, and dilation of the ureter and intrarenal collecting system are frequently present in ureteral obstruction. One major additional advantage to CT is the ability to identify alternative explanations for the cause of a patient's acute flank pain. In fact, as many as one-third of all patients originally felt to have ureteral stones are shown by CT to have an alternative diagnosis (Fig. 9–34). At this point, MR imaging performs little role in the evaluation of stone disease.

Bladder stones may occur secondary to transport from the ureter or arise de novo. Most cases of bladder stones are secondary to urinary stasis such as occurs with bladder outlet obstruction from neurogenic bladders or prostatic enlargement. The diagnosis of bladder stones is similar to those in the upper urinary tract. Finally, urethral stones occur and in males the vast majority are present as a result of passage from the bladder or above. In women, urethral stones are most frequently the result of urethral diverticula, which can result in urinary stasis and stone formation.

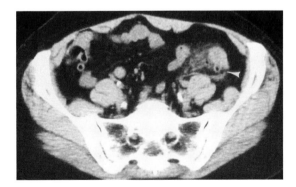

Fig. 9–34. CT scan in a patient who presented with acute left abdominal pain. The study shows inflammatory stranding surrounding the descending colon on the left with a few colonic diverticula evident (*arrowhead*). The findings are typical for diverticulitis. No stones were seen along the course of the ureters.

EXERCISE 9-4: BLADDER MASS

Clinical Histories:

Case 9-10. A 65-year-old male presents with hematuria. A plain film from a urogram is shown in Fig. 9–35.

Case 9-11. A 65-year-old male presents with microscopic hematuria. A coned-down view of the bladder from an IVU is shown in Fig. 9–36.

Questions:

9-10. In Case 9-10, the most likely diagnosis is
    A. squamous cell carcinoma
    B. a bladder stone
    C. transitional cell carcinoma
    D. blood clot

9-11. In Case 9-11, the most likely diagnosis is
    A. squamous cell carcinoma
    B. a bladder stone
    C. transitional cell carcinoma
    D. prostatic hypertrophy

Radiographic Findings:

9-10. In this case, the coned film of the bladder shows a filling defect (*arrow*) in the upper leftward aspect of the urinary bladder. The lesion appears to arise from the bladder mucosa, whereas blood clots and bladder stone have intraluminal locations. (*B* and *D* are incorrect.) Although squamous cell carcinomas are the second most common bladder mucosal neoplasm, they are much less common than transitional cell carcinoma. Additionally they often

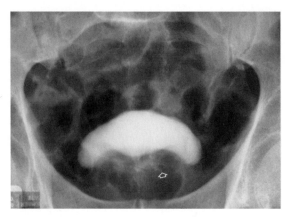

Fig. 9–36.

are associated with calcifications and recurrent infections. (*A* is incorrect.) Thus, the lesion is highly suggestive of transitional cell carcinoma, the most common malignancy of the urinary tract. (*C* is the correct answer to Question 9-10.) Therefore, further evaluation is required. Cystoscopy, which allows for direct visualization and biopsy, remains the gold standard for evaluation of bladder masses.

9-11. In this case, the radiograph shows symmetrical enlarged prostate with calcifications (*arrow*) indenting the bladder base. This is commonly seen in elderly men with benign prostatic hypertrophy. (*D* is the correct answer to Question 9-11.)

Discussion:

Transitional cell carcinoma (TCC) is the most common neoplasm of the urinary collecting system and represents up to 90% of all neoplasms of the bladder itself. Although they can occur anywhere that there is transitional epithelium, from the renal collecting system to the urethra, they are most commonly found in the urinary bladder. This is felt to be due to several factors, including the large surface area of the bladder. In addition, it has been well documented that TCC is associated with numerous chemical carcinogens as well as cigarette smoking. Also, because the bladder acts as a temporary storage site prior to excretion, carcinogens remain in contact with the epithelium of the bladder for a longer period of time than they do with that of the remainder of the urinary tract. Bladder TCC usually presents with hematuria. A transitional cell carcinoma can obstruct the vesicoureteral junction and cause obstructive symptoms as well. Transitional cell carcinoma of the bladder spreads by local invasion and by lymphatic and hematogenous spread. Most are superficial at presentation, with only about 1 in 4 displaying muscle

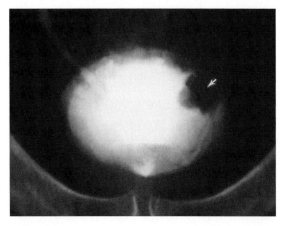

Fig. 9–35.

invasion and 1 in 20 having distant metastases at the time of diagnosis.

Plain radiographs are most often unremarkable in TCC of the bladder, with less than 1% displaying some stippled calcifications. Transitional cell carcinomas can be seen as filling defects in a contrast-filled bladder, particularly when greater than 1 cm in size. Filling defects within the bladder on IVU or cystogram are somewhat nonspecific with considerations including tumor, radiolucent stones, fungus balls, and blood clots. However, transitional cell cancers have a characteristic stippled and frond-like appearance. It is important to note that IVU is fairly insensitive for detecting bladder TCC and a negative study does not exclude the lesion. Ultrasound can show exophytic soft-tissue lesions within the bladder. CT is useful for evaluation of possible bladder masses, because the size of the mass itself, as well as the extent of invasion through the bladder wall into adjacent pelvic structures, can be evaluated. Also important is evaluation of abdominal and pelvic lymph nodes, and post-treatment examination for tumor recurrence. CT generally demonstrates a soft-tissue mass with occasional calcification arising from the bladder wall (Fig. 9–37). Although early, MR imaging may prove useful for evaluating bladder tumor invasion. While the above imaging findings strongly suggest the diagnosis of transitional cell carcinoma, cystoscopy is important to confirm the histologic diagnosis and evaluate for other, smaller lesions not visible on imaging.

Other tumors can be seen in the bladder as well, including malignancies such as squamous cell carcinoma

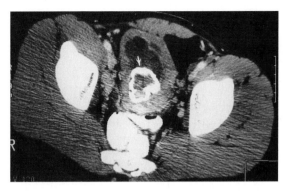

Fig. 9–38. Pheochromocytoma. CT scan at the level of the urinary bladder shows soft-tissue mass (*arrow*) with extensive rounded peripheral calcification within the posterior wall of the bladder.

and adenocarcinoma, uncommon benign lesions, and some inflammatory processes may appear mass-like. Pheochromocytomas can rarely be seen (Fig. 9–38) arising from the bladder wall. Despite the rarity, the classic symptomatology of hypertension, headache, and flushing occurring during micturiction should suggest the diagnosis of a catecholamine-producing tumor. On imaging, these are reported to have characteristic thick, circumferential calcifications.

Benign prostatic hypertrophy is seen in elderly men older than 60 years of age. The hypertrophied prostatic lobes extend upward and impress on the bladder base. However, prostatic hypertrophy can be present without uplifting of the bladder base. During IVU, the enlarged prostate may also elevate the interureteric ridge, causing a "J-shaped" appearance of the distal ureters. However, an enlarged prostate indenting the bladder base is nonspecific because prostate cancer must be included in the differential diagnosis.

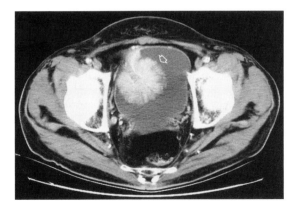

Fig. 9–37. CT scan at the level of the urinary bladder obtained 60 seconds after contrast material administration. CT scan shows an enhancing, pedunculated mass (*arrow*) arising from the anterior wall of the urinary bladder.

BIBLIOGRAPHY

Dalrymple NC. Pearls and pitfalls in the diagnosis of ureterolithiasis by unenhanced helical CT. *Radiographics.* 2000;20:439–447.

Dunnick NR, Korobkin M. Imaging of adrenal incidentalomas: current status. *AJR.* 2002;179:559–568.

Dyer RB, Chen MY, Zagoria RJ. Abnormal calcifications in the urinary tract. *Radiographics.* 1998;16:123–142.

Dyer RB, Chen MY, Zagoria RJ. Intravenous urography: technique and interpretation. *Radiographics.* 2001;21:799–824.

Ornstein DK, Arcangeli CF, Andriole GL. Renal masses: urologic management. *MRI Clin North Am.* 1997;5:1.

Zagoria RJ. Imaging of small renal masses: a medical success story. *AJR.* 2000;175:945.

Gastrointestinal Tract

10

David J. Ott

Imaging of the hollow organs of the gastrointestinal tract began more than a century ago with the use of the heavy-metal salts of bismuth and barium. By the first decades of the 20th century, barium sulfate suspensions emerged as the contrast agent of choice for opacification and radiographic examination of the gastrointestinal tract. By the 1970s, other imaging modalities, including fiber-optic endoscopy and computed tomography (CT), were invented and developed into alternate ways of imaging the hollow gastrointestinal organs.

The emergence of the newer techniques has had a dramatic impact on the use of luminal contrast examinations of the gastrointestinal tract. In this chapter, I describe the current radiographic techniques available to examine the gastrointestinal tract with contrast materials, emphasizing the use of barium suspensions and illustrating normal anatomy. Patient preparation, selection of these techniques and imaging options are also discussed. Finally, a series of exercises will show the most common pathologic lesions of the gastrointestinal tract relative to specific clinical presentations.

TECHNIQUES AND NORMAL ANATOMY

Luminal Contrast Examinations

Luminal contrast examinations of the gastrointestinal tract can be performed with a variety of contrast materials. Barium sulfate suspensions are the preferred material for most examinations. A variety of barium sulfate suspensions are available commercially and many are formulated for specific examinations depending on their density and viscosity. Water-soluble contrast agents, which contain organically bound iodine, are materials used less often and primarily to demonstrate perforation of a hollow viscus or to evaluate the status of a surgical anastomosis in the gastrointestinal tract.

UPPER GASTROINTESTINAL TRACT

The organs that can be examined in the upper gastrointestinal tract include the pharynx, esophagus, stomach, and duodenum. The pharynx and esophagus may be evaluated separately or as part of more complete examinations of the upper gastrointestinal tract. Various techniques are available to assess the function and structure of the pharynx depending on the indications for the examination. Videotape recording of pharyngeal function and filming of pharyngeal structures are often combined for a more thorough examination. Also materials of variable viscosity can be used in patients to determine dietary needs.

Pharyngeal function is complex and is best evaluated with motion-recording techniques that allow slow motion review of the recording. Filming of the pharynx is usually done with the patient in the frontal and lateral positions (Fig. 10–1). In the frontal view, the paired valleculae and piriform sinuses are separated. The lateral view of the pharynx superimposes these structures, but permits better visualization of the base of the tongue, hyoid bone, and epiglottis anteriorly, and the posterior pharyngeal wall and cervical spine posteriorly.

The esophagus, stomach, and duodenum are usually examined together as part of the upper gastrointestinal

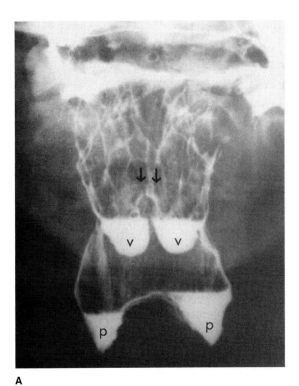
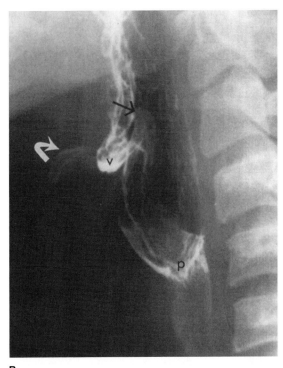

A

B

Fig. 10–1. Frontal **A** and lateral **B** views of the pharynx. In the frontal position, the paired valleculae (v) and piriform sinuses (p) have a symmetric appearance and are seen separately. On the lateral projection, the valleculae (v) and piriform sinuses (p) are superimposed. The upright epiglottis (*arrows both views*) lies posterior to the valleculae, which are posterior to the hyoid bone (*curved arrow*).

series. A variety of radiographic techniques are used and usually combined to optimize the upper gastrointestinal examination. Techniques include observation of esophageal motility, which may also be recorded on videotape; filming of the organs with varying amounts of barium suspension, gas, or air; and obtaining views of the mucosal surfaces. An upper gastrointestinal examination may be done with a moderately dense barium suspension using the natural amount of air present in the upper gastrointestinal tract; this is usually called a *single-contrast upper gastrointestinal series* (Fig. 10–2). Another method involves the use of a high-density barium suspension plus gas-producing crystals and is called a *double-contrast upper gastrointestinal series* (Fig. 10–3).

The esophagus consists mainly of a tubular portion with a bell-shaped termination called the *esophageal vestibule* (Fig. 10–4). The esophagogastric junction normally lies within or below the esophageal hiatus. When the esophagogastric junction lies above the hiatus, hiatal hernia is present, which is the most common

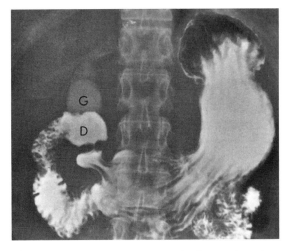

Fig. 10–2. Prone frontal radiograph of stomach and duodenum from a single-contrast upper gastrointestinal examination. The duodenal bulb (D) is attached to the gastric antrum by the pyloric channel. The gallbladder (G) is also opacified from an oral cholecystogram.

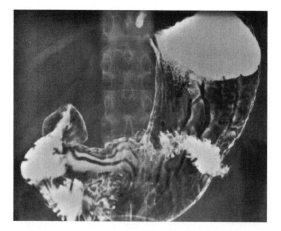

Fig. 10–3. Supine frontal film of the stomach and duodenum from a double-contrast upper gastrointestinal examination in which a high-density barium suspension and gas crystals (CO_2) are used. Compared to the previous figure, the stomach is better distended primarily by the generated gas.

structural abnormality found on the upper gastrointestinal examination. The esophageal mucosal surface has a smooth appearance when distended and shows smooth, thin longitudinal folds when the organ is collapsed. Esophageal peristalsis can be observed by having the patient swallow single volumes of barium suspension.

The stomach has a complex shape that varies considerably depending on the degree of distention. When the stomach is collapsed, the rugal folds are seen prominently and may mimic focal or diffuse gastric disorders. With gastric distention, the rugal folds are flattened and the mucosal surface of the stomach is seen more effectively (Fig. 10–5). A fine reticulated mucosal pattern of the stomach called the *areae gastricae* may be appreciated, especially when high-density barium sus-

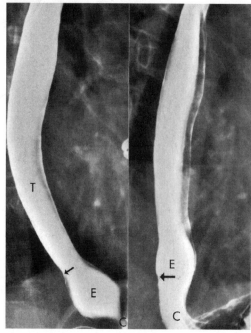

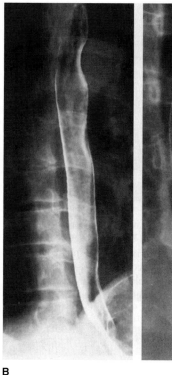

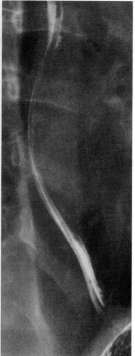

A   B

Fig. 10–4. A Full-column radiograph of the normal esophagus (*left*) with the patient drinking barium rapidly in the prone oblique position. The tubular esophagus (T) joins the esophageal vestibule (E) at the tubulovestibular junction (*arrow*). The lower end of the esophageal vestibule is constricted (C) at the level of the diaphragmatic hiatus. In another patient (*right*), the esophagogastric junction (*arrow*) lies above the level of the diaphragmatic hiatus (C), indicating the presence of hiatal hernia (E = esophageal vestibule). **B** Double-contrast (*left*) and mucosal relief (*right*) films of the esophagus. Multiple radiographic techniques are combined to evaluate the esophagus to optimize the efficacy of the examination.

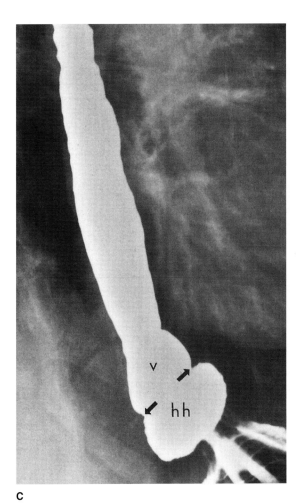

C

Fig. 10–4. **C** Hiatal hernia (hh) protruding above the diaphragmatic hiatus and demarcated from the esophageal vestibule (v) at the esophagogastric junction (*arrows*).

pensions are used. Barium studies of the upper gastrointestinal tract evaluate gastric function poorly; radionuclide gastric emptying studies are more effective for this purpose.

The duodenum is attached to the stomach at the narrow pylorus and consists of the duodenal bulb and the descending and ascending portions, although a horizontal segment is often added (Fig. 10–6). The duodenum terminates at the duodenojejunal flexure, which is attached to the ligament of Treitz. The duodenal bulb has a triangular or heart-shaped appearance normally tapering to the apex of the bulb with its junction with the descending portion. The bulbar mucosal surface is normally smooth. The duodenum assumes a C-shape

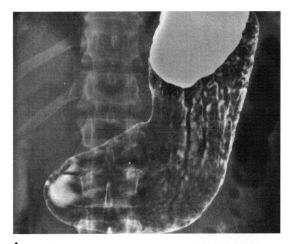

A

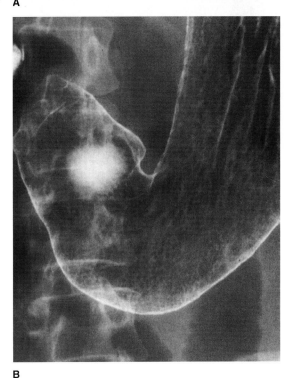

B

Fig. 10–5. **A** Double-contrast radiograph of the stomach with the patient in the supine position. In the body of the stomach, posterior wall rugal folds are seen as long lucent defects surrounded by the barium suspension, and anterior rugal folds are etched by a coating of the contrast material. **B** Double-contrast film of the lower gastric body and antrum. The areae gastricae are seen as a fine reticulated pattern, especially in the lowest portion of the stomach, while larger and linear rugal folds are present in the upper gastric body.

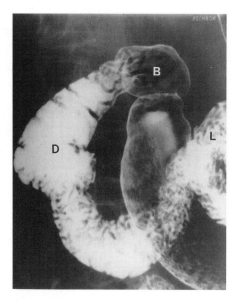

Fig. 10–6. Radiograph of the duodenum showing the duodenal bulb (B) attached to the gastric antrum. The descending duodenum (D) extends from the apex of the bulb to the inferior duodenal flexure. The horizontal and ascending portions of the duodenum terminate at the duodenojejunal junction (L), which is attached to the ligament of Treitz.

configuration within the upper abdomen and the mucosal folds have a circumferential and symmetric appearance throughout its length.

SMALL INTESTINE

The radiographic examination of the small bowel evaluates the mesenteric portion of the organ, which consists of the jejunum and ileum. The following three methods can be used to examine the small intestine: (1) peroral small bowel series, (2) enteroclysis, and (3) various retrograde techniques. The peroral small-bowel series is most commonly used and is often done immediately following an upper gastrointestinal series. The patient ingests 16 to 24 ounces of an appropriate barium suspension and serial films of the abdomen are obtained in a timely order (Fig. 10–7). In addition, smaller films with pressure on the abdomen (i.e., compression) are used to separate and visualize all of the loops of the small bowel; the entire small bowel, including the terminal ileum, is filmed in this fashion.

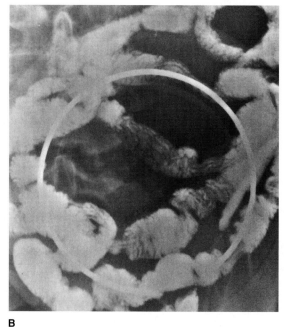

A   B

Fig. 10–7. A Large film of the abdomen from a peroral small-bowel examination with the entire small intestine opacified with barium suspension. On the left side of the abdomen, the jejunum shows a more typical "feathery" pattern of the mucosal folds compared to the ileum, which is smaller in caliber and has fewer folds in the right lower abdomen. The appendix (*arrow*) is also visualized. **B** Compression film (balloon paddle is identified by the circular metallic ring) of the small bowel from a peroral examination with separation and clear visualization of the small bowel loops.

Enteroclysis is an intubated examination of the small intestine and can be done by several techniques. The small intestine is intubated by a nasal or oral route with a small-bore enteric tube, which is directed with fluoroscopic guidance into the distal duodenum or proximal jejunum (Fig. 10–8). In the single-contrast method, a dilute barium suspension is used and allowed to flow into the small bowel by gravity. Other techniques include the use of a dense and more viscous barium suspension along with water, air, or a methylcellulose solution to produce a double-contrast effect. Compared to the peroral small-bowel examination, the enteroclysis techniques permit better control of small-bowel distention and more exact visualization of small-bowel loops.

Retrograde examination of the small bowel involves filling of the organ from the opposite direction. A variety of techniques are used depending on the patient's anatomy (Fig. 10–9). Reflux of the small intestine through the ileocecal valve can be done as part of a barium enema. If the patient has an ileostomy, various devices can be introduced into the ostomy site and a barium suspension instilled directly.

The length of the mesenteric small bowel in adults averages about 20 feet but varies considerably among individuals. The jejunum comprises just over one-third of the length and the ileum the remainder although no discrete transition is seen between the two segments. The normally distended small bowel has a caliber of 2 to 3 cm being slightly larger more orad in the jejunum. Depending on the degree of distention, the mucosal folds (valvulae conniventes) may have a feathery appearance or may be transversely oriented across the intestinal lumen with more complete distention. The mucosal folds are more numerous in the jejunum and gradually decrease in number and size in the ileum.

LARGE INTESTINE

The radiographic examination of the large bowel evaluates the entire organ from the rectum to the cecum. Reflux of barium suspension into the ileum and the appendix, if present, occurs commonly. As with the upper gastrointestinal examinations, the colon can be evaluated by the following techniques: (1) single-contrast

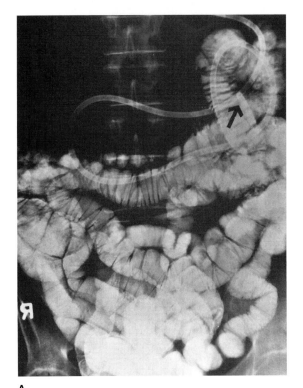

A

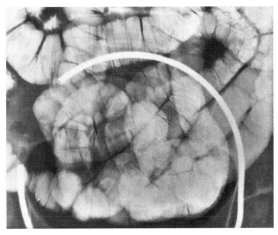

B

Fig. 10–8. **A** Large film of the abdomen from an enteroclysis examination of the small intestine. The small bowel is intubated with the tip of the tube (*arrow*) in the jejunum. Compared to the peroral examination, the small-bowel loops are distended more fully, causing the mucosal folds to assume a transverse orientation. **B** Compression film (ring of balloon paddle) of the small-bowel loops in the pelvis with the patient in a prone position. Although the loops are overlapped, the "see-through" effect using a dilute barium suspension permits their clear visualization.

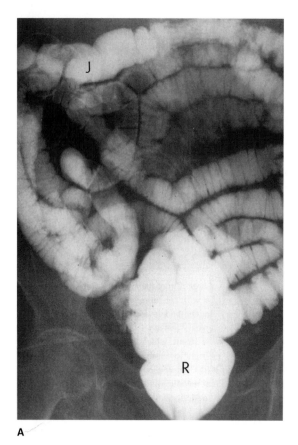

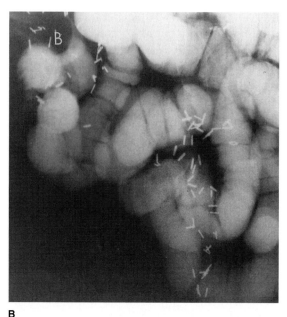

A

B

Fig. 10–9. **A** Reflux examination of most of the small intestine from a barium enema (R = rectum) in a patient following a right hemicolectomy for colon carcinoma who presents with rectal bleeding. The ileocolic junction (J) is located in the right upper abdomen. **B** Reflux study of the small bowel via an ileostomy in a patient following total colectomy for ulcerative colitis. A Foley catheter was inserted into the ileostomy and the balloon (B) distended with air to prevent leakage at the cutaneous site.

barium enema or (2) double-contrast barium enema. Both examinations require insertion of a rectal tip for installation of the examining materials. The single-contrast barium enema is performed using a low-density barium suspension that flows into the colon through the rectal tip (Fig. 10–10). Small films with abdominal pressure applied to the area of interest are exposed as each segment of the colon is opacified. A series of larger films is also obtained with the patient in various frontal and oblique positions.

The double-contrast barium enema is performed with a special rectal tip that allows installation and removal of a dense, viscous barium suspension and also installation of air. The double-contrast effect is produced by the combined use of the barium suspension and the

air (Fig. 10–11). As with the single-contrast method, all segments of the colon are examined with the patient in various positions, and both large and small films are obtained.

The large intestine consists of the rectum, sigmoid colon, descending colon, splenic flexure, transverse colon, hepatic flexure, ascending colon, and cecum. The length of the colon varies considerably among adults depending mainly on the length and redundancy of the sigmoid colon and the colic flexures. The colon varies in caliber depending on the location and degree of luminal distention. The mucosal surface has a smooth appearance and the colonic contour is indented by the haustra, which are less numerous in the descending portion of the colon (Fig. 10–12). The rectal valves of Houston are

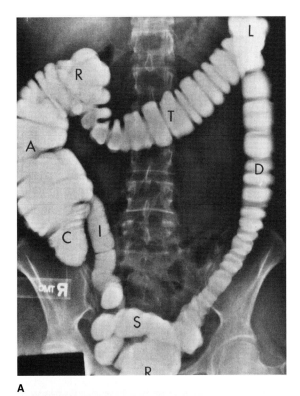

A

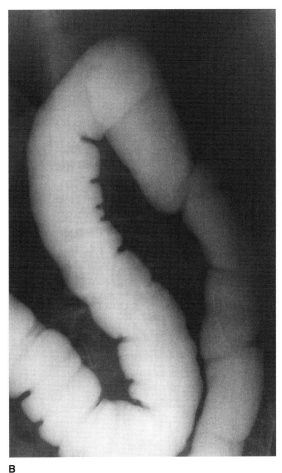

B

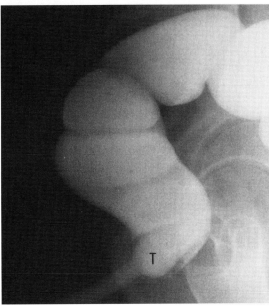

C

Fig. 10–10. **A** Large film of the abdomen from a single-contrast barium enema with the patient in the supine position. The rectum (R), descending colon (D), left colic flexure (L; also known as the splenic flexure), transverse colon (T), right colic flexure (R; also known as the hepatic flexure), ascending colon (A), and cecum (C) are visualized. The sigmoid colon (S) and colic flexures are not seen well in this position and require additional films. The terminal ileum (I) has refluxed from the colon. **B** Left colic flexure from a single-contrast examination with the patient turned to the right shows clear separation of the upper descending colon and distal transverse colon. **C** Lateral radiograph of the rectum from a single-contrast barium enema. The rectal tip (T) is located in the lower rectum. The valves of Houston are seen as transverse folds crossing the lumen of the rectum.

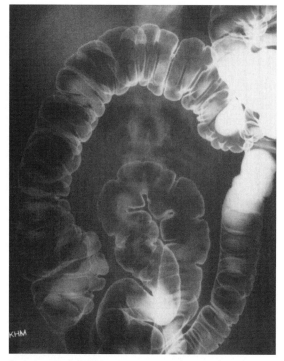

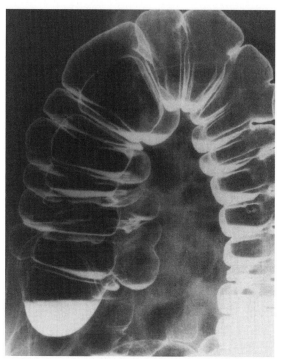

A

B

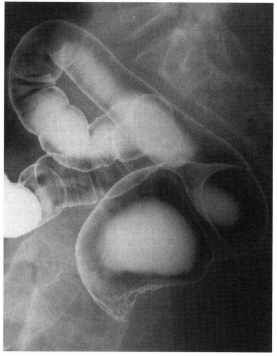

Fig. 10–11. **A** Large film of abdomen from a double-contrast barium enema with the patient in the supine position. The double-contrast effect is produced by coating the mucosal surface of the colon with a moderately dense, viscous barium suspension and distending the organ with air; a specially designed enema tip is needed for the examination. **B** Double-contrast radiograph of the right colic or hepatic flexure with the patient turned toward the left with separation of the ascending colon and proximal transverse colon to improve visualization. **C** Double-contrast film of the rectum and a portion of the sigmoid colon with the patient in a lateral position.

C

often seen, especially on the double-contrast barium enema. The ileocecal valve has a variety of appearances and may appear large if infiltrated with fat, mimicking a neoplasm.

Other Imaging Modalities

Fiber-optic gastrointestinal endoscopy and newer cross-sectional imaging techniques have affected the number and types of traditional luminal contrast examinations performed on the gastrointestinal tract. In addition to

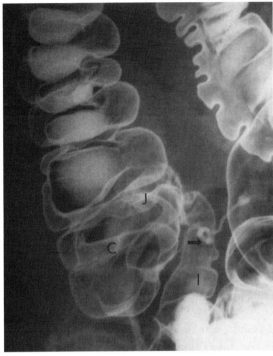

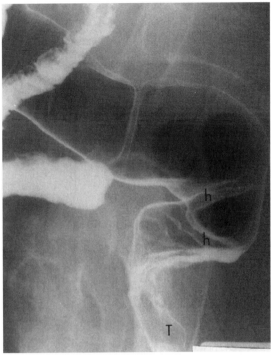

A **B**

Fig. 10–12. **A** Double-contrast view of the right side of the colon showing the cecum (C), ileocecal junction (J), refluxed terminal ileum (I), and the appendix (*arrow*). The multiple haustrations of the colon are seen well and are produced by the teniae coli. **B** Double-contrast appearance of the rectum with the patient in the lateral position. The valves of Houston (h) are shown clearly. The rectal tip (T) has migrated into the anal canal.

endoscopy, these newer techniques include CT imaging, abdominal ultrasound, and magnetic resonance (MR) imaging. Each of these imaging modalities is briefly discussed next to illustrate their impact on luminal contrast radiology.

ENDOSCOPY

Upper gastrointestinal endoscopy visualizes the mucosal surfaces of the esophagus, stomach, and duodenum. The pharynx and often the distal portion of the duodenum are not evaluated. Also, endoscopy does not assess functional abnormalities of these organs. The major advantage of endoscopy compared to barium examination of the upper gastrointestinal tract is a better demonstration of milder inflammatory processes, such as small peptic ulcers and erosions.

Endoscopy of the mesenteric portions of the small intestine has become possible in recent years. A variety of enteroscopes are available to examine the jejunum and ileum; however, complete endoscopic visualization

of the entire mesenteric small intestine remains difficult. Enteroscopy can be used to evaluate patients with diffuse small-bowel disease, especially if biopsy is needed, and those with unexplained gastrointestinal bleeding.

Colonoscopy is both a diagnostic and therapeutic modality. Inflammatory and neoplastic diseases of the colon are evaluated accurately. Biopsies can be obtained when needed. Using various techniques, the majority of colonic polyps can be removed through the colonoscope. When compared to the barium enema, colonoscopy is associated with more complications, including colonic perforation, and a higher cost and mortality.

CT IMAGING

CT imaging of the chest and abdomen can portray the various organs of the gastrointestinal tract. Mucosal disease, such as ulcers, and small neoplasms will not be shown with this imaging modality. Larger gastrointestinal neoplasms, thickening of the walls of the hollow organs, and extrinsic processes can be detected with CT imaging. A major role of CT scanning, especially in the esophagus and colon, is staging malignancy of these organs. In the colon, for example, CT examination is used for initial staging, especially of distant metastases, and for evaluation of recurrence following surgery. Recurrent masses appearing after surgery may also be biopsied percutaneously.

ABDOMINAL ULTRASOUND

Abdominal ultrasound has had an increasing impact on evaluation of the hollow organs of the gastrointestinal tract, although their location and gas interfering with transmission of sound remain technical problems. An ultrasound can be used to assess for inflammatory disorders, such as acute appendicitis. Endoluminal ultrasound using blind probes or those attached to an endoscope have been used in the upper gastrointestinal tract and the colorectum to stage malignancy.

MAGNETIC RESONANCE IMAGING

MR imaging is the newest modality developed for cross-sectional imaging of the body and nearly all organ systems can be evaluated with this technique. MR imaging of the hollow organs of the gastrointestinal tract is being used to evaluate and stage malignancies, especially of the esophagus and rectum, and also to assess inflammatory and obstructive bowel disease.

TECHNIQUE SELECTION

Patient Preparation

Preparation of the patient is needed for contrast examinations of the gastrointestinal tract and varies with the organ system being evaluated. The upper gastrointestinal tract and small bowel require minimal preparation when compared to the colon. No preparation is needed if only the pharynx and esophagus are being examined. For an upper gastrointestinal or small-bowel examination, the patient should have nothing orally after midnight or the next morning preceding the radiographic study. Fluid and food in the stomach and small intestine degrade the examination by interfering with good mucosal visualization and causing artifacts that may mimic disease. Also, if patients are to have other imaging examinations that may introduce fluid into the upper gastrointestinal tract, such as an abdominal CT study in which oral contrast material is used, the examinations must be scheduled on separate days.

Preparation for the barium enema examination is much more complicated and more strenuous on the patient, but must be performed properly to obtain an accurate evaluation of the colon by this method. The presence of even small amounts of residual stool in the large bowel may mimic colonic disease, or a filling defect in the colon may be passed off as stool but be a neoplasm. Various colonic preparations have been recommended and usually combine the use of dietary changes, oral fluids, and several cathartics the day preceding the barium enema examination. At our institution, the standard preparation includes (1) a 24-hour clear liquid diet, (2) oral hydration, (3) a saline cathartic (e.g., magnesium citrate) in the afternoon, (4) an irritant cathartic (e.g., castor oil) in the early evening, and (5) a tap-water cleansing enema the morning of the radiographic examination 30 to 60 minutes before the barium enema is performed. Other cleansing options for the colon can be suggested if indicated clinically; for example, magnesium containing cathartics is avoided in patients with renal failure.

Specific Contrast Examinations

A variety of radiographic techniques are available to examine the gastrointestinal tract. Selection of an appropriate technique will depend on the clinical indications for the examination, the efficacy of the various techniques, and the age and physical condition of the patient being examined. Indications and efficacy of the specific contrast examinations will be emphasized. However, the age and physical condition of the patient will also impact on the quality of the study performed and on the types of examinations that can be done optimally.

UPPER GASTROINTESTINAL TRACT

The main indications for radiographic examination of the upper gastrointestinal tract include dysphagia, odynophagia, chest pain, pyrosis, suspicion of esophageal varices, dyspepsia, upper gastrointestinal bleeding, and evaluation of obstruction. Dysphagia may be of oropharyngeal or esophageal origin; a modified examination of the oral cavity and pharynx may be required in some patients. The most common diseases causing these symptoms that may be diagnosed by radiographic evaluation are esophageal and gastric malignancies, reflux esophagitis and peptic stricture, infectious esophagitis, lower esophageal mucosal ring, and peptic ulcers and erosions of the stomach and duodenum. Many of these diseases are illustrated and discussed in the chapter exercises.

The efficacy of the radiographic examination of the upper gastrointestinal tract depends on the quality of the study performed and on the types of diseases being evaluated. The diseases that are detected most effectively include malignancies, peptic stricture, esophageal mucosal ring, moderate to severe reflux and infectious esophagitis, and peptic ulcers that are greater than 5 mm in size regardless of their location. The limitations of this examination are detection of milder inflammations, such as mild reflux esophagitis or early infectious esophagitis, small gastric and duodenal ulcers (i.e., less than 5 mm), and erosive gastritis and duodenitis.

SMALL INTESTINE

The more specific indications for small-bowel examination include gastrointestinal bleeding that is not localized to the other organs of the gastrointestinal tract, diarrhea or more specifically steatorrhea, inflammatory bowel disease, intestinal obstruction, intra-abdominal malignancy, and abdominal fistula. The small bowel is not a common site for disease and less specific symptoms, such as vague abdominal pain, do not warrant performance of a small-bowel study. The diseases that can cause small-bowel bleeding include Meckel's diverticulum, Crohn's disease, ischemic enteritis, and primary and secondary neoplasms. Small-bowel obstruction is usually due to adhesions, external hernias, or intrinsic or extrinsic neoplasms. Rare diseases leading to malabsorption, such as sprue, are other considerations.

As with the upper gastrointestinal tract, the efficacy of radiographic examination of the small bowel depends on the type and quality of examination performed and on the types of diseases being evaluated. The enteroclysis examination is often preferred for evaluating small-bowel obstruction or potential focal lesions of the small intestine, such as Meckel's diverticulum. Most diseases of the small bowel are detected effectively by a properly performed radiographic examination. Limitations of small-bowel studies, depending on the thoroughness of the examination done, include early inflammatory disease, localization of obstruction, focal structural disease, and peritoneal adhesions. Many of these diseases are illustrated and discussed in the chapter exercises.

LARGE INTESTINE

The major indications for radiographic examination of the colon are rectal bleeding, suspicion of inflammatory bowel disease, question of neoplastic disease, and evaluation of colonic obstruction. The most common diseases causing colonic bleeding are diverticulosis, idiopathic colitis, larger colonic polyps and carcinoma, and ischemic colitis. Common causes of colonic obstruction include diverticulitis, colonic malignancy, volvulus of the large bowel, and extrinsic disorders, especially pelvic malignancy invading the rectosigmoid region of the colon. Most of these diseases are illustrated and discussed in the chapter exercises.

As with the other studies discussed, the efficacy of the radiographic examination of the large bowel depends on the type and quality of examination performed and on the diseases being evaluated. The diseases that are detected most effectively include diverticular disease and its complications, more severe forms of idiopathic and ischemic colitis, larger colonic polyps (i.e., greater than 1 cm in size), and colonic carcinoma. The limitations of the barium enema include smaller colonic polyps less than 1 cm in size and mild inflammatory bowel disease, although the double-contrast examination of the colon is more effective than the single-contrast method in detecting these more subtle abnormalities. An important limitation of the barium enema in older patients is evaluation of vascular malformations. Finally, regarding active gastrointestinal bleeding, the radiographic examination can demonstrate lesions that may be bleeding but will not localize the exact site of bleeding; angiography or radionuclide studies are needed to pinpoint the bleeding site.

EXERCISES

EXERCISE 10-1: DYSPHAGIA

Clinical Histories:

Case 10-1. A 55-year-old man presents with intermittent dysphagia for solid food (Fig. 10–13).

Case 10-2. A 35-year-old woman who recently developed dysphagia presents with gastroesophageal reflux symptoms (Fig. 10–14).

Case 10-3. A 65-year-old man presents with both dysphagia and odynophagia (Fig. 10–15).

Case 10-4. A 30-year-old woman presents with dysphagia and regurgitation (Fig. 10–16).

Questions:

10-1. What is the most likely cause for the symmetric narrowing at the lower end of the esophagus (*arrows*) in Fig. 10–13?
  A. Carcinoma of the esophagus
  B. Peptic esophageal stricture
  C. Lower esophageal mucosal ring
  D. Achalasia of the esophagus
  E. None of the above

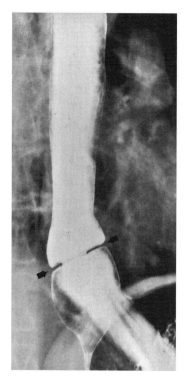

Fig. 10–13.

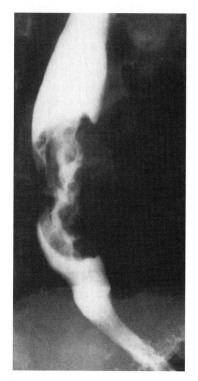

Fig. 10–15.

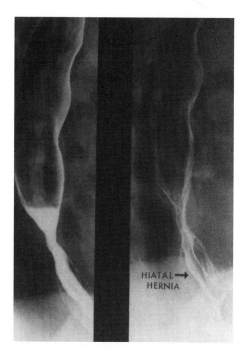

HIATAL →
HERNIA

Fig. 10–14.

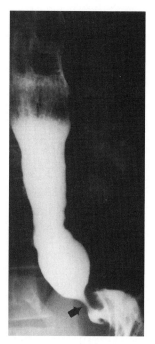

Fig. 10–16.

10-2. In Case 10-2, the smooth stricture above the hiatal hernia in Fig. 10–14 is most likely due to
   A. candida esophagitis.
   B. reflux esophagitis.
   C. herpetic esophagitis.
   D. caustic esophagitis.
   E. esophageal malignancy.

10-3. The most likely cause of the focal, irregular esophageal narrowing shown in Fig. 10–15 is
   A. squamous cell carcinoma.
   B. adenocarcinoma.
   C. carcinoma complicating Barrett's esophagus.
   D. benign peptic stricture from reflux disease.
   E. stricture from caustic esophagitis.

10-4. In Case 10-4 (Fig. 10–16), aperistalsis of the esophagus was present associated with smooth narrowing at the lower end of the esophagus (*arrow*) suggesting
   A. stricture in Barrett's esophagus.
   B. stricture in sclerodermic esophagus.
   C. peptic stricture from reflux esophagitis.
   D. achalasia of the esophagus.
   E. secondary achalasia due to gastric carcinoma.

Radiologic Findings:

10-1. Figure 10–13 shows a smooth, symmetric, thin annular narrowing at the lower end of the esophagus, which is a lower esophageal mucosal ring. (*C* is the correct answer to Question 10-1.)

10-2. Figure 10–14 demonstrates a smooth, tapered narrowing in the lower esophagus associated with a hiatal hernia that is typical for a peptic stricture. (*B* is the correct answer to Question 10-2.)

10-3. Figure 10–15 shows an annular, irregular squamous cell carcinoma of the esophagus. (*A* is the correct answer to Question 10-3.)

10-4. Figure 10–16 represents idiopathic achalasia. (*D* is the correct answer to Question 10-4.)

Discussion:

Dysphagia is a frequent indication for radiographic examination of the esophagus. The most common esophageal causes of dysphagia are shown in the case presentations in this exercise.

The lower esophageal mucosal ring is an acquired thin, annular membrane of unknown cause that demarcates the esophagogastric junction and is a sign of hiatal hernia. More importantly, the mucosal ring is probably the most important cause of solid food dysphagia seen in adults. Fifty years ago, Schatzki described the association of the mucosal ring, which often bears his name, with dysphagia and determined that the prevalence of dysphagia related to the caliber of the ring. Rings greater than 20 mm in diameter cause symptoms rarely; those less than 14 mm in caliber are nearly always symptomatic, whereas mucosal rings 14 to 20 mm in diameter cause dysphagia in about half of patients. The mucosal ring is best detected radiographically and the use of a solid bolus, such as a portion of a marshmallow, optimizes detection of these rings and verifies the structure as a cause of dysphagia (Fig. 10–17).

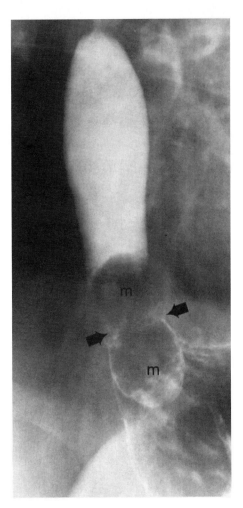

Fig. 10–17. Patient with solid food dysphagia and a mucosal ring measuring 16 mm in caliber. A one-half portion of a marshmallow (m) impacted at the level of the ring (*arrows*) and reproduced dysphagia.

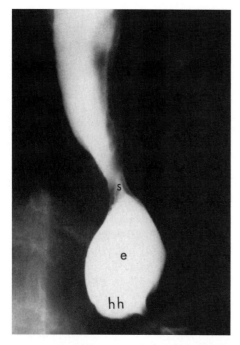

Fig. 10–18. Peptic stricture (s) above a normal intervening segment of esophagus (e) associated with a small hiatal hernia (hh). The esophagus between the hernia and stricture was lined by columnar epithelium at endoscopic examination.

Peptic stricture of the esophagus is a complication of reflux esophagitis and is the second most common benign cause of dysphagia. Reflux strictures typically occur at the esophagogastric junction and are associated with a hiatal hernia in virtually all patients. Peptic strictures show a variety of morphologic appearances from a smooth, tapered appearance to an annular configuration that may resemble a mucosal ring. Irregularity of the stricture margin may also be seen and must be differentiated from an esophageal malignancy. Barrett's esophagus is another complication of gastroesophageal reflux disease and is suggested radiographically when a peptic stricture is located above the esophagogastric junction (Fig. 10–18).

Squamous cell carcinoma is the most common primary malignancy of the esophagus accounting for about 70% to 80% of esophageal cancers. The usual appearance of this malignancy is a focal, irregular narrowing with abrupt upper and lower margins, which rarely mimics a peptic stricture. Squamous cell carcinomas of the esophagus occur in older patients who often have a history of tobacco and alcohol abuse; this malignancy may also be multifocal and associated with similar

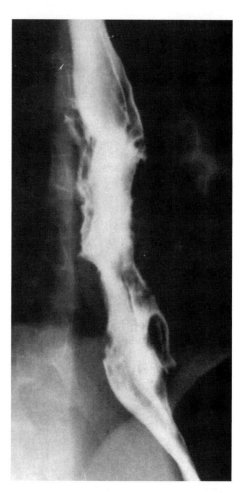

Fig. 10–19. Patient with Barrett's esophagus complicated by an irregular adenocarcinoma, which may be difficult to distinguish from the accompanying changes of esophagitis and stricture. Adenocarcinoma occurs in about 5% to 10% of patients who have Barrett's esophagus and periodic endoscopic surveillance is usually recommended.

lesions in the upper aerodigestive tract. Adenocarcinoma of the esophagus is now seen more frequently and has increased dramatically in incidence recently. It is typically found in conjunction with Barrett's esophagus (Fig. 10–19).

Idiopathic achalasia is a primary motility disorder of the esophagus of unknown cause that presents with dysphagia, regurgitation, and weight loss occasionally. The findings on esophageal manometry include total absence of primary esophageal peristalsis and a dysfunctional lower esophageal sphincter (i.e., failure of

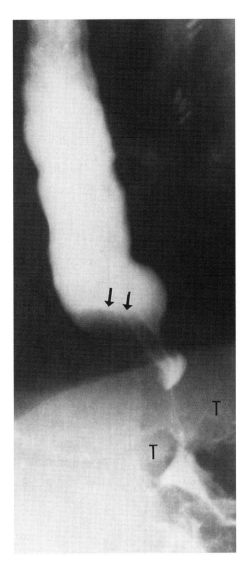

Fig. 10–20. An older patient with an abrupt onset of dysphagia and odynophagia. Narrowing and mass effect (*arrows*) are present at the lower end of the esophagus, which was also aperistaltic. These changes mimic idiopathic achalasia, but the tumor mass (T) in the proximal stomach proved to be a gastric adenocarcinoma causing secondary achalasia.

relaxation). The radiographic features mirror the manometric findings; aperistalsis is observed and the lower end of the esophagus has a smooth, tapered or "beak-like" appearance. In achalasia, hiatal hernia is an uncommon observation, which is usually seen in patients with peptic stricture or scleroderma of the esophagus.

An important differential diagnosis is secondary achalasia due to an infiltrative gastric adenocarcinoma (Fig. 10–20); patients are usually older and have a more abrupt onset of symptoms, which often includes odynophagia.

EXERCISE 10-2: UPPER GASTROINTESTINAL BLEEDING

Clinical Histories:

Case 10-5. A 28-year-old man presents with epigastric pain and occult blood in his stools (Fig. 10–21).

Case 10-6. A 63-year-old woman presents with epigastric pain, weight loss, and anemia (Fig. 10–22).

Case 10-7. A 32-year-old alcoholic man presents with severe epigastric pain and hematemesis (Fig. 10–23).

Case 10-8. A 44-year-old woman presents with postprandial epigastric pain that is relieved with meals and occult blood in the stools (Fig. 10–24).

Questions:

10-5. What is the most likely cause of the gastric lesion (*arrowhead*) shown in Fig. 10–21?
   A. Malignant gastric ulcer
   B. Gastric diverticulum
   C. Lymphoma of the stomach
   D. Polypoid carcinoma of the stomach
   E. Benign gastric ulcer

10-6. In Case 10-6, an irregular polypoid lesion (Fig. 10–22, *arrows*) projects into the anterior body of the stomach (F, fundus; A, antrum; D, duodenal bulb). What is the least likely cause of this abnormality?
   A. Benign gastric ulcer
   B. Polypoid gastric carcinoma
   C. Gastric lymphoma
   D. Leiomyosarcoma of the stomach
   E. Secondary malignancy of the stomach

10-7. What is the best possibility for the nodular appearance of the duodenal bulb in Fig. 10–23 (P, pylorus)?
   A. Duodenal ulcer
   B. Erosive duodenitis
   C. Brunner's gland hyperplasia
   D. Duodenal carcinoma
   E. Multiple swallowed olive pits

10-8. In Case 10-8, what is the most likely cause of the barium collection seen in Fig. 10–24 in

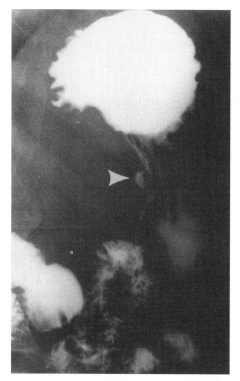

Fig. 10–21.

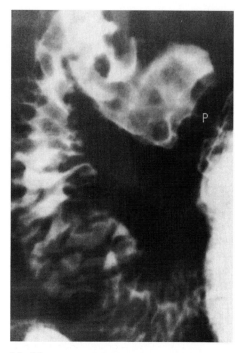

Fig. 10–23.

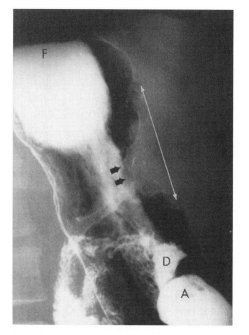

Fig. 10–22.

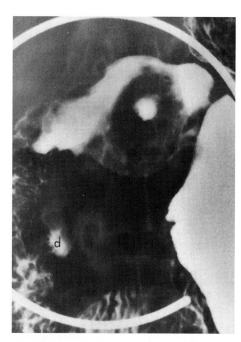

Fig. 10–24.

the duodenal bulb with the patient in the prone position (d, duodenal diverticulum)?

A. Benign duodenal ulcer on posterior wall
B. Malignant duodenal ulcer
C. Benign duodenal polyp
D. Benign duodenal ulcer on anterior wall
E. None of the above

Radiologic Findings:

10-5. Figure 10–21 shows a small, smooth collection of barium projecting from the lesser curvature of the stomach associated with a lucent collar at the neck of the collection. This combination of findings indicates a benign gastric ulcer. (*E* is the correct answer to Question 10-5.)

10-6. Figure 10–22 shows an irregular, polypoid mass arising from the anterior wall of the stomach and projecting into the gastric lumen. A neoplasm of the stomach is the most likely cause, which in this patient was a primary adenocarcinoma. A benign gastric ulcer is the least likely explanation. (*A* is the correct answer to Question 10-6.)

10-7. Figure 10–23 is a close-up film of the duodenal bulb and loop. Multiple nodules, some with central collections of barium, are present within the bulb and represent duodenal erosions. (*B* is the correct answer to Question 10-7.)

10-8. Figure 10–24 demonstrates a smooth collection of barium within the central portion of the duodenal bulb, which was an anterior wall duodenal ulcer. (*D* is the correct answer to Question 10-8.)

Discussion:

Many causes of upper gastrointestinal bleeding can be detected on a radiographic examination of this portion of the gastrointestinal tract. As illustrated in the cases of this exercise, gastric or duodenal erosions and ulcers and carcinoma of the stomach are the most important causes.

The radiographic features that suggest a benign gastric ulcer include (1) projection from the lumen of the stomach, (2) smooth lucent line (Hampton's line) or collar (as in this case) at the neck of the ulcer, (3) normal rugal folds that radiate to the edge of the ulcer collection, and (4) complete and permanent healing of the ulcer on repeat radiographic or endoscopic examination of the stomach. If at least two or more of these findings are present, a confident radiographic diagnosis of benign gastric ulcer is possible. A malignant gastric ulcer, which represents a small minority of all ulcers seen in the stomach, is suggested when the collection of barium within the ulcer is irregular and projects within the gastric lumen (i.e., within a neoplastic mass), a smooth line or

collar at the ulcer margin is not present, or the rugal folds are nodular and terminate abruptly (Fig. 10–25). Lack of healing of a gastric ulcer is not a specific sign of malignancy.

Adenocarcinoma is the most common primary malignancy of the stomach but has decreased in incidence recently in the United States. Gastric adenocarcinoma comprises about 95% of all primary malignancies of the stomach; lymphoma and leiomyosarcoma account for most of the remainder although Kaposi's sarcoma is seen in patients with AIDS. The morphologic types of gastric carcinoma include ulcerative forms, polypoid or nodular lesions (Fig. 10–26), and focal or diffuse infiltrative processes, especially if the histologic subtype is a scirrhous carcinoma (Fig. 10–27). A properly performed radiographic examination of the stomach will detect virtually all gastric carcinomas.

Erosions in the stomach and duodenum are a common cause of upper gastrointestinal bleeding. Because these erosions may be few in number and small in size, endoscopic examination of the stomach and duodenum is more sensitive in their detection than radiologic evaluation. The radiographic features of duodenitis depend on the severity of the disease and include thickening and nodularity of the duodenal folds or the presence of erosions, which appear as punctate collections of barium centered on a nodule. Brunner's gland hyperplasia may have an appearance similar to duodenitis but erosions are not seen and patients may not be symptomatic. Carcinoma of the duodenal bulb is extremely rare and does

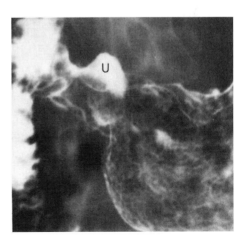

Fig. 10–25. An irregular ulcer (U) in the gastric antrum that does not project from the lumen nor show a smooth ulcer margin. Fixed antral narrowing is present and the mucosal surface is distorted adjacent to the ulcer. An ulcerated adenocarcinoma of the stomach was found on biopsies from an endoscopic examination.

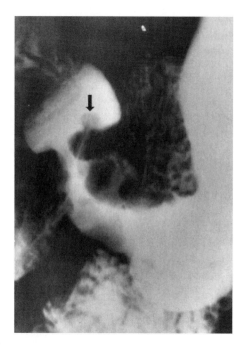

Fig. 10–26. Nodular fixed narrowing of the gastric antrum associated with a small nodule at the base of the duodenal bulb (*arrow*). Although gastric carcinoma would be a likely possibility, lymphoma of the stomach was diagnosed at surgery.

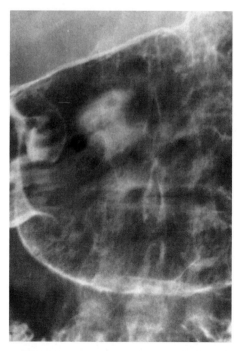

Fig. 10–28. Close-up double-contrast radiograph of the gastric antrum showing multiple erosions, which appear as small nodular defects with a central punctate collection of barium. On endoscopic examination, erosions present as reddened nodules with a central yellow exudate at the site of mucosal disruption.

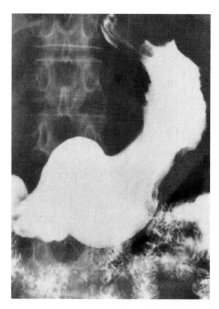

Fig. 10–27. Mildly irregular narrowing of the proximal half of the stomach due to scirrhous carcinoma, which may mimic benign narrowing of the stomach.

not typically enter the differential diagnosis of inflammatory lesions in this anatomic region. Gastric erosions also appear as nodular defects, usually within the antrum of the stomach (Fig. 10–28).

Approximately 95% of duodenal ulcers occur within the duodenal bulb and have about an equal distribution on the anterior and posterior walls of the duodenum. The remaining 5% of duodenal ulcers are located near the apex of the bulb. On radiographic examination, a duodenal ulcer is seen as a round or oval collection of barium that should maintain a fixed size and shape on multiple images of the collection; inconsistent collections of barium, often seen in the duodenal fornices or at the apex or in the presence of bulbar deformity, may be mistaken for an active ulcer. Anterior wall duodenal ulcers are best visualized with the patient in the prone position (as in this case), whereas posterior wall ulcers are seen well with the patient supine (Fig. 10–29). As with duodenal carcinomas, polyps in the bulb are rare and would appear as lucent filling defects and not as a collection of barium.

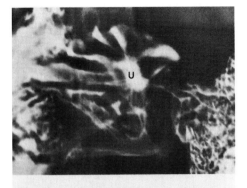

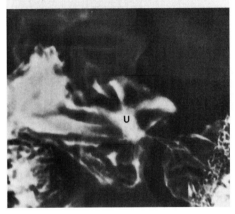

Fig. 10–29. Two views of the duodenal bulb with the patient in a supine position demonstrating a posterior wall ulcer (u) with radiating folds extending around the circumference of the barium collection.

EXERCISE 10-3: SMALL-BOWEL BLEEDING

Clinical Histories:

Case 10-9. A 24-year-old woman presents with intermittent abdominal pain, diarrhea, and anemia (Fig. 10–30).

Case 10-10. A 48-year-old man presents with rectal bleeding but no other symptoms (Fig. 10–31).

Case 10-11. A 72-year-old woman presents with sudden onset of abdominal pain and occult rectal bleeding (Fig. 10–32).

Case 10-12. A 58-year-old man presents with abdominal pain, anemia, and intermittent rectal bleeding (Fig. 10–33; used with permission from Chen MYM, Zagoria RJ, Ott DJ, Gelfand DW. *Radiology of*

the Small Bowel. New York: Igaku-Shoin; 1992).

Questions:

10-9. Radiographic examination of the small bowel in Case 10-9 (Fig. 10–30) is suggestive of which disease?
A. Crohn's disease
B. Tuberculosis
C. Whipple's disease
D. Lymphoma of small bowel
E. Small bowel metastases

10-10. In Fig. 10–31, which is the most likely explanation of the saccular structure (x) seen in the distal small bowel?
A. Normal loop of small bowel
B. Large ulcer of small bowel
C. Meckel's diverticulum
D. Ulcerated small-bowel malignancy
E. None of the above

10-11. What is the least likely explanation for the diffuse fold thickening in the central small bowel in Fig. 10–32?
A. Ischemic enteritis
B. Small-bowel hemorrhage
C. Radiation enteritis
D. Small-bowel edema
E. Malignancy of small bowel

10-12. Select the least likely possibility to explain the irregular, ulcerated small bowel lesion shown in Fig. 10–33.
A. Leiomyosarcoma
B. Ulcerated lymphoma
C. Metastatic ulcerated mass
D. Large benign small-bowel ulcer
E. Ulcerated adenocarcinoma

Radiologic Findings:

10-9. Figure 10–30 demonstrates multifocal segments of narrowed and nodular small bowel most consistent with Crohn's disease. (*A* is the correct answer to Question 10-9.) Tuberculosis could appear similar but is rare and neoplasms of the bowel typically present as focal masses.

10-10. Figure 10–31 shows a smooth, saccular structure of the distal small bowel that proved to be a Meckel's diverticulum. (*C* is the correct answer to Question 10-10.) Benign ulcers of the small bowel are rare and ulcerated malignancies are usually irregular in appearance.

10-11. Figure 10–32 illustrates a long segment of small bowel of normal caliber with smooth thickening of the folds (i.e., valvulae conniventes). This appearance is usually due to submucosal infiltration of fluid (i.e., edema) or blood and can be seen in all of the choices given

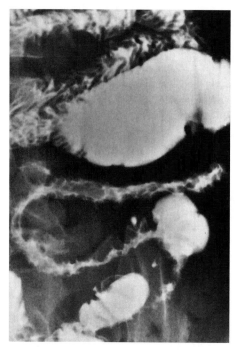

Fig. 10–30.

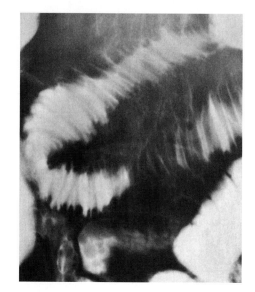

Fig. 10–32.

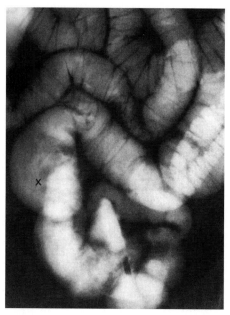

Fig. 10–31.

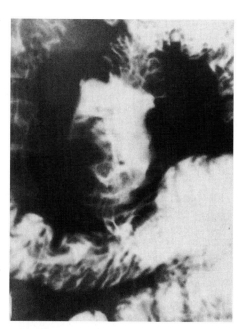

Fig. 10–33.

except a small-bowel malignancy. (*E* is the correct answer to Question 10-11.) This patient had ischemic enteritis.

10-12. Figure 10–33 shows an expansible ulcerated mass of the small bowel, which usually occurs in an ulcerated malignancy of various histologic types including metastatic neoplasms. In this case the cause was lymphoma. As stated previously, benign small-bowel ulcers are extremely rare. (*D* is the correct answer to Question 10-12.)

Discussion:

Small-bowel bleeding and obstruction can be caused by a wide assortment of diseases, some of which may present with both signs. Crohn's disease and ischemia of the small bowel are likely the two most common causes in younger and older patients, respectively.

Crohn's disease is an inflammatory disorder of the gastrointestinal tract of unknown etiology. The small bowel and the ileocecal region are the most common sites of involvement. Crohn's disease may affect a single segment, often the terminal ileum, or multiple areas of the small bowel with normal intervening loops (i.e., skip segments). The involved bowel is usually narrowed with a nodular mucosal surface due to criss-crossing transverse and longitudinal ulcerations. Deeper ulcerations can progress to sinus tracts and fistulas with adjacent organs. Marked narrowing of the bowel lumen from inflammation and spasm may mimic stricture and cause partial small-bowel obstruction (Fig. 10–34).

Meckel's diverticulum is one of the most common anomalies of the gastrointestinal tract and occurs in about 2% to 3% of the general population. The diverticulum is usually asymptomatic and is found incidentally, but may be a cause of intestinal bleeding if the structure contains ulcerated ectopic gastric mucosa. When shown on radiographic examination of the small bowel, especially using the enteroclysis technique, Meckel's diverticulum appears as a changeable saccular outpouching along the antimesenteric border of the bowel within a short distance from the terminal ileum. A rarer complication of a Meckel's diverticulum is inversion into the lumen of the small bowel with subsequent obstruction (Fig. 10–35).

Ischemic disease of the small intestine can be caused by nonobstructive hypoperfusion of the organ or result from thrombotic or embolic vascular disease. The radiographic findings are variable depending on the extent and severity of the underlying process and its duration and promptness of treatment. Small-bowel dilatation from ileus or narrowing due to spasm and submucosal edema and hemorrhage are opposite appearances that may be seen. Submucosal infiltration of the small bowel as seen in ischemic enteritis may occur in other disorders and have identical appearances; small-bowel hemorrhage related to anticoagulants,

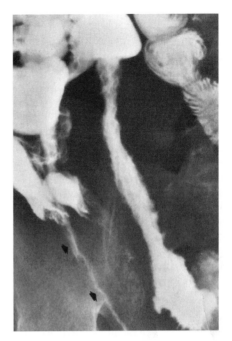

Fig. 10–34. Another patient with Crohn's disease of the distal small bowel with narrowing and irregularity of several segments. The terminal ileum (*arrows*) is severely narrowed, an appearance called the "string-sign," which is often due to spasm.

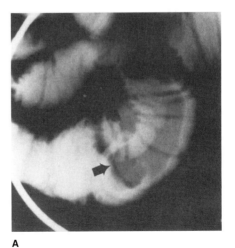

A

Fig. 10–35. **A** Inverted Meckel's diverticulum (*arrow*) appearing as a luminal filling defect in the ileum and simulating a polypoid neoplasm.

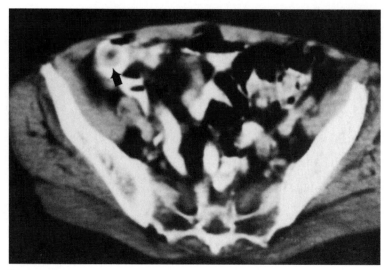

Fig. 10–35. B CT of inverted Meckel's diverticulum showing a central fat density (*arrow*). (Used with permission from Chen YM et al. Inverted Meckel's diverticulum. *Comput Med Imaging Graph.* 1989;13:477–479.)

B

trauma, hemophilia, or vasculitis from many causes are other considerations; also, edematous conditions (e.g., hypoproteinemia and heart or renal failure) are further causes. Small-bowel ischemia may resolve spontaneously or progress to perforation; stricture is a late complication (Fig. 10–36).

Primary small-bowel neoplasms are rare. Benign neoplasms of the small intestine are less often symptomatic compared to malignancies. Adenomas, lipomas, and leiomyomas are the most common benign neoplasms but comprise only 60% of the benign total due to a large number of miscellaneous lesions. Symptomatic small-bowel neoplasms are usually malignant and nearly all are adenocarcinoma, lymphoma, carcinoid tumor, or leiomyosarcoma. These malignancies, along with metastatic neoplasm to the small bowel (Fig. 10–37), show a wide spectrum of

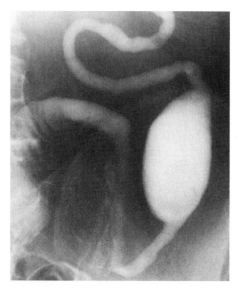

Fig. 10–36. Another patient with small-bowel ischemia that progressed to diffuse multifocal strictures, evident by smooth narrowings of the intestine.

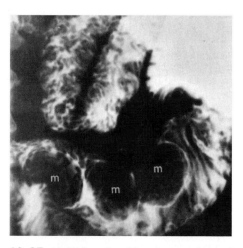

Fig. 10–37. Multiple polypoid metastases (m) to the small bowel from a malignant melanoma. (Used with permission from Chen MYM, Zagoria RJ, Ott DJ, Gelfand DW. *Radiology of the Small Bowel.* New York: Igaku-Shoin; 1992.)

appearances varying from polypoid and ulcerated masses (as in this case) to multifocal and infiltrative processes.

EXERCISE 10-4: SMALL-BOWEL OBSTRUCTION

Clinical Histories:

Case 10-13. A 38-year-old woman with previous abdominal surgery presents with distention of the abdomen and vomiting (Fig. 10–38).

Case 10-14. A 68-year-old man presents with abdominal pain, vomiting, and mass in the abdomen on physical examination (Fig. 10–39; used with permission from Chen MYM, Zagoria RJ, Ott DJ, Gelfand DW. *Radiology of the Small Bowel.* New York: Igaku-Shoin; 1992).

Case 10-15. A 56-year-old man has epigastric pain and nausea (Fig. 10–40; used with permission from Chen MYM, Zagoria RJ, Ott DJ, Gelfand DW. *Radiology of the Small Bowel.* New York: Igaku-Shoin; 1992).

Case 10-16. A 42-year-old woman with a gynecologic malignancy presents with abdominal distention and vomiting (Fig. 10–41).

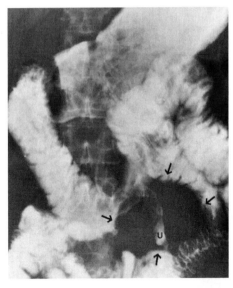

Fig. 10–39.

Questions:

10-13. Barium enema (Fig. 10–38; C, cecum) with reflux into a normal terminal ileum (TI) shows a small-bowel obstruction (*arrow*) and a lucent band (*connected arrows*) that are most likely due to

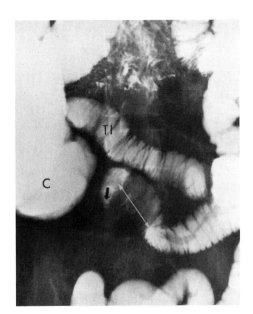

Fig. 10–38.

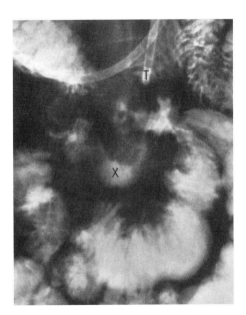

Fig. 10–40.

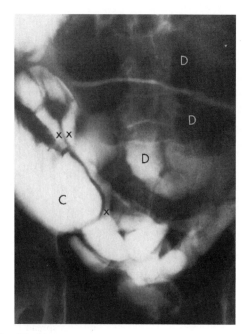

Fig. 10–41.

A. ileocolic intussusception.
B. obstructing adhesions.
C. Meckel's diverticulum.
D. small-bowel volvulus.
E. polypoid malignancy.

10-14. What is the least likely cause for the small-bowel mass (*arrows*) with central ulceration (u) causing obstruction in Fig. 10–39?
A. Lymphoma of the small bowel
B. Ulcerated leiomyosarcoma
C. Leiomyoma with central ulceration
D. Metastatic mass with ulceration
E. Adenocarcinoma of small bowel

10-15. Enteroclysis (Fig. 10–40; T, tip of tube) shows an angulated small-bowel mass (X) in the proximal jejunum. What is the least likely cause for this mass?
A. Carcinoid tumor
B. Metastatic mass
C. Small-bowel lymphoma
D. Polypoid mass with intussusception
E. Adenocarcinoma of small bowel

10-16. Barium enema (Fig. 10–41; C, cecum) shows reflux in the small bowel with multiple areas of ileal narrowing (x) and proximal small-bowel dilatation (D) that are most likely due to

A. peritoneal adhesions.
B. primary small-bowel carcinomas.
C. peritoneal metastases.
D. radiation enteritis.
E. small-bowel intussusceptions.

Radiologic Findings:

10-13. Figure 10–38 shows obstruction of the distal small bowel with a lucent band caused by adhesions. (*B* is the correct answer to Question 10-13.)

10-14. Figure 10–39 demonstrates an ulcerated small-bowel mass that is most likely a primary or metastatic malignancy. Lymphoma and leiomyosarcoma (the diagnosis in this patient) would be the most likely considerations. Adenocarcinoma usually does not present as a large mass displacing adjacent small-bowel loops. (*E* is the correct answer to Question 10-14.)

10-15. Figure 10–40 displays an angulated mass in the proximal small bowel that is most likely a primary or metastatic neoplasm. Adenocarcinoma would more likely cause focal narrowing and may have this appearance, although in this patient a carcinoid tumor was found at surgery. A polypoid neoplasm with intussusception would present with focal dilatation. (*D* is the correct answer to Question 10-15.)

10-16. Figure 10–41 shows obstruction of the distal small bowel at multiple sites on a reflux examination. With a history of gynecologic malignancy, peritoneal metastases with serosal implants causing obstruction is a common occurrence. (*C* is the correct answer to Question 10-16.)

Discussion:

The most common causes of small-bowel obstruction are adhesions, hernias, and primary or secondary neoplasms of the small intestine. External hernias (e.g., inguinal canal) causing bowel obstruction are seen less often in recent decades and internal hernias remain uncommon.

Peritoneal adhesions are most often the cause of small-bowel obstruction in adults. Previous abdominal surgery is the usual explanation for development of peritoneal adhesions. The patient described in Case 10-13 had previous abdominal surgery and presented with suspected small-bowel obstruction on plain films of the abdomen. A nasogastric tube had been placed and injection of contrast material into the stomach caused further vomiting; also, dilution of the contrast material in a dilated, fluid-filled jejunum degraded the examination. Consequently, a barium enema was performed with the main purpose being to reflux the distal small bowel to the level of obstruction, which was accomplished. Whether to perform an antegrade (i.e., peroral examination or enteroclysis) or retrograde study of the small bowel in suspected obstruction is not easily decided and is often based on clinical correlation and findings on plain films of the abdomen. Focal small-bowel obstruction is diagnosed on contrast examination by demonstrating an area of caliber transition from dilated to normal caliber bowel. If angulated loops are seen at a caliber transition in the absence of a mass effect, adhesions are a likely cause of the obstruction (Fig. 10–42).

Small-bowel malignancies were discussed briefly in the previous exercise. Adenocarcinomas of the small bowel occur most often in the duodenum and jejunum and are much less common in the ileum. The morphologic appearance of adenocarcinomas of the small intestine consists of polypoid, ulcerative, stenosing, and infiltrative forms, which are similar to their counterparts in the stomach and colon. Primary lymphomas of the small bowel are a heterogeneous group of tumors and controversy persists regarding definition of primary and secondary forms of this neoplasm. Lymphomas may involve any level of the small intestine but are most common in the ileum; the gross pathologic patterns include nodular or polypoid masses, constricting lesions that resemble carcinoma, or a more diffusely infiltrative process.

Leiomyosarcoma and carcinoid tumor are the other two primary malignancies seen in the small bowel. Leiomyosarcomas (Fig. 10–43) usually occur as single lesions and are most often found in the jejunum and ileum. Pathologically, this tumor typically presents as a polypoid lesion with an intraluminal and extramural component; a bulky, irregular mass is common and ulceration with central necrosis can occur. Carcinoid tumors arise from enterochromaffin or similar-type cells and more than 90% originate in the gastrointestinal tract. Most carcinoid tumors of the small bowel are located in the ileum. Their radiologic appearances reflect their broad pathologic morphology and may present as single or multiple polypoid lesions or as focal stenosis leading to partial obstruction; angulation and kinking of bowel loops may occur with a desmoplastic reaction and cause a mass that is best seen on cross-sectional imaging (Fig. 10–44).

Secondary malignancies involving the small bowel are more common than the primary types. The three routes of secondary malignancy that can spread to the small intestine include (1) hematogenous metastases, with carcinoma of breast, lung, and melanoma being the most common; (2) intraperitoneal seeding of tumor

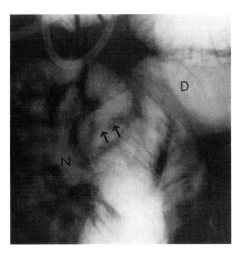

Fig. 10–42. Enteroclysis examination (tube in upper left corner) in a patient with suspected small-bowel obstruction. Caliber transition is seen between dilated (D) and normal (N) bowel with angulated loops (*arrows*). At surgery, peritoneal adhesions were found to be the cause of the obstruction.

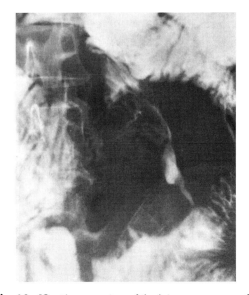

Fig. 10–43. Close-up view of the leiomyosarcoma of the small bowel in Case 10-14 that better demonstrates the central ulceration often seen in this malignancy. (Used with permission from Chen MYM, Zagoria RJ, Ott DJ, Gelfand DW. *Radiology of the Small Bowel.* New York: Igaku-Shoin; 1992.)

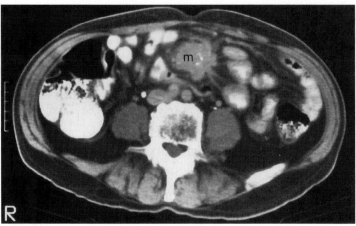

Fig. 10–44. CT image of the carcinoid tumor in Case 10-15 shows a mass (m) associated with the neoplasm that was not appreciated fully on the contrast examination of the small bowel. (Used with permission from Chen MYM, Zagoria RJ, Ott DJ, Gelfand DW. *Radiology of the Small Bowel*. New York: Igaku-Shoin; 1992.)

from elsewhere within the abdomen; and (3) direct contiguous invasion of bowel (most often seen with pelvic malignancies). Carcinoma of the cervix, endometrium, and ovary often affect the distal small bowel by intraperitoneal seeding or direct invasion; the colon may

also be involved and radiographic evaluation of these patients may be best performed with a barium enema with one goal being reflux into the ileum (Fig. 10–45*A,B*).

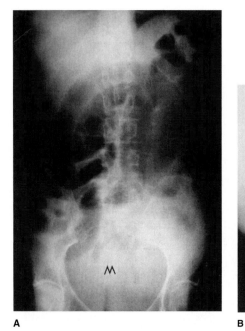

A

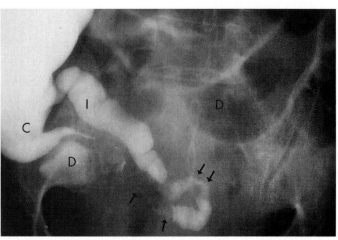

B

Fig. 10–45. A A 55-year-old woman with advanced ovarian carcinoma presents with a large pelvic mass (M) and small-bowel distention on plain film of the abdomen. **B** Barium enema in this patient did not show colonic involvement, but reflux into a normal caliber terminal ileum (I) demonstrated angulated obstruction (*arrows*) of the small bowel due to the pelvic malignancy with more proximal dilated (D) bowel loops (C, cecum).

EXERCISE 10-5: COLONIC BLEEDING

Clinical Histories:

Case 10-17. A 52-year-old woman presents with intermittent bright red rectal bleeding (Fig. 10–46).

Case 10-18. A 64-year-old man presents with melena and right-sided abdominal pain (Fig. 10–47).

Case 10-19. A 34-year-old woman presents with bloody diarrhea and tenesmus (Fig. 10–48).

Case 10-20. A 74-year-old man presents with cardiac disease and abrupt onset of hematochezia (Fig. 10–49).

Questions:

10-17. In Fig. 10–46, what is the most likely cause of the large polypoid lesion (*arrows*) in the sigmoid colon of this patient?
   A. Annular carcinoma
   B. Benign lipoma
   C. Polypoid carcinoma
   D. Pedunculated benign adenoma
   E. Hyperplastic polyp

10-18. The irregular, focal narrowing in the ascending colon of this patient (Fig. 10–47) represents
   A. polypoid carcinoma.
   B. annular carcinoma.

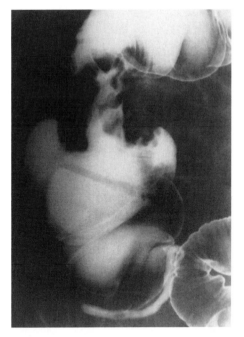

Fig. 10–47.

   C. inflammatory stricture.
   D. surgical anastomosis.
   E. large lipoma.

10-19. In Fig. 10–48, the double-contrast radiograph of the rectosigmoid region suggests what disease?
   A. Ischemic colitis
   B. Pseudomembranous colitis
   C. Lymphogranuloma venereum
   D. Crohn's colitis
   E. Ulcerative colitis

10-20. The irregular narrowing of the descending colon in Fig. 10–49 is most likely due to

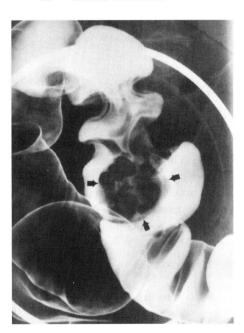

Fig. 10–46.

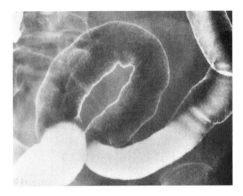

Fig. 10–48.

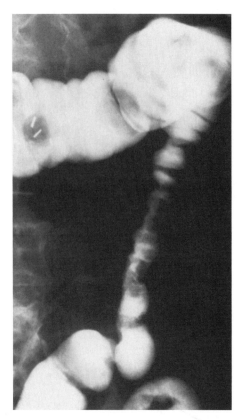

Fig. 10–49.

- **A.** ischemic colitis.
- **B.** granulomatous colitis.
- **C.** ulcerative colitis.
- **D.** amebic colitis.
- **E.** pseudomembranous colitis.

Radiologic Findings:

10-17. Figure 10–46 shows a large, lobulated (i.e., irregular surface) polypoid mass of the sigmoid colon, which was a carcinoma. (*C* is the correct answer to Question 10-17.)

10-18. Figure 10–47 demonstrates an annular carcinoma of the ascending colon. (*B* is the correct answer to Question 10-18.)

10-19. Figure 10–48 shows a diffuse, irregular mucosal pattern (i.e., granularity) of the rectosigmoid colon most consistent with ulcerative colitis. (*E* is the correct answer to Question 10-19.)

10-20. Figure 10–49 represents a patient with ischemic colitis. (*A* is the correct answer to Question 10-20.) Granulomatous colitis (i.e., Crohn's disease) would be a second choice, but unlikely at the age and with the presentation of this patient.

Discussion:

Rectal bleeding can result from a multitude of abnormalities throughout the gastrointestinal tract. In this exercise, the more important colonic causes of rectal bleeding are illustrated. Another common cause of rectal bleeding is diverticular disease of the colon, which can be shown on barium enema examination. A further consideration, especially in older patients, is vascular malformations (e.g., angiodysplasia) of the right side of the colon, which is not seen on the barium enema study. In general, contrast studies of the gastrointestinal tract can detect many abnormalities that may be a source of bleeding but cannot determine if the lesion is bleeding actively; angiography and radionuclide studies are helpful to demonstrate bleeding.

The two most common polypoid lesions of the colon are the hyperplastic and neoplastic polyps. Most hyperplastic polyps are less than 5 mm in diameter, are sessile and smooth, and may resemble small neoplastic polyps of similar size. Neoplastic polyps have a broad pathologic spectrum, which includes (1) benign adenomas (tubular, tubulovillous, and villous types), (2) adenomas with focal carcinoma, and (3) polypoid carcinoma. Consequently, the radiologic appearances of neoplastic colonic polyps are varied and benign and malignant neoplasms may appear similar. Neoplastic polyps can be sessile or pedunculated and smooth or lobulated (Fig. 10–50).

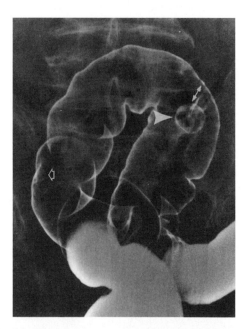

Fig. 10–50. Double-contrast radiograph of the rectosigmoid region shows a small, smooth, sessile adenoma (*arrow*) and a larger pedunculated (*interconnected arrows*) adenoma (*arrowhead*) more proximally.

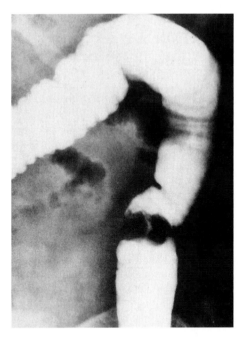

Fig. 10–51. Radiograph from a single-contrast barium enema showing an annular carcinoma of the descending colon.

Ulcerative and Crohn's colitis are the two common idiopathic inflammatory diseases of the colon. Other causes of colitis include infections of various types, drug-related types (i.e., antibiotic colitis), radiation-induced colitis (usually proctitis), ischemic colitis, and miscellaneous disorders. A number of these disorders may mimic the idiopathic types and clinical correlation and exclusion of colonic infection are important. Radiographic differentiation between ulcerative and Crohn's colitis is usually possible in most patients. The features most suggestive of ulcerative colitis are continuous disease with rectal involvement, ahaustral shortening of the colon, and a finely ulcerated or granular mucosal surface (as seen in Case 10-19). The more specific findings of Crohn's colitis include discontinuous disease (i.e., skip areas) with ileitis, eccentric wall involvement, discrete (i.e., aphthoid ulcers) or deep ulceration, intramural fissuring, and formation of fistula to adjacent organs (Fig. 10–52). Complications that may occur in idiopathic colitis include toxic megacolon, carcinoma, sclerosing cholangitis, and abnormalities of the eyes, skin, and joints. Toxic megacolon and complicating carcinoma are more common in ulcerative colitis.

Size is an important radiologic criterion to estimate the risk of malignancy in a sessile colonic polyp; a polyp less than 1 cm in size has only a 1% chance of malignancy, a 1- to 2-cm polyp about a 10% risk, and a polyp over 2 cm at least a 25% or more chance of malignancy. The finding of a pedicle is important, regardless of the size of the head of the polyp, because even if malignancy is present, invasion down the pedicle into the adjacent colonic wall is rare. Lobulation is a less important indicator of malignancy; however, if a large colonic polyp has a smooth surface, a lipoma is a likely consideration.

Adenocarcinoma of the colon is the second most common malignancy that affects both sexes. About 95% of colonic carcinomas occur in patients older than 40 years of age with a peak in the late seventh decade. As with adenocarcinomas elsewhere in the gastrointestinal tract, a variety of morphologic forms are seen, including polypoid carcinoma (malignant potential discussed previously), ulcerative and infiltrative types, and the annular carcinoma (as in Case 10-18); the latter is also called the "apple-core" lesion. In the colon of an adult patient, an irregular constricting lesion having an abrupt transition with the normal colonic wall is nearly always an adenocarcinoma (Fig. 10–51). Inflammatory strictures and surgical anastomoses typically have a smooth and often tapered appearance.

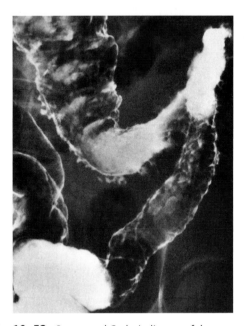

Fig. 10–52. Segmental Crohn's disease of the transverse and descending portions of the colon, showing multiple deep ulcers projecting from the margins of the affected colon and small "aphthoid" ulcers appearing like erosions seen in the upper gastrointestinal tract.

Ischemic colitis usually affects older patients and, like ischemic disease of the small bowel, may result from nonobstructive causes or from thrombotic or embolic disease. The most common location for ischemic involvement of the colon is the region of the splenic flexure and descending colon, which is the vascular "watershed" area for the superior and inferior mesenteric arteries. Other regions of the colon can be affected although ischemic disease of the rectum is rare. The radiologic features of ischemic disease of the colon depend on the location of involvement, severity and duration of its cause, and temporal changes during recovery of the colon. In the severest form, colonic infarction and perforation may occur, often with dire consequences for the patient. The most common appearances relate to submucosal hemorrhage, which causes narrowing of the affected colon associated with irregular, smooth margins often called *thumbprinting* (as in Case 10-20); complete healing and return to normal may occur (Fig. 10–53) or progression to a smooth, tapered stricture can result.

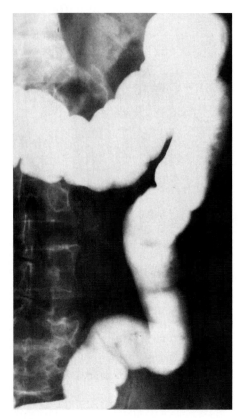

Fig. 10–53. Same patient as in Fig. 10–49; 6 weeks following the acute onset of ischemic colitis in which the previously affected colon has returned to normal.

EXERCISE 10-6: COLONIC OBSTRUCTION

Clinical Histories:

Case 10-21. A 47-year-old man presents with left lower abdominal pain and change in bowel habits (Fig. 10–54).

Case 10-22. A 69-year-old woman presents with rectal bleeding and obstipation (Fig. 10–55).

Case 10-23. A 70-year-old man presents with acute abdominal distention and obstipation (Fig. 10–56; used with permission from Ott DJ, Chen MYM. Specific acute colonic disorders. *Radiol Clin North Am.* 1994;32:871–884).

Case 10-24. A 33-year-old woman presents with cyclic lower abdominal pain, change in bowel habits, and rectal bleeding (Fig. 10–57).

Questions:

10-21. The radiograph in Fig. 10–54 of the sigmoid-descending colon affected by diverticula shows an area of long narrowing most likely caused by

    A. an annular carcinoma.

    B. ischemic colitis.

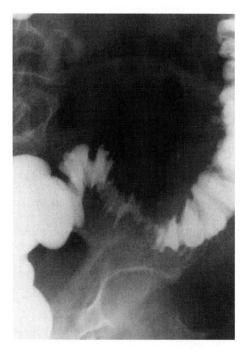

Fig. 10–54.

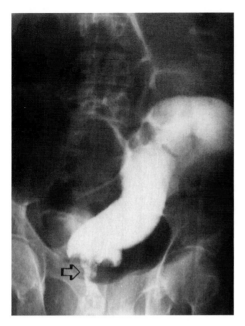

Fig. 10–55.

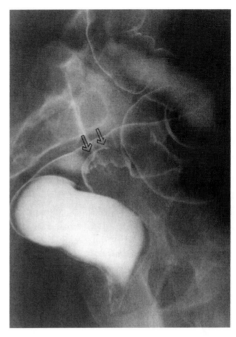

Fig. 10–57.

C. ulcerative colitis.
D. sigmoid diverticulitis.
E. peritoneal metastases.

10-22. The limited single-contrast barium enema (Fig. 10–55) shows an obstructing rectal

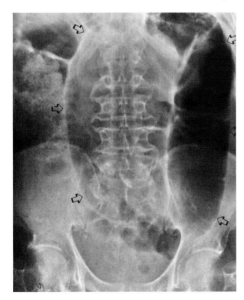

Fig. 10–56.

process (*arrow*), causing colonic obstruction that is likely due to

A. rectal carcinoma.
B. lymphoma of the rectum.
C. crohn's proctitis.
D. infectious proctitis.
E. invasive carcinoma of the cervix.

10-23. What is the most likely explanation of the two adjacent loops of distended colon (*arrows*) in Fig. 10–56?

A. Right colon volvulus
B. Sigmoid volvulus
C. Ileocecal intussusception
D. Functional colonic ileus
E. Internal colonic hernia

10-24. In Fig. 10–57, a smooth mass (*arrows*) partially obstructing the anterior rectosigmoid region is likely due to

A. a polypoid colon carcinoma.
B. rectosigmoid diverticulitis.
C. pelvic endometriosis.
D. invasive endometrial carcinoma.
E. posterior cul-de-sac metastases.

Radiologic Findings:

10-21. Figure 10–54 shows an area of long narrowing in the sigmoid colon associated with diverticula, which was caused by an acute diverticulitis. (*D* is the correct answer to Question 10-21.) Crohn's disease of the sigmoid colon may simulate diverticulitis. An annular carcinoma would not involve such a long segment and would also demonstrate mucosal destruction.

10-22. Figure 10–55 shows an annular rectal carcinoma causing distal colonic obstruction. (*A* is the correct answer to Question 10-22.) Rectal lymphoma is rare and the other possibilities listed do not typically cause circumferential narrowing of the rectum.

10-23. Case 10-23 (Fig. 10–56) is a patient with sigmoid volvulus. (*B* is the correct answer to Question 10-23.) Sigmoid involvement is most likely because the involved loops are pointing inferiorly into the pelvis.

10-24. Case 10-24 (Fig. 10–57) is a woman with pelvic endometriosis that has invaded the rectosigmoid junction anteriorly. (*C* is the correct answer to Question 10-24.) The location is rare for diverticulitis, and the patient is rather young for the other options offered.

Discussion:

Colonic obstruction when seen in adults is usually caused by diverticulitis or carcinoma of the colon. Volvulus of the colon is much less common. However, extrinsic involvement of the rectum or sigmoid colon from pelvic malignancies is an important consideration in the middle-aged or older patient.

Diverticulitis is always a differential consideration in the adult patient with a suspected obstruction of the distal colon. Diverticulitis is usually due to perforation of a single diverticulum, with subsequent formation of a paracolic abscess, and typically is located in the sigmoid colon (as in Case 10-21). The radiographic findings suggesting diverticulitis on contrast enema of the colon include (1) extravasation into an abscess (most definitive finding), (2) eccentric or circumferential narrowing of the colon, and (3) transverse or longitudinal sinus tracts (also seen in Crohn's disease). Complications of sigmoid diverticulitis are obstruction (Fig. 10–58), fistula formation (especially to the bladder), and development of a stricture. Free communication with the peritoneal cavity is rare. CT examination of the pelvis is often preferred in the evaluation of diverticulitis; also, percutaneous drainage of a diverticular abscess can be performed using CT guidance.

Adenocarcinoma of the colon was discussed in the previous exercise as a common source of rectal bleeding but is also an important cause of colonic obstruction. The location and morphologic type of colonic carcinoma will impact on the clinical presentation of the patient. Carcinomas of the right side of the colon are often polypoid, may grow to a large size, and more often present clinically with localized pain, palpable mass, and melena. In the left side of the colon, carcinomas usually present at an earlier stage because obstructive symptoms are more common, often due to an annular carcinoma (Fig. 10–59). Although

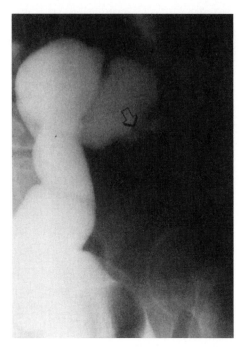

Fig. 10–58. Another patient with sigmoid diverticulitis causing near complete colonic obstruction (*arrow*).

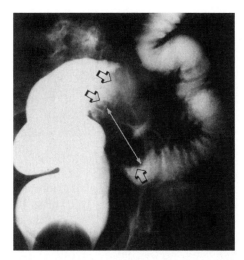

Fig. 10–59. Obstructing sigmoid carcinoma (*interconnected arrows*) near the rectosigmoid junction. Diverticulitis would be the main differential diagnosis; however, the abrupt, irregular areas of transition (*arrows*) favor a malignancy.

carcinomas of the colon have shown a rightward shift in location in recent decades, about half of these malignancies still originate in the rectum or sigmoid colon.

Sigmoid volvulus is a closed-loop colonic obstruction due to twisting along the mesenteric or long axis of the bowel. Although colonic volvulus is not common, about 90% occur in the sigmoid colon. On plain abdominal films, the sigmoid volvulus forms an inverted U-shaped structure with the twisted sigmoid loops lying adjacent and having an oval appearance called the "coffee bean" sign (as in Case 10-23). On barium enema examination, tapered obstruction of the sigmoid colon is found (Fig. 10–60). Cecal volvulus results from a twisting obstruction of the right side of the colon and rarely involves the cecum only. The dilated proximal colon may be seen as an oval structure in the midabdomen or in the left upper quadrant, but rarely points into the pelvis (Fig. 10–61A). Barium enema examination will locate the obstruction to the right side of the colon (Fig. 10–61B).

The anterior wall of the rectosigmoid colon is a common site for involvement of the colon by extrinsic inflammatory or neoplastic diseases. Inflammatory processes may spread into the posterior cul-de-sac and secondarily involve the colon; endometriosis can arise

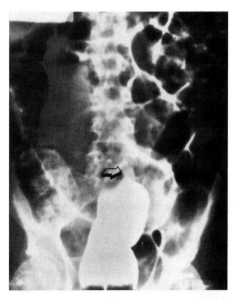

Fig. 10–60. Barium enema in same patient as in Fig. 10–56 showing obstruction at the rectosigmoid junction (*arrow*) due to sigmoid volvulus. (Used with permission from Ott DJ, Chen MYM. Specific acute colonic disorders. *Radiol Clin North Am.* 1994;32:871–884.)

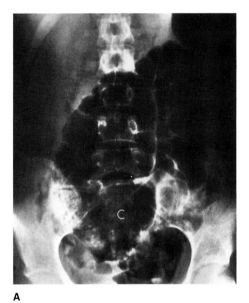

A

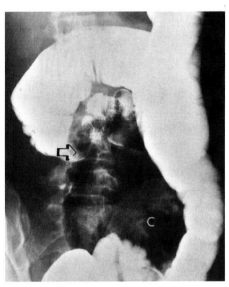

B

Fig. 10–61. **A** Plain abdominal radiograph of right colon volvulus (C, cecum). **B** Barium enema is same patient shows near complete obstruction (*arrow*) in the ascending colon (C, cecum). (Used with permission from Ott DJ, Chen MYM. Specific acute colonic disorders. *Radiol Clin North Am.* 1994;32:871–884.)

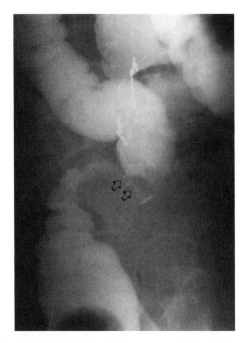

Fig. 10–62. A 54-year-old woman with advanced carcinoma of the uterine cervix that has invaded posteriorly, causing obstruction at the rectosigmoid junction (*arrows*).

in this same area, implant on the colonic serosa, and invade into the colonic wall as occurred in Case 10-24. However, pelvic malignancies related to the uterine cervix, endometrium, ovary, bladder, and prostate are the most common neoplastic processes that can affect the rectosigmoid colon. Circumferential narrowing may occur with these extrinsic malignancies and mimic a primary carcinoma of the colon (Fig. 10–62).

BIBLIOGRAPHY

Chen MYM, Zagoria RJ, Ott DJ, Gelfand DW. *Radiology of the Small Bowel.* New York: Igaku-Shoin; 1992.

Gelfand DW. *Gastrointestinal Radiology.* New York: Churchill-Livingstone; 1984.

Gore RM, Levine MS, eds. *Textbook of Gastrointestinal Radiology.* 2nd ed, Vol. 1. Philadelphia: Saunders; 2000.

Halpert RD, Feczko PJ. *Gastrointestinal Radiology: The Requisites.* 2nd ed. St. Louis: Mosby; 1999.

Ott DJ. Radiology of the oropharynx and esophagus. In: Castell DO, Richter JE, eds. *The Esophagus.* 3rd ed. Philadelphia: Lippincott Williams & Wilkins; 1999:45–87.

Ott DJ, Gelfand DW, Chen MYM. *Manual of Gastrointestinal Fluoroscopy.* Springfield, Ill.: Charles C Thomas; 1996.

Liver, Biliary Tract, and Pancreas

11

Robert E. Bechtold

The diagnosis of diseases of the liver, biliary tract, and pancreas optimally depends on using both clinical and radiographic data. Understanding the proper use of these data and ordering radiographic studies in the optimal sequence are helpful for making the diagnosis most efficiently. Frequently, the clinical presentation and associated laboratory work provide most of the clues for diagnosis. Physical examination, history, and pertinent laboratory values are often helpful in making the diagnosis or at least in providing clues for selecting the optimal radiographic studies. If clinical information is insufficient or if radiographic confirmation is necessary, plain films and contrast studies may be performed. Upright and supine plain radiographs are helpful for the detection of free air, calcifications, and other abnormalities. Contrast studies such as endoscopic retrograde cholangiopancreatography (ERCP) and percutaneous transhepatic cholangiography (PTC) are often helpful in analyzing diseases of the liver, biliary tree, and pancreas. For instance, pancreatic or biliary ductal systems, fistulae from these ductal systems, and associated abnormalities such as encasing tumors can be diagnosed by cholangiography.

Digital cross-sectional imaging, nuclear medicine (NM) and an important form of NM called positron emission tomography (PET), and angiography have provided considerable information in analyzing diseases of these organs, which cannot be directly visualized with plain radiography, even using traditional contrast material, i.e., barium. Cross-sectional techniques consist of ultrasound (US), computed tomography (CT), and magnetic resonance (MR) imaging. This chapter reviews the use of cross-sectional imaging and, where pertinent, nuclear medicine and angiography to evaluate abnormalities of the liver, biliary tract, and pancreas.

TECHNIQUES AND NORMAL ANATOMY

Ultrasonography

Ultrasonography utilizes a high-frequency sound wave transmission through the body. A transducer is used both to emit and to receive a very high-frequency sound (3.5–12 MHz). The technique employs a radar-like detection of objects within the beam, in which the high-frequency sound waves are bounced off the objects and detected by the transducer. These signals are relayed to a computer, which displays a two-dimensional image in whatever plane is defined by the orientation of the transducer. The term for the different shades of gray seen within an US image is *echogenicity*.

Vascular flow can be visualized by US with Doppler imaging, which consists of three types: color, spectral, or power Doppler imaging. In color Doppler imaging, a color-coded display creates color maps of the vessels. Color shade and color intensity reflect blood flow direction and velocity, respectively. Spectral Doppler imaging is portrayed as a sine-wave form in which peaks represent increasing velocity and valleys represent decreasing velocity of flow. This is often combined with color Doppler imaging and together is called *duplex imaging*. An alternate form of Doppler imaging employing color mapping is *power Doppler imaging*. Power Doppler imaging is more sensitive than color Doppler to flow velocity, but unlike color Doppler, cannot indicate flow direction.

Nuclear Medicine

Nuclear medicine techniques utilize the administration of radioactively labeled substances chemically bonded to physiologic agents. These combined substances are administered to the patient and travel to the organs that concentrate the physiologic agents. The radioactivity within the labeled substances is then detected with a camera sensitive to the presence of radioactive emissions. A more recent application of NM is PET, in which positrons emitted, often from radioactive sugar-containing compounds, are detected and imaged. The sugar-containing compounds are metabolized more actively by growing malignant tissue as compared to surrounding normal tissue and are, therefore, visible as areas of greater emissions. The term for different shades within a nuclear medicine image is *activity*.

Computed Tomography

Computed tomography utilizes x-rays and a ring-shaped structure called a *gantry*. The gantry contains an x-ray tube, which is directed toward a row of detectors on the other side of the gantry. The patient is placed on a table that is incrementally (axial CT) or continuously (spiral CT) shifted through the opening of the gantry. The x-ray tube rotates around the patient, emitting a focused beam that passes through the patient. The attenuated beam is received by the detectors. These signals are transmitted to a computer, which reconstructs a series of two-dimensional images in a transverse plane through the body, much like cutting a loaf of bread.

Blood vessels can be demonstrated by using intravenously injected iodinated contrast material, and the bowel can be demonstrated by means of an orally administered contrast agent. These images can be reconstructed in other planes, termed *multiplanar reconstruction*, or MPR, or in a three-dimensional, or 3-D, image. Most existing CT scanners have a single detector system that permits the acquisition of a single image at a time with each gantry rotation. Newer CT scanners, called *multidetector CT scanners*, or MDCT scanners, employ 4 to 16 adjacent detectors, which allow the simultaneous acquisition of multiple images with one gantry rotation.

MDCT scanners scan extremely quickly and provide markedly improved image quality by reducing motion artifacts and by permitting the acquisition of much thinner sections. These newer scanners also greatly facilitate the performance of MPR and 3-D scanning. The term for different shades within a CT image is *attenuation* or *density*.

Angiography

In angiography, contrast agents are administered intravascularly, and complex radiographic machines trace the injected contrast material through the blood vessels by a rapid sequence of x-ray films or with digital imaging techniques. The term for different shades within an angiographic image is *density*.

Magnetic Resonance Imaging

Magnetic resonance imaging is a very complex technique that evaluates magnetism within the patient. The device is outwardly similar to a CT unit. The patient is placed on table that carries the patient into a cylinder, which contains a magnet. The magnet emits a radio-frequency pulse that causes the protons of the atoms within the body to line up together. The magnet then emits another radio-frequency pulse, which perturbs the orientation of the protons so that as a group they are flipped to the side. The protons then return to their original orientation, and their return is accompanied by a release of energy. The rate at which the protons return to normal orientation and release energy is defined by the characteristics of the tissue, which in turn are defined by the relaxation times, T_1 and T_2, of the protons. Blood flow and proton density also affect the image. Signals from this process are sent to a computer, which reconstructs either a two-dimensional image in any plane or a 3-D image.

MR imaging has superb contrast resolution, but historically required long data acquisition times. More recently, faster MR imaging techniques have brought imaging times toward alignment with those of CT and are fast enough to reduce or eliminate motion artifacts. Generalized parenchymal lesion detection and characterization, together with MR angiography, or MRA, have been further improved greatly with the use of MR imaging-specific intravenous contrast agents, especially gadolinium, Gd. The term for different shades within an MR image is *signal intensity*. Flow is identified by signal intensity changes in the blood vessels.

Normal Anatomy

With US, normal organs are displayed as structures of different echogenicity. In general, fluid is *anechoic* (i.e., has no echoes). Soft tissue has echoes of mild to moderate intensity. Bone has extremely strong echoes. Abnormal organs are displayed as areas of diffuse inhomogeneity or as focal regions of decreased or increased echogenicity within the organ. The normal appearances of the liver, biliary system, and pancreas have been well established. The liver is second to the pancreas in echogenicity among organs in the upper abdomen. The liver typically has homogeneous parenchymal detail (Fig. 11–1). Numerous intrahepatic vessels including portal veins and hepatic veins are easily seen within the liver. The gallbladder appears as an anechoic pear-shaped structure along the inferior aspect of the liver (Fig. 11–2). It normally has a thin, homogeneous wall less than 3 mm thick. The degree of distention of the gallbladder varies with postprandial intervals. The biliary ducts are thin tubes, the walls of which are 1.5 mm or less. The ducts increase in caliber as they extend from the liver to the sphincter of Oddi (Fig. 11–3). The upper limit in caliber of the extrahepatic biliary ducts increases with age. The pancreas is the most echogenic organ in the abdomen (Fig. 11–4). It is homogeneous, comma shaped, and parallel to splenic vein and extends from the left upper quadrant caudally and to the right. In anteroposterior dimension the pancreatic head is 3 cm, the body 2.5 cm, and the tail 2 cm.

With NM techniques, normal organs are displayed as regions of homogeneous activity conforming to the general shape of the organ. Abnormal organs are displayed as diffuse inhomogeneity or as focal areas of reduced or

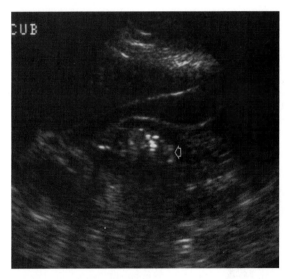

Fig. 11–2. Longitudinal US image of the normal gallbladder, showing the anechoic lumen and smooth, thin walls of the gallbladder. Air-filled, echogenic duodenum is seen immediately behind the gallbladder (*open arrow*).

increased activity. In the past, the liver was most commonly studied with NM with technetium-labeled sulfur colloid. However, this technique has largely been

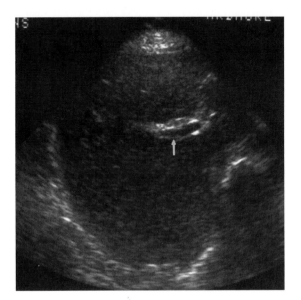

Fig. 11–1. Transverse US image of the normal liver, showing homogeneous parenchymal detail, the hyperechoic hemidiaphragmatic surface, the linear portal vein, and the parallel biliary duct (*arrow*).

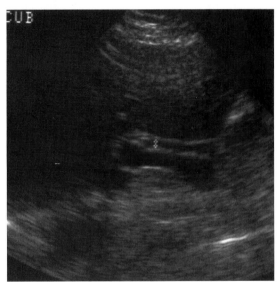

Fig. 11–3. Longitudinal US image of the normal biliary duct, showing the narrow caliber and the thin, uniform ductal walls (cursors denote the internal walls of the duct).

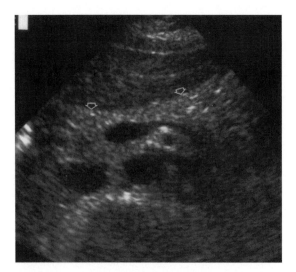

Fig. 11–4. Transverse US image of the normal pancreas, showing the homogeneous, echogenic pancreatic head, body and tail (*open arrows*), lying in front of the splenic and superior mesenteric veins.

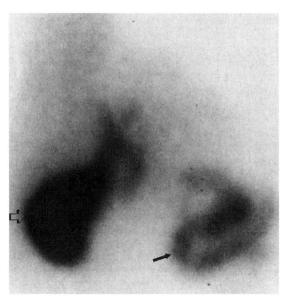

Fig. 11–5. Hepatobiliary NM scan, showing the presence of radiopharmaceutical within the gallbladder lumen (*open arrow*) and duodenum (*closed arrow*), demonstrating the patency of both cystic and common bile duct. (Courtesy of Robert Cowan, M.D., Winston-Salem, NC.)

replaced by CT, US, and MR imaging. The most common NM study of the liver today utilizes technetium-labeled red blood cells to evaluate for cavernous hemangioma. Evaluation of the biliary system is a common application for NM studies. Technetium-labeled hepatobiliary imaging iminodiacetic acid derivatives, especially disophenin and mebrophenin, are taken up by the liver, excreted into the bile, carried to the biliary tree and gallbladder, and from there travel to the bowel through the extrahepatic ducts (Fig. 11–5). Depending on the exact agent used, these are termed *hepatic iminodiacetic acid,* (HIDA) scans. Currently no practical imaging of the pancreas is done by means of NM techniques.

With CT, normal organs are displayed as regions of differing attenuation. Abnormal organs are displayed as diffuse inhomogeneity or as focal areas of decreased or increased attenuation. The liver, biliary system, and pancreas are well demonstrated by CT (Fig. 11–6). The liver is the most dense organ in the abdomen. The normal liver parenchyma appears homogeneous, just as in an US image. The portal and hepatic vessels and the biliary ductal system are likewise easy to identify. Overall measurements of wall thickness and biliary duct caliber are the same as for US. The pancreas is easily identified on CT, and the pancreatic duct is frequently well seen.

At angiography, normal organs enhance to variable extents. Abnormal organs either inhomogeneously enhance or have focal areas of decreased or increased enhancement. Although the parenchyma of the normal organs is rarely demonstrated, the blood vessels of these organs are seen in exquisite detail (Fig. 11–7). In the liver, both the hepatic artery and all of its branches can be seen. Delayed studies through the liver in the venous

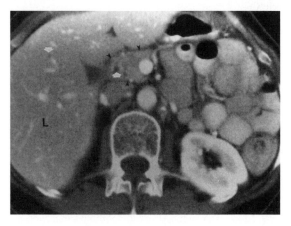

Fig. 11–6. CT showing normal liver (L), pancreas (*arrowheads*), and biliary tree, in both the liver and pancreas (*arrows*).

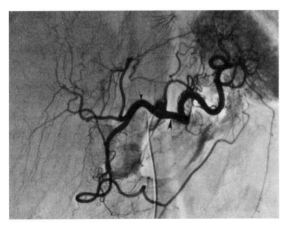

Fig. 11–7. Celiac arteriogram, showing normal distribution of the splenic (*large arrowhead*) and hepatic (*small arrowhead*) arteries, and the normal homogeneous stain of the spleen in the left upper quadrant.

phase demonstrate the portal vein. The cystic artery and any collateral vessels can be angiographically demonstrated. Angiographic studies of the pancreas can demonstrate major pancreatic branches, as well as encasement, displacement, stenosis, or occlusion.

On MR imaging, normal organs have homogeneous signal intensity or well-recognized variations in signal intensity. Abnormal organs have inhomogeneous signal intensity or areas of increased or decreased signal intensity. The normal liver, biliary system, and pancreas are well demonstrated on MR imaging (Fig. 11–8). The liver has a homogeneous signal intensity that is usually higher than that of muscle and lower than that of the spleen. The biliary system is normally demonstrated as an area of low signal intensity on T_1-weighted images and high signal intensity on T_2-weighted images. This appearance reflects the fluid bile within the gallbladder and biliary tree. Magnetic resonance cholangiopancreatography, or MRCP, demonstrates the biliary system as very high signal intensity structures against a very low signal intensity background of surrounding solid tissues (Fig. 11–9). The pancreas is of intermediate signal on both T_1- and T_2-weighted images and may be hard to differentiate from bowel if no oral contrast agent is administered to the patient. As in CT and US, the normal fatty change within the pancreas that occurs with age is visible.

TECHNIQUE SELECTION

Diseases of the liver, biliary system, and pancreas can be conveniently, if arbitrarily, separated into the following categories to help illustrate the optimal sequences of imaging techniques: diffuse hepatocellular disease, focal hepatic diseases, abdominal trauma, inflammatory disease of the biliary tract, and pancreatic inflammation or neoplasm.

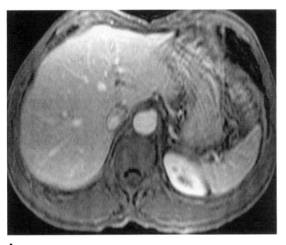

A

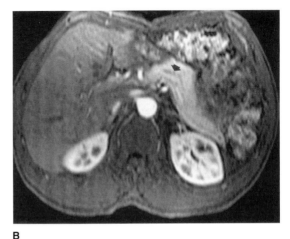

B

Fig. 11–8. **A** Dynamic gadolinium-enhanced T_1-weighted gradient echo image of the upper abdomen, taken at the level of the midliver, demonstrating homogeneous liver, with interspersed intrahepatic vessels, and spleen. **B** Dynamic gadolinium-enhanced T_1-weighted gradient echo image of the upper abdomen, taken at the level of the pancreas and kidneys, demonstrating the homogeneous pancreatic body and tail with pancreatic duct (*arrow*), and the corticomedullary differentiation in the kidneys.

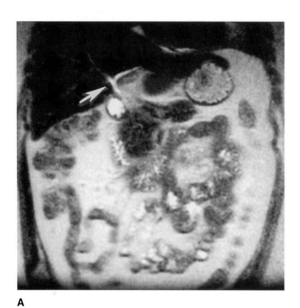
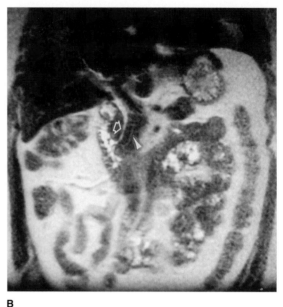

A

B

Fig. 11–9. **A** MRCP of the normal biliary ducts, taken at the level of the porta hepatis, demonstrating the branching proximal intrahepatic ducts (*arrow*). **B** MRCP of the normal biliary ducts, taken at the level of the distal extrahepatic bile duct, demonstrating the intrapancreatic passage of the biliary (*arrow*) and pancreatic (*arrowhead*) ducts, entering the duodenum.

Diffuse Hepatocellular Disease

In diffuse hepatocellular disease, CT is probably the first study used to survey the liver because it is moderately sensitive to liver lesions and is also helpful for evaluating surrounding organs. Ultrasound may have application unless fatty liver is present, because fat attenuates the US beam. NM has only infrequent applications. MR imaging may be the most sensitive modality for detecting and characterizing diffuse diseases of the liver, including cirrhosis and hemochromatosis, especially when combined with contrast agents. Angiography may be used to study collateral formation in cirrhosis.

Focal Hepatic Diseases

In focal diseases of the liver, US is often used first, because it is inexpensive, widely available, and moderately sensitive to localized lesions in the absence of preexisting diffuse diseases, such as cirrhosis. It is, however, of limited value in obese patients and whenever air is present, for example, when air-filled bowel obscures the liver. CT is a pivotal examination, often employed after US. It is used as a survey of the entire body, is easy to compare in serial studies, and is sensitive to disease. Air and bone do not interfere with CT examinations. Contrast-enhanced MDCT scanners can be used to perform CT angiography, or CTA, which is

a noninvasive means of producing images depicting vessels much like conventional angiography. NM techniques can be used to analyze a focal lesion within the liver for possible cavernous hemangioma. MR imaging is used frequently to characterize focal lesions within the liver, especially those discovered during survey techniques like US or CT.

NM and MR imaging are considered the optimal means for evaluating the liver for cavernous hemangioma, and both are highly accurate (approximately 95%) in evaluating the liver for cavernous hemangioma. In the opinion of some authorities, MR imaging is the optimal means for both detection and characterization of focal liver lesions of all types. Newer MR pulse sequences, contrast agents, and fast scanning techniques arguably make MR imaging the optimal means for both detection and characterization of focal liver lesions of all types. Angiography is primarily used to provide a vascular road map in planning surgery for focal liver lesions.

Abdominal Trauma

CT is the only commonly accepted means for analyzing abdominal trauma, particularly of the liver. CT is reasonably accurate in the detection of trauma-related abnormalities of the liver, biliary system, and pancreas. US may be useful if CT is not available or to quickly identify intraperitoneal hemorrhage in patients who are in the emergency department and are going directly to the operating room. Angiography may be useful to embolize persistently bleeding arteries in the liver or spleen when surgery is not possible. Currently, NM and MR imaging have no application in studying the liver, biliary tract, or pancreas in trauma.

Pancreatic Inflammation or Neoplasm

Ultrasound is often the initial means to study pancreatic inflammation or neoplasm. It is effective in evaluating the pancreas if not interrupted by surrounding bowel gas. If ileus is present, or if a lesion has already been detected by US and additional confirmation is required, CT is the method of choice. NM has no major current application in studying the pancreas. MR imaging may be useful to study endocrine tumors of the pancreas. Recent advances in MR imaging, especially MRCP, have brought MR imaging further to the forefront of pancreatic and biliary duct evaluation. This latter technique highlights fluid-containing structures such as biliary or pancreatic ducts, and voids nearly all signal intensity from background solid structures. Angiography is useful to identify bleeding arteries as a source of hemorrhagic pancreatitis but is occasionally used to identify encasement of arteries in a pancreatic neoplasm.

Patient Preparation for Radiographic Techniques

Generally, these radiographic techniques require little patient preparation. This is convenient, especially in evaluation of trauma. Ideally, a patient should fast after midnight before an US examination. As a minimum, the patient should fast for 6 hours. Patients ideally should fast before CT examinations as well, but this requirement is not crucial. Dilute oral contrast medium for CT is administered at least 2 hours in advance and again just before the examination begins. Intravenous contrast material is often given as a bolus by a power injector immediately prior to the study. Proper laboratory evaluation of renal function, including serum creatinine below 1.5 mg/dL, is usually required before administering iodinated intravenous contrast material since it can be nephrotoxic. Ideally, NM is also performed after fasting. Preparation for angiography again requires fasting and laboratory evaluation of renal function and possible coagulopathy. Proper preparation of patients for MR imaging is controversial. However, some authorities advise administering an iron-containing oral contrast agent and an agent to relax the bowel, such as glucagon, before scanning. No assessment of renal function is necessary because MR contrast agents are not nephrotoxic.

Conflicts Among Examinations

These examinations may interfere with each another. No barium should be administered before US or CT. Oral contrast agents may generate bowel gas, decompress the gallbladder, and hinder US. The oral contrast agent administered prior to a CT examination interferes with angiography by obscuring the abdomen. Intravenous contrast material interferes with any subsequent NM tests studying iodine metabolism such as those involving the thyroid gland because intravenous contrast agents contain iodine. Previous angiography usually requires that a CT examination be postponed for a day or two so that residual contrast material within the kidneys can be excreted. Usually, there are no conflicts between these examinations and NM or MR imaging.

EXERCISES
EXERCISE 11-1: DIFFUSE LIVER DISEASE
Clinical Histories:

Case 11-1. A 55-year-old American patient presents with abdominal swelling (Fig. 11–10).

Case 11-2. A 33-year-old long-time diabetic patient presents with right upper quadrant "mass" (Fig. 11–11).

Case 11-3. A 65-year-old patient presents with fever and increased liver function tests (Fig. 11–12).

Case 11-4. An 80-year-old patient presents without symptoms referable to the abdomen (Fig. 11–13).

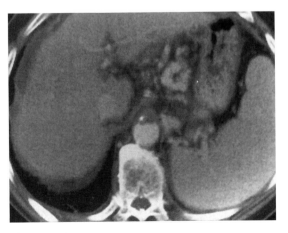

Fig. 11–10.

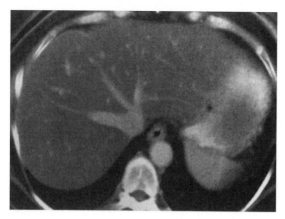

Fig. 11–11.

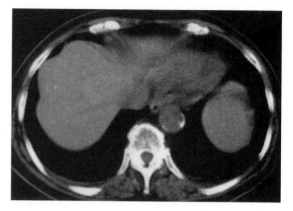

Fig. 11–13.

Questions:

11-1. The most likely diagnosis in Case 11-1 (Fig. 11–10) is
  A. cirrhosis.
  B. diffuse liver tumor.
  C. Budd-Chiari syndrome.
  D. schistosomiasis.

11-2. The most likely diagnosis in Case 11-2 (Fig. 11–11) is
  A. cirrhosis.
  B. fatty liver.
  C. hepatic iron overload.
  D. old granulomatous disease.

11-3. The most likely diagnosis in Case 11-3 (Fig. 11–12) is
  A. cirrhosis.
  B. thorotrast-induced liver disease.
  C. hepatitis.
  D. hepatic iron overload.

11-4. The most likely diagnosis in Case 11-4 (Fig. 11–13) is
  A. cirrhosis.
  B. old granulomatous disease.
  C. fatty liver.
  D. Osler-Weber-Rendu disease.

Radiologic Findings:

11-1. In this case (Fig. 11–10), the overall liver size is small, especially the right lobe, with disproportionate enlargement of the left and caudate lobes; multiple collaterals are present around the stomach and in the central upper abdomen; and ascites is present—all findings of cirrhosis. (*A* is the correct answer to Question 11-1.)

11-2. In this case (Fig. 11–11), the overall liver size is large, the predominant finding is marked low density throughout entire liver, and no mass effect is present on any vessel—all findings of fatty liver. (*B* is the correct answer to Question 11-2.)

11-3. In this case (Fig. 11–12), the overall liver size is enlarged and attenuation inhomogeneous and mildly reduced. Also, no focal mass is present. These are findings of hepatitis. (*C* is the correct answer to Question 11-3.)

11-4. In this case (Fig. 11–13), multiple small, highly attenuating, punctate lesions are scattered throughout liver and spleen, characteristic of calcifications from old granulornatous disease, without any other predominant finding. (*B* is the correct answer to Question 11-4.)

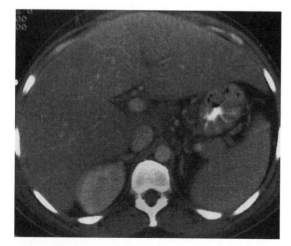

Fig. 11–12.

Discussion:

Differentiation of liver disease into diffuse or focal disease is an artificial but convenient way to analyze liver disorders radiographically. Diffuse hepatocellular diseases are a common diagnostic problem. Although historical, physical, and laboratory testing are the first means for identifying these diseases, imaging may be required as a part of the overall assessment of the patient.

Cirrhosis is a chronic disease of the liver. It is characterized by injury and regeneration of hepatic parenchymal cells and is accompanied by formation of connective tissue within the liver. In the United States, the most common cause of cirrhosis is alcoholism, whereas in Asia, the most common cause is viral hepatitis. Cirrhosis results in disproportionate diminution of the right lobe compared to the left lobe and caudate lobe of the liver (Fig. 11–14). Nodular regeneration of the liver results in a nodular edge of the liver and inhomogeneity of the parenchyma. The process is accompanied by, first, increased resistance to normal hepatopetal (toward the liver) flow and, finally, the development of hepatofugal (away from the liver) flow. The increased resistance in the portal vein secondarily enlarges the spleen. This process also creates enlarged collateral venous channels to reroute blood around the liver (Fig. 11–10). These portosystemic collaterals are visible frequently on cross-sectional imaging studies, most commonly in paraumbilical veins, coronary veins, and even spontaneous splenorenal shunts. Ascites is nearly always present. Most authorities are increasingly convinced that MR imaging is the most sensitive imaging modality for examination of the liver in cirrhosis and other diffuse diseases of the liver. MR im-

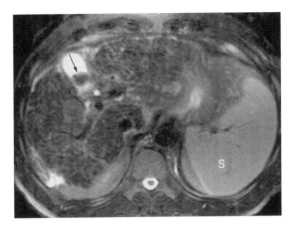

Fig 11–15. T_2-weighted MR image demonstrating cirrhosis, consisting of diffuse heterogeneity due to innumerable tiny low signal intensity nodules, regenerative nodules containing fibrous tissue and iron. Also note cholelithiasis (*arrow*) and splenomegaly (*S*).

aging can demonstrate not only the contour changes and collateral formation visible with CT, but also the more subtle intraparenchymal nodular changes consequent to formation of regenerative and dysplastic nodules characteristic of cirrhosis within the complex fibrotic and inflamed host hepatic tissue (Fig. 11–15). Importantly, MR imaging is considered to be a sensitive imaging means in the diagnosis of tumor such as hepatoma superimposed on a background of cirrhosis (Fig. 11–16).

Diffuse tumor in the liver can occur in patients with certain primary malignancies (Fig. 11–17), particularly breast carcinoma. It is usually distributed randomly throughout the left and caudate lobes. Collateral veins normally are not found. Portal venous or intrahepatic biliary radicles may be compromised or displaced, although portal vein thrombosis is uncommon.

Budd-Chiari syndrome is a condition involving obstruction of the hepatic veins or the intrahepatic inferior vena cava (IVC). It is due to hypercoagulable states that produce thrombosis; tumors of the liver, kidneys, adrenal glands, or IVC; trauma (the "three T's"; i.e., thrombosis, tumors, trauma); pregnancy; and even webs or membranes in the lumen of the IVC. This syndrome produces a marked congestion of the liver resulting from resistance to flow out of the liver, which consequently enlarges and becomes edematous. The liver has a mottled appearance on CT that is due to the interstitial edema, especially after administration of intravenous contrast material (Fig. 11–18).

Schistosomiasis is one of the world's most common parasitic diseases and is rarely seen in persons living outside

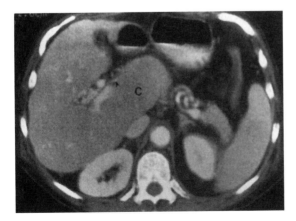

Fig. 11–14. CT in cirrhosis showing the disproportionate enlargement of the caudate lobe (C), as well as multiple collateral venous channels in the porta hepatis (*arrowhead*).

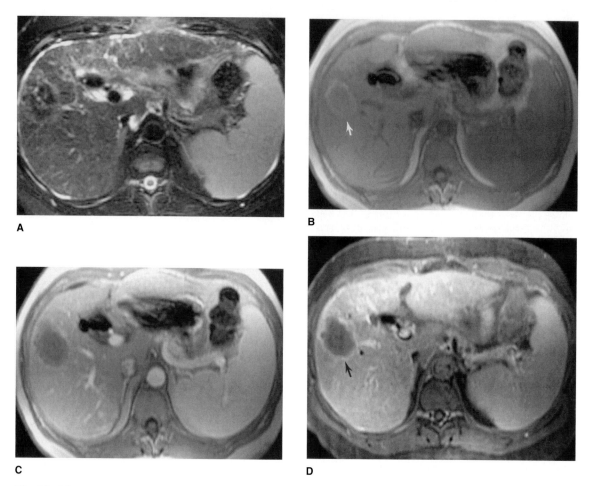

Fig. 11–16. **A** T$_2$-weighted scan showing heterogeneous parenchyma, with superimposed focal mass in the right hepatic lobe. Splenomegaly is present and small amounts of ascites surround the liver. **B** Preinfusion T$_1$-weighted MR imaging showing background of cirrhosis and the high signal intensity of the periphery of the lesion (*arrow*) before contrast administration. **C** Immediate postinfused T$_1$-weighted MR imaging showing the absence of contrast enhancement in the lesion, including the absence of puddling of contrast. **D** Delayed postinfused T$_1$-weighted MR imaging showing the lack of centripetal contrast accumulation of contrast within the lesion (*arrow*); thus, it is not a cavernous hemangioma; the lesion is compatible with a hepatoma.

the endemic areas of China, Japan, the Middle East, and Africa; it does occur, however, in immigrants to the United States. The larvae are hosts that enter the human gastrointestinal system, pass into lymphatic channels, migrate into mesenteric veins and portal veins, and, as adult worms, deposit ova that embolize to the portal system. This process leads to a granulomatous inflammation, periportal fibrosis, portal vein occlusion, varices, and splenomegaly. Imaging studies demonstrate periportal fibrosis. The fibrosis enhances on CT after con-

trast material administration and appears on US as increased echogenicity of the periportal sheath surrounding the portal veins.

Fatty liver, or steatosis, is a common disorder. It is found in up to 50% of patients who are diabetic or alcoholic, and has been found in up to 25% of nonalcoholic, healthy adults who die accidentally. The many causes of fatty liver, besides diabetes and alcoholism, include (1) obesity, (2) chronic illness, (3) corticosteroid excess, (4) parenteral nutrition, and (5) hepatotoxins,

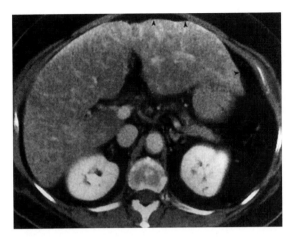

Fig. 11–17. CT in diffuse tumor showing diffuse, coarse inhomogeneity of the liver parenchyma, with a nodular border (*arrowheads*). Note absence of caudate lobe hypertrophy.

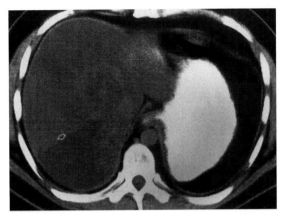

Fig. 11–19. CT in geographic fatty infiltration of the liver showing well-marginated, focal, low-density portion of the liver posteriorly (*arrow*).

including chemotherapy. Fatty liver may be distributed evenly or focally. When distributed uniformly, fatty liver is recognizable as a pattern of homogeneous increased echogenicity on US, decreased attenuation on CT (Fig. 11–11), or increased signal intensity on T_1-weighted MR images. When distributed nonuniformly, it resembles focal disease of the liver in that normal islands of liver tissue are seen against the background of lower density fatty liver (Fig. 11–19). Specialized MR imaging scans, NM studies, or biopsy may be required to differentiate among the possibilities.

Hepatic iron overload can be due to deposition in hepatocytes or reticuloendothelial cells. Parenchymal iron deposition occurs in primary idiopathic hemochromatosis, secondary hemochromatosis, cirrhosis, or intravascular hemolysis; the iron overload in these conditions is generally referred to as *hemochromatosis*. Reticuloendothelial iron deposition occurs in transfusional iron overload or rhabdomyolysis; the iron overload in these conditions is referred to as *hemosiderosis*. The liver, including the right lobe, is enlarged greatly unless cirrhosis is present. On CT, the density of the liver is very high (Fig. 11–20),

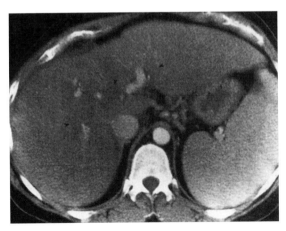

Fig. 11–18. CT in Budd-Chiari syndrome showing subtle, diffuse mottled appearance of liver (*arrowheads*).

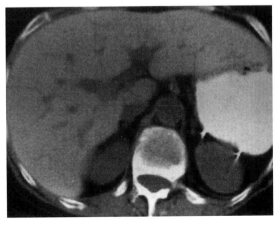

Fig. 11–20. CT in iron overload showing dense liver in relationship to the lower density intrahepatic portal vessels.

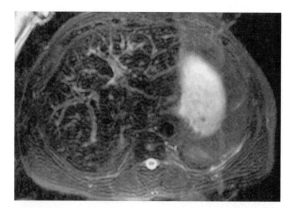

Fig. 11–21. T_2-weighted MR imaging showing almost completely "black" liver, due to the deposition of intra-hepatic iron. Note that the liver, which usually has higher signal intensity than muscle, is isointense to paraspinous muscle.

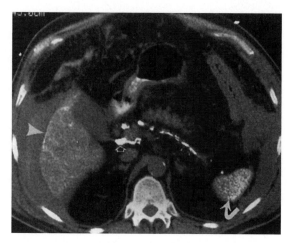

Fig. 11–22. CT in Thorotrast administration showing the presence of high-density. Thorotrast in the liver (*arrowhead*), lymph nodes (*open arrow*), and spleen (*curved arrow*).

and on MR imaging the liver has extremely low signal on both T_1- and T_2-weighted images (Fig. 11–21). Patients with hepatic iron overload may develop hepatocellular carcinoma.

Old granulomatous disease is a disorder in which prior granulomatous inflammation, usually caused by *Histoplasma capsulatum*, involves the liver. Other granulomatous inflammatory conditions that could be involved include sarcoidosis, Wegener's granulomatosis, and certain toxins. The granuloma tends to undergo necrosis, and dystrophic calcification forms within the lesion. This gives the lesion its most characteristic form, multiple punctate calcifications. The granuloma is visible on US as focal, extremely hyperechoic, shadowing lesions, and on CT as extremely high-density punctate lesions (Fig. 11–13).

Thorotrast, a thorium-containing contrast agent, was used in the early 20th century for angiography and other purposes. Unfortunately, Thorotrast emits alpha and beta radiation, has a biologic half-life of 400 years since it is not excreted, and therefore has been responsible for the development of several malignancies of the liver and spleen, including angiosarcoma and hepatoma. The particles are taken up by liver, spleen, lymphatics, and bone marrow. They appear on CT studies as large, dense particles in the liver, spleen, and peripancreatic and periportal lymph nodes (Fig. 11–22). US shows typical calcifications.

Hepatitis is a diffuse inflammation of the liver, occurring as either acute or chronic disease. Patients with acute hepatitis have hepatocellular necrosis. In chronic cases, periportal inflammation and even

fibrosis may occur. In acute hepatitis, the echogenicity of the parenchyma is decreased as a result of the edema, and the portal radicles are more evident; this has been termed the "starry sky" appearance. In chronic hepatitis, the texture of the liver is coarsened as a result of the fibrotic change in the periportal space, and this may decrease the visibility of the portal vein radicles. Findings on CT include hepatomegaly and decreased density (Fig. 11–12). Most commonly, no important findings except hepatomegaly occur on CT in hepatitis. On MR imaging, the liver has low signal intensity on T_1-weighted images and high signal intensity on T_2-weighted images because of the edema and inflammation.

Osler-Weber-Rendu disease, or hereditary hemorrhagic telangiectasia, affects many organs and is seen predominantly, but not exclusively, in skin and the gastrointestinal tract. In the liver, it produces either telangiectasias, cirrhosis, or both. Multiple small aneurysms may be present, and hematomas may occur if the aneurysms bleed. These aneurysms and any consequent hematomas from aneurysmal rupture can be visible on both US and CT. Angiography can demonstrate enlarged hepatic arteries and early but not immediate hepatic vein opacification.

EXERCISE 11-2: FOCAL LIVER DISEASES

Clinical Histories:

Case 11-5. A 44-year-old American patient presents with right upper quadrant pain and fever (Fig. 11–23).

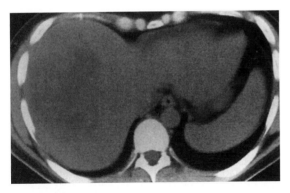

Fig. 11–23.

Case 11-6. A 45-year-old female presents with incidentally discovered liver lesion (Fig. 11–24*A,B*).

Case 11-7. A 65-year-old female presents with a long history of a pancreatic mass (Fig. 11–25).

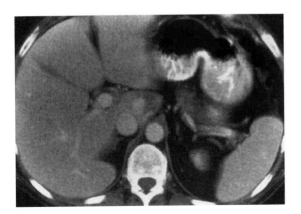

A

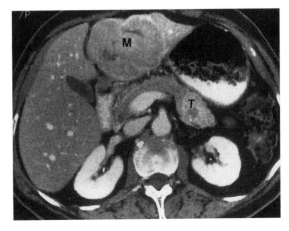

Fig. 11–25.

Case 11-8. A 61-year-old male presents with upper abdominal pain (Fig. 11–26).

Questions:

11-5. The most likely diagnosis in Case 11-5 (Fig. 11–23) is
   A. pyogenic liver abscess.
   B. echinococcal disease.
   C. candidiasis.
   D. amoebic abscess.

11-6. The most likely diagnosis in Case 11-6 (Fig. 11–24) is
   A. hemangioma.
   B. metastatic disease.
   C. angiosarcoma.
   D. focal nodular hyperplasia.

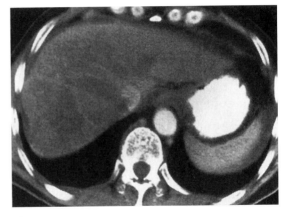

B

Fig. 11–24.

Fig. 11–26.

11-7. The most likely diagnosis in Case 11-7 (Fig. 11–25) is
  A. hemangioma.
  B. hepatocellular carcinoma.
  C. metastatic disease.
  D. liver cell adenoma.

11-8. The most likely diagnosis in Case 11-8 (Fig. 11–26) is
  A. metastatic disease.
  B. hepatocellular carcinoma.
  C. liver cell adenoma.
  D. abscess.

Radiologic Findings:

11-5. In this case, Fig. 11–23 shows an inhomogeneous liver lesion with central necrosis and a peripheral rim of edema. Although this could conceivably represent an echinococcal or amoebic abscess in this patient with fever, the patient is from the United States rather than a foreign country, thus, the most likely diagnosis is a pyogenic abscess. (*A* is the correct answer to Question 11-5.) As more individuals from other countries, especially Third World nations, immigrate to the United States, more echinococcal or amoebic liver abscesses will be seen.

11-6. In this case, Fig. 11–24 shows a focal lesion in the caudate lobe of the liver, which enhances early and fills in later with contrast material. This early peripheral and nodular-appearing distribution of intravenous contrast within the lesion, and eventual centripetal accumulation of contrast material to fill in the lesion is characteristic of cavernous hemangioma. (*A* is the correct answer to Question 11-6.)

11-7. In this case, Fig. 11–25 shows a focal lesion occupying the left lobe of the liver (M), and there is a focal enhancing mass in the pancreatic tail (T), representing a pancreatic neoplasm metastatic to the liver. (*C* is the correct answer to Question 11-7.)

11-8. In this case, Fig. 11–26 shows a focal lesion within the right lobe of the liver, which is associated with a clot entering the hepatic vein and even the inferior vena cava, findings typical for hepatocellular carcinoma. (*B* is the correct answer to Question 11-8.)

Discussion:

Recognition of the focal or diffuse nature of liver disease is helpful for sorting out the possible causes. The two can overlap, especially since one may lead to another, e.g., cirrhosis can cause hepatoma.

Pyogenic liver abscesses are relatively common focal inflammatory lesions of the liver caused by bacteria. These lesions have high morbidity and mortality, if undiscovered. They are multiple in many cases, involving

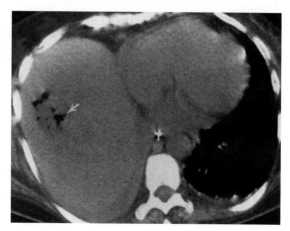

Fig. 11–27. CT in pyogenic abscess showing the presence of gas within the lesion (*arrow*).

both hepatic lobes. These abscesses create a severe leukocytosis. Pyogenic abscesses occur when collections of leukocytes undergo necrosis and become walled off. The imaging studies, while not definitive, provide helpful findings. On US, these lesions often are well demarcated, may be multiloculated, and have fluid centers and irregular walls. Gas within an abscess creates an echogenic structure with shadowing. On CT, the abscess appears as a low-density lesion. Intra-abscess gas occurs in approximately 50% of abscesses (Fig. 11–27), and enhancement of the border of the lesion after intravenous contrast infusion also occurs in approximately 50% of abscesses. Low-density edema may surround the abscess (Fig. 11–23). Rapid enhancement of the edge of an abscess after bolus injection of contrast material may be helpful. On ^{99m}Tc-sulfur colloid scans, the abscess appears as a defect within the liver. MR imaging demonstrates signs of an irregular, fluid-containing lesion, i.e., low signal intensity on T_1-weighted examinations and high signal intensity on T_2-weighted examinations. Edema may be visible surrounding the lesion on T_2-weighted images.

Echinococcal disease is a parasitic infestation that involves multiple organs, most commonly the liver. It is endemic in several regions around the world. The most common form is due to *Echinococcus granulosis*, which, after being ingested by humans, is carried into the gut, transmitted to the portal circulation, and eventually deposited in the liver, where it develops into large, occasionally multiloculated, cysts, which may calcify. On US, these lesions appear as well-defined cysts with regular borders, which may contain swirling debris and multiple septae. Smaller, "daughter" cysts often surround them. Small calcifications are present. CT shows

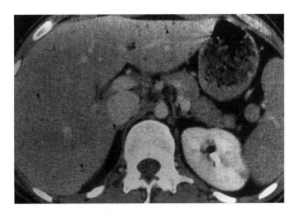

Fig. 11–28. CT in candidiasis showing multiple small, low-density lesions scattered throughout the liver (*arrowheads*), representing multifocal fungal abscesses.

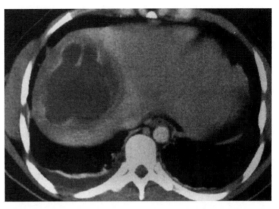

Fig. 11–29. CT in amoebic abscess showing the presence of an irregular peripherally enhancing lesion within the liver. This is indistinguishable from a pyogenic abscess.

similar morphologic findings, as well as enhancement of the wall after intravenous contrast material infusion. Calcifications are crescentic, corresponding to the membranes. MR imaging shows a cystic mass with a rim-like periphery of low signal intensity on both T_1- and T_2-weighted images and with a central matrix of high signal intensity.

Candidiasis is a fungal disease. It affects the liver primarily in renal transplant patients and patients who have been immunocompromised by malignancy or chemotherapy for the malignancy. The organism forms multiple microabscesses, which create the characteristic appearance on imaging studies. US shows several patterns, the most common being multiple small, hypoechoic structures containing a hyperechoic central spot, the "bull's-eye" lesion. Other patterns may occur. CT shows similar multiple small abscesses (Fig. 11–28), including the bull's-eye lesion.

Amoebic abscesses are caused by a parasite, *Entamoeba histolytica*, and the liver is the most commonly involved organ. The leukocytosis is much less severe than with a pyogenic abscess. Unlike pyogenic abscesses, which require drainage, amoebic abscesses can often be cured by medical treatment. Like echinococcal abscesses, amoebic abscesses start when organisms reach the liver through the portal circulation from the bowel. The abscesses may rupture into the peritoneal cavity or even into the thorax. Imaging studies, including NM, US, and CT, are usually nonspecific and demonstrate focal defects within the liver (Fig. 11–29). The lesions can resemble echinococcal abscesses. One helpful finding is intraperitoneal or intrathoracic fluid, if rupture has occurred.

Hemangioma is the most common benign tumor of the liver and is second only to metastases as the most common tumor overall within the liver. Symptomatic tumors are more often found in women, probably because of bleeding. Hemangiomas are often peripherally located in the liver, less than 2 cm in diameter, and not associated with abnormalities in liver function tests. They are most commonly single. On US they are usually homogeneous and hyperechoic (Fig. 11–30*A*), but an important variant is the isoechoic mass with hyperechoic periphery. They are often peripheral, with posterior acoustic enhancement. Some large lesions have central scars. CT shows homogeneous, low-attenuation lesions, which enhance after intravenous contrast material administration, have nodular peripheral enhancement (called "puddling" of contrast material), and accumulate contrast material centripetally over a period of several minutes (Fig. 11–24). This finding is most useful when the patient has no known primary tumor; otherwise, this pattern is more likely due to a metastasis. Technetion-99m-labeled red blood cell scans are diagnostic for hemangioma when early vascular-phase images show decreased activity and delayed blood-pool scans demonstrate increased activity at the lesion site (Fig. 11–30*B*). MR imaging demonstrates lesions with low signal intensity on T_1-weighted scans, which is typical for most lesions. However, T_2-weighted MR imaging demonstrates high signal intensity similar to that of fluid, which is considered diagnostic of hemangioma or cyst. Intravenous Gd "puddles" in cavernous hemangioma and gradually migrates centripetally toward the center of the lesion (Fig. 11–31), analogous to the distribution of iodinated contrast material in cavernous hemangioma on CT, and likewise is considered diagnostic of cavernous hemangioma. This puddling in cavernous hemangioma is different from the more curvilinear or

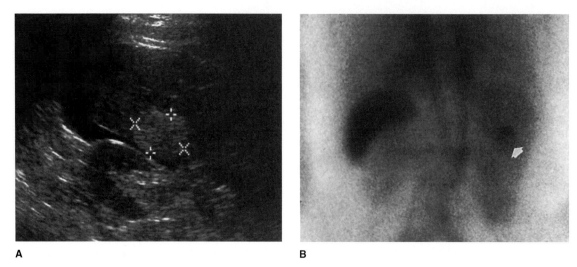

A

B

Fig. 11–30. **A** Transverse US in cavernous hemangiorna showing a hyperechoic, well-defined, homogeneous lesion at the posterior edge of the liver (*cursors*). **B** Tagged red blood cell NM scan showing the presence of a region of increased activity within the liver (*arrow*). Note that the image was obtained over the posterior aspect of the patient, so the liver is on the left side of the image. (Courtesy of Nat Watson, M.D., Winston-Salem, NC.)

heterogeneous distribution of contrast accumulation seen in malignant tumor. Angiography can be very helpful, because it shows punctate collections of contrast material shortly after injection, analogous to puddling seen in CT or MR imaging (Fig. 11–32*A*). These collections become denser, usually within a minute, because contrast puddles in the vascular spaces of the tumor (Fig. 11–32*B*).

Although typically diffuse, steatosis of the liver can present as focal deposits of fat. Furthermore, sometimes steatosis can present as the reverse, namely, residual focal islands of hepatic tissue unaffected by fatty deposition. Both of these conditions can be confusing since they may resemble focal solid masses including tumor on CT or US. MR imaging is the most accurate means to identify

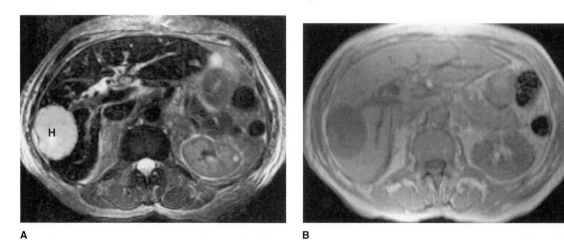

A

B

Fig. 11–31. **A** T$_2$-weighted scan demonstrating the markedly high signal intensity and well circumscribed margin of a cavernous hemangioma (H). **B** Preinfusion T$_1$-weighted MR imaging of cavernous hemangioma, showing the dark signal of the lesion.

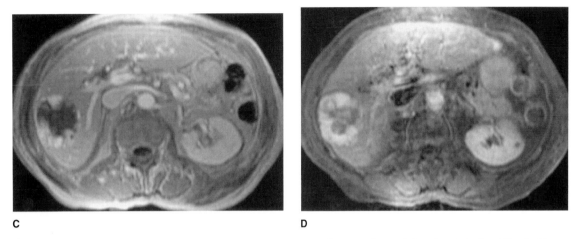

C   D

Fig. 11–31. **C** Immediate postinfused T₁-weighted MR imaging showing the peripheral nodular "puddling" of intravenous contrast material. **D** Delayed postinfused T₁-weighted MR imaging showing the centripetal filling in toward the center of the lesion.

sites of focal fat or focal fatty sparing. In particular, a pulse sequence called *out-of-phase T₁-weighted imaging*, which emphasizes the presence of fat intermixed with any host water-containing tissue, is very sensitive in the detection of the presence or absence of fat within focal fat or focal fatty sparing, respectively. Wherever fat is intermixed with water-containing parenchyma, there is loss of signal intensity on out-of-phase images. Therefore, focal fatty infiltration appears as sites of relative signal loss, whereas focal fatty sparing appears as sites of relative signal gain (Fig. 11–33). This imaging technique is the most sensitive and specific cross-sectional modality for characterizing focal fatty distribution, a very common condition.

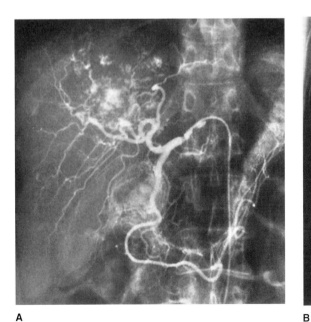

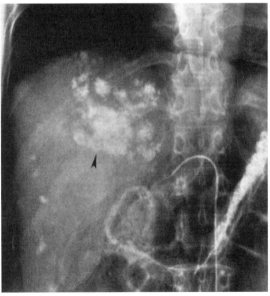

A   B

Fig. 11–32. Capillary **A** and venous **B** phase hepatic arteriogram in cavernous hemangioma showing the dense and persistent stain of the lesions (*arrowhead*).

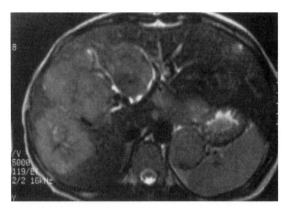

Fig. 11–36. T_2-weighted transverse MR imaging in liver metastasis showing the presence of intermediately high signal intensity liver lesions.

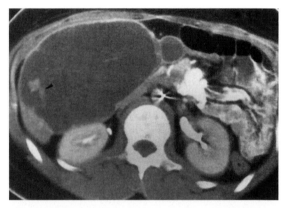

Fig. 11–38. CT in FNH showing a low-density lesion occupying the majority of the right lobe of the liver, and demonstrating a central scar (*arrowhead*).

Focal nodular hyperplasia (FNH) and liver cell adenoma are easily confused. Both are histologically benign liver disorders that produce single or multiple lesions. Both processes can occur in young adults. On imaging studies, they can resemble primary or metastatic liver tumors. However, some important differences pertain. FNH is probably a hamartoma of the liver, i.e., a localized overgrowth of mature cells that are identical to the types constituting the liver and contain fibrous tissue, blood vessels, bile ducts, and occasional well-differentiated hepatocytes. Adenoma is a true benign tumor composed of one tissue element of the liver, the hepatocyte. FNH often contains a central fibrotic scar.

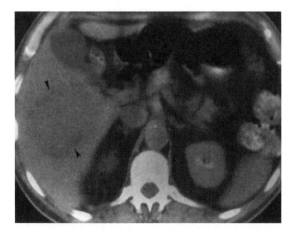

Fig. 11–37. CT in angiosarcoma showing a low-density lesion in the right lobe of the liver (*arrowheads*). This is indistinguishable from any other liver neoplasm.

Adenoma is associated with the use of oral contraceptives, whereas FNH probably is not. Adenoma, unlike FNH, tends to undergo hemorrhage, and thus to present as acute abdominal pain. US is nonspecific in studying FNH. Adenoma is usually hyperechoic but heterogeneous. On CT, FNH is transiently but markedly and uniformly hypervascular, and the central scar may be seen (Fig. 11–38). Adenoma usually shows low density, may hemorrhage as high-density collections on preinfusion scans, and enhances variably. On Tc-sulfur colloid NM scans, FNH can show either increased, decreased, or normal activity compared to that of liver. Adenoma usually shows no increased uptake in NM studies, but this varies. FNH has low signal intensity on T_1-weighted MR imaging and slightly high signal intensity on T_2-weighted images (Fig. 11–39). If the central scar is present, it may exhibit high signal intensity on T_2-weighted images. Adenoma, like many lesions, has a nonspecific appearance of low signal intensity on T_1-weighted examinations and slightly high signal intensity on T_2-weighted examinations. Hemorrhage is recognizable as high signal intensity on T_1-weighted images. Angiographically, FNH is hypervascular with radiating branches that produce a "spoke-wheel" appearance. Adenoma has a variable angiographic appearance but is generally less vascular than FNH.

Hepatocellular carcinoma, or hepatoma, is a primary malignancy of the liver. It is found in older cirrhotic patients in the United States and in younger patients in areas of the Far East and Africa, where it is endemic. Chronic hepatitis B and C infection and exposure to aflatoxin predispose to formation of hepatoma. On imaging studies, hepatoma appears as (1) a single predominant lesion (most common form), (2) a predominant lesion with multiple, smaller, surrounding

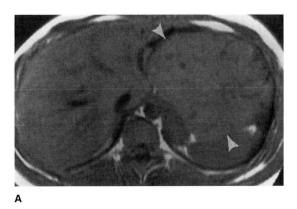 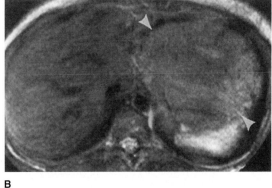

A   **B**

Fig. 11–39. **A** T$_1$-weighted MR image showing FNH in the left lobe with a nonspecific appearance of low signal intensity (*arrowheads*). **B** T$_2$-weighted image showing FNH with mildly high signal intensity (*arrowheads*).

daughter lesions, or (3) diffuse tumor. Portal vein invasion by the tumor in any form is relatively common and can aid in distinguishing hepatoma from other lesions. On US, hepatoma is most commonly a discrete lesion with increased, similar, or decreased echogenicity in comparison to that of liver. On CT, lesions are most commonly of low density and may enhance if fast scans in the arterial phase are performed after contrast material administration (Fig. 11–40). Portal venous thrombosis can be seen, and preexisting cirrhosis or Thorotrast can be demonstrated. MR imaging findings are similar to those of CT, but as with CT, the lesion is inhomogeneous.

EXERCISE 11-3: UPPER ABDOMINAL TRAUMA

Clinical Histories:

Case 11-9.   A 45-year-old motor vehicle accident victim presents with upper abdominal pain (Fig. 11–41).

Case 11-10.   A 57-year-old man presents who was beaten in the abdomen with a baseball bat (Fig. 11–42).

Questions:

11-9.   The most likely diagnosis in Case 11-9 (Fig. 11–41) is
   A.   hepatic contusion.
   B.   hepatic laceration.
   C.   uncomplicated ascites.
   D.   hemoperitoneum.

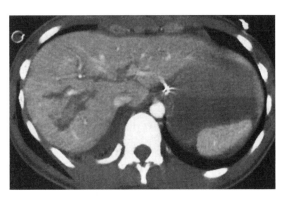

Fig. 11–41.

Fig. 11–40. CT in hepatoma showing the presence of an inhomogeneous lesion that enhances mildly in its periphery (*arrow*).

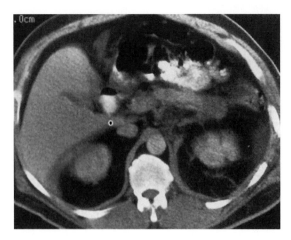

Fig. 11–42.

11-10. The most likely diagnosis in Case 11-10 (Fig. 11–42) is
  A. pancreatic trauma.
  B. bowel injury.
  C. mesenteric injury.
  D. hepatic laceration.

Radiologic Findings:

11-9. In this case (Fig. 11–41), the liver has an irregularly linear lesion in its central aspect, representing a liver laceration. (*B* is the correct answer to Question 11-9.)

11-10. In this case (Fig. 11–42), there is a low-density bulbous enlargement of the pancreatic tail, representing a pancreatic injury. (*A* is the correct answer to Question 11-10.)

Discussion:

Hepatic injury is common after blunt trauma. Hepatic injuries may be life threatening as a result of bleeding and shock, but more often surgery is not required. Observation and systemic support may be the only treatment necessary. Like trauma to any other organ, injury to the liver varies from mild to severe. A mild injury of the liver produces a localized collection of traumatized liver tissue and an interstitial hematoma, like a bruise, which is termed a *contusion*. More severe injuries that involve complete disruption of the tissue into fracture planes, perhaps involving the hepatic veins, inferior vena cava, or portal veins, and are called *lacerations*.

Most blunt abdominal trauma in the United States is radiographically evaluated with CT. Angiography is used to a lesser extent. US, NM, and MR imaging are of little or no value in a general survey of abdominal trauma. On CT, hepatic contusion is seen as a low-

attenuation lesion, perhaps with mass effect on surrounding hepatic vessels. Associated hemoperitoneum is not usually seen. On CT, hepatic laceration appears as an irregular, stellate, or linear lesion through the liver parenchyma (Fig. 11–41), sometimes extending to the porta, liver capsule, or IVC (Fig. 11–43). A hallmark of severe trauma to upper abdominal organs is accompanying hemoperitoneum, which appears as a collection of high-density material at the site of bleeding and is termed the *sentinel clot*. Acute blood that has migrated away from the site of active bleeding, or old hemoperitoneum at any site, often has the attenuation of simple or near-simple fluid and can resemble intraperitoneal fluid, or ascites, from a number of causes.

Ascites is a nonspecific reaction of the peritoneal space to a variety of causes, including tumor, inflammation, trauma, increased systemic venous resistance (e.g., congestive heart failure), renal or hepatic insufficiency, and many other conditions. It is characterized by the production of intraperitoneal fluid. This fluid can be simple, a transudate, in which case it has fluid density (Fig. 11–44) and is free to move to the dependent portion of the abdominal or pelvic cavity with patient movement. Alternatively, it can be complex, an exudate, in which case it is denser than simple fluid, is accompanied by solid tissue (e.g., tumor deposits in peritoneal metastases) or layered material (e.g., blood from trauma or inflammatory cellular debris in peritonitis), and often is *loculated*, or unable to move freely throughout the intraperitoneal cavity (e.g., abscess).

Pancreatic injury is uncommon, but potentially serious. Mortality from pancreatic injuries is nearly 20%. Being crushed against the spine probably accounts for the frequency of injury to the body of the pancreas. Pancreatic trauma may or may not be associated with increased amylase. Usually caused by blunt trauma, pancreatic trauma is often associated with injuries to other organs, such as liver and bowel. These injuries produce intraperitoneal blood

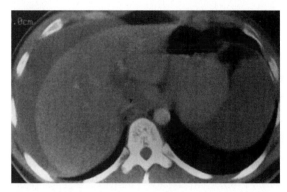

Fig. 11–43. CT in liver laceration showing the extension of the laceration into the IVC (*arrowheads*).

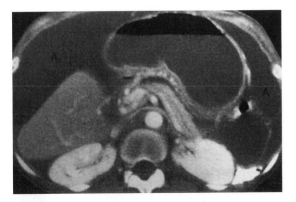

Fig. 11–44. CT in ascites showing fluid diffusely distributed throughout the abdomen (A).

and fluid, and interstitial mesenteric edema, which can be confusing. As with hepatic trauma, CT is usually the modality of choice to evaluate pancreatic trauma, but even on CT, the diagnosis can be difficult. On CT, the pancreas may be ill defined, enlarged, or even disrupted, i.e., fractured.

Bowel and mesenteric injuries are found in approximately 5% of all patients undergoing laparotomy after motor vehicle accidents. Injuries of the bowel and mesentery frequently accompany injury to the liver or pancreas. These injuries can result in massive intraperitoneal bleeding from disruption of mesenteric vessels or peritonitis from bowel perforation. As elsewhere, CT is the modality of choice to evaluate patients for possible bowel or mesenteric injuries, but these injuries, like those to the pancreas, can be difficult to detect. On CT,

injuries of the bowel and mesentery include free air with the intraperitoneal or retroperitoneal spaces (Fig. 11–45), free intra-abdominal fluid, circumferential or eccentric bowel wall thickening, enhancement of the bowel wall, streaky soft-tissue infiltration of the mesenteric fat, free mesenteric hematoma, and especially sentinel clot. Angiography may demonstrate free extravasation of contrast material in injuries of the mesenteric vessels, and percutaneous embolization may stop bleeding when surgery is not possible.

EXERCISE 11-4: BILIARY INFLAMMATION

Clinical Histories:

Case 11-11.   A 53-year-old male presents with acute right upper quadrant pain, fever, pain on palpation over the gallbladder, and elevated liver function tests (Fig. 11–46).

Case 11-12.   A 22-year-old HIV-positive female presents with debiliatating and chronic illness with vague right upper quadrant pain, but no tenderness on palpation over the gallbladder (Fig. 11–47).

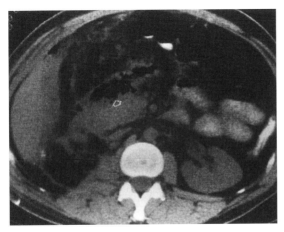

Fig. 11–45. CT in bowel injury showing the presence of extraluminal gas (*arrow*) due to bowel perforation.

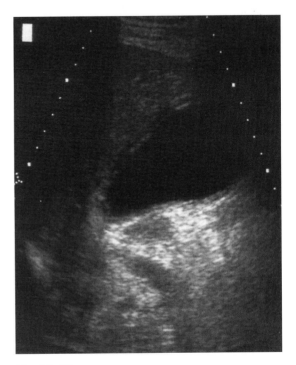

Fig. 11–46.

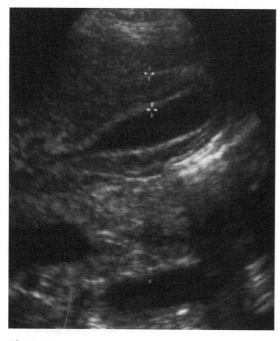

Fig. 11–47.

Case 11-13. An 84-year-old male presents with right upper quadrant pain, marked fever, and suspicion of sepsis (Fig. 11–48).

Case 11-14. A 53-year-old male presents with history of cholecystectomy, upper abdominal pain, jaundice, and fever (Fig. 11–49).

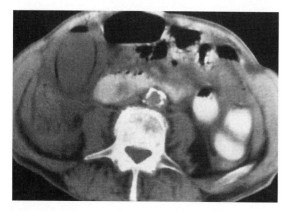

Fig. 11–48.

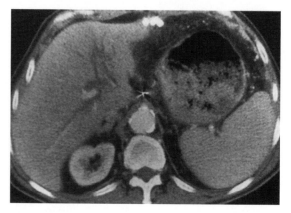

Fig. 11–49.

Questions:

11-11. The most likely diagnosis in Case 11-11 (Fig. 11–46) is
   A.   acute cholecystitis.
   B.   uncomplicated cholelithiasis.
   C.   chronic cholecystitis.
   D.   porcelain gallbladder.

11-12. The most likely diagnosis in Case 11-12 (Fig. 11–47) is
   A.   oriental cholangiohepatitis.
   B.   AIDS-associated cholangiopathy.
   C.   choledocholithiasis.
   D.   porcelain gallbladder.

11-13. The most likely diagnosis in Case 11-13 (Fig. 11–48) is
   A.   acute cholecystitis.
   B.   emphysematous cholecystitis.
   C.   porcelain gallbladder.
   D.   hydrops of gallbladder.

11-14. The most likely diagnosis in Case 11-14 (Fig. 11–49) is
   A.   choledocholithiasis.
   B.   ascending cholangitis.
   C.   acute cholecystitis.
   D.   emphysematous cholecystitis.

Radiologic Findings:

11-11. In this case, Fig. 11–46 shows that the gallbladder is distended, and the wall is thickened, measuring more than 5 mm, and has multiple lamina, indicating gallbladder wall inflammation from acute cholecystitis. (*A* is the correct answer to Question 11-11.)

11-12. In this case (Fig. 11–47), the gallbladder wall is markedly thickened, measuring over 1 cm., with multiple lamina, but was not tender to palpation, findings seen often with AIDS cholangiopathy. (*B* is the correct answer to Question 11-12.)

11-13. In this case (Fig. 11–48), gas within the gallbladder wall and lumen is the primary abnormality, indicating emphysematous cholecystitis. (*B* is the correct answer to Question 11-13.)

11-14. In this case, Fig. 11–48 shows that the biliary ducts are distended and irregular, which in the clinical presentation of fever and jaundice most strongly suggests cholangitis. (*B* is the correct answer to Question 11-14.)

Discussion:

Calculi are a common problem in the gallbladder and biliary ducts. Cholelithiasis is one of the most common abdominal disorders overall and is the most common cause of cholecystitis, as well as the most common indication for abdominal surgery. Gallstones develop when the composition of bile, which includes bile salts, lecithin, and cholesterol, varies from normal and creates supersaturation of cholesterol, which then precipitates. Historically, patients thought to be harboring gallstones on the basis of clinical criteria were examined by oral cholecystography, which shows filling defects in the gallbladder lumen opacified by orally ingested iodinated contrast material. However, this examination has been largely replaced by sonography, occasionally supported by other imaging information. On US, gallstones usually appear as mobile, intraluminal, echogenic foci that cast a well-defined acoustic shadow (Fig. 11–50). Two other possible appearances are echogenic foci in the gallbladder fossa without visible surrounding bile when the gallbladder is contracted, and small, mobile, echogenic foci that do not cast a shadow. On CT, gallstones appear as dense, well-defined, intraluminal structures (Fig. 11–51), but their density can vary from fat density to near bone density, depending on the relative concentration of calcium and cholesterol. MR imaging of the biliary system, especially MRCP, has become more important in biliary imaging, including the detection of calculi of the gallbladder and biliary tree. Although US remains the primary and initial means of identifying biliary calculi, MRCP can be used as a supplementary technique, especially in ductal calculi, because imaging of the biliary tree by US may be suboptimal when obscured by bowel gas. MRCP can depict the biliary system, filling defects within the biliary tree (Fig. 11–52), and congenital variants of the biliary ducts, and is about as accurate as ERCP in displaying a biliary "road map." It can also be used to evaluate the biliary ducts when ERCP is impossible to perform such as when the patient has undergone a Billroth procedure, interrupting the continuity of the upper gastrointestinal

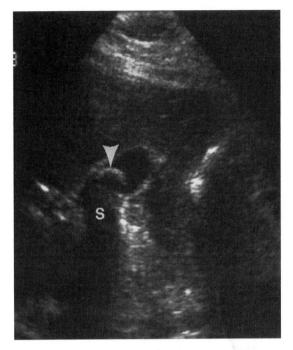

Fig. 11–50. Transverse US in cholelithiasis showing an echogenic structure (*arrowhead*) casting an acoustic shadow (S).

tract. NM and angiography have no major role at this time in assessment of gallstones.

Choledocholithiasis occurs when calculi pass from the gallbladder into the biliary ducts or when calculi develop originally within the ductal system. Regardless of origin, they may obstruct the biliary ducts, cause biliary colic, and lead to cholangitis. Common duct stones are usually evaluated with US and CT and by direct visualization with ERCP. On US, choledocholithiasis appears as echogenic foci within the lumen of the biliary duct. Sonographically, common duct stones are detected less readily than gallbladder stones, and meticulous technique is required. Choledocholithiasis can cause acoustic shadows, but for technical reasons they are detected less frequently than cholelithiasis (Fig. 11–53). On CT, choledocholithiasis appears as intraluminal biliary ductal foci, which, like gallbladder stones, may vary in density from hypodense to isodense to hyperdense to bile, depending on their composition (Fig. 11–54).

Cholecystitis is inflammation of the gallbladder that is almost always caused by obstruction of the cystic duct, usually by an impacted calculus. The inflammation may be acute or chronic, uncomplicated or complicated,

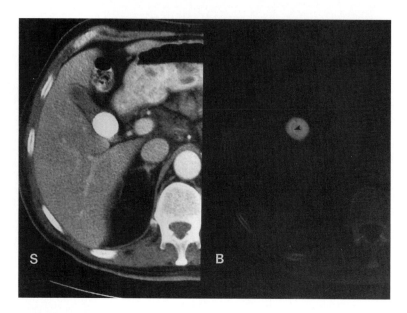

Fig. 11–51. CT in cholelithiasis using both soft-tissue windows (S) and bone windows (B) showing an extremely dense structure lying in the gallbladder. Note the laminated architecture of the gallstone on the bone windows (*arrowhead*).

calculous or acalculous. As the gallbladder continues to accumulate bile, intraluminal pressure increases and vascular insufficiency of the wall occurs, causing ischemia, necrosis, and often supervening inflammation. The gallbladder distends, the gallbladder wall thickens from edema, and the patient is tender to palpation over the gallbladder (positive Murphy's sign).

Both ultrasound and hepatobiliary NM studies are the modalities of choice to evaluate possible cholecysti-

tis. Sonographic signs of acute cholecystitis include cholelithiasis, gallbladder wall thickening (greater than 3 mm), irregular or linear hypoechoic structures within the gallbladder wall, a positive Murphy's sign, and marked gallbladder distention (Fig. 11–55). A combination of these signs is a good positive predictor of acute cholecystitis. In marked chronic cholecystitis, US shows persistent gallbladder wall thickening or sludge, stones, and contraction of the gallbladder. However, in the presence of

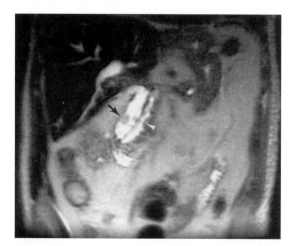

Fig. 11–52. Coronal MRCP demonstrating choledocholithiasis, appearing as filling defects (*arrow*) in the distal bile duct. Note the parallel pancreatic duct (*arrowhead*).

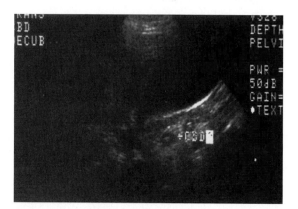

Fig. 11–53. Transverse US in choledocholithiasis showing the presence of an intraductal stone (CBD). Note that it does not cast an acoustic shadow, which, unlike gallbladder stones, is typical of intraductal stones.

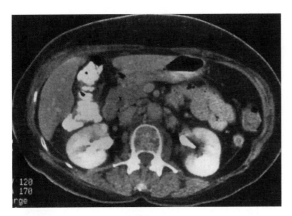

Fig. 11–54. CT in choledocholithiasis showing the presence of a stone within the common bile duct (*arrowheads*). Note that it is soft-tissue density, which is often, though not always, the case with intraductal stones.

cholelithiasis, the gallbladder almost always shows signs of chronic inflammation histologically, even without symptoms or sonographic findings.

Hepatobiliary NM HIDA scans depict acute cholecystitis as an absence of filling of the gallbladder with the radionuclide once it is excreted by the liver into the biliary ducts; this absence of filling is due to the obstruction of the cystic duct lumen by inflammatory edema of

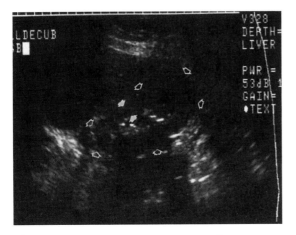

Fig. 11–55. Longitudinal US in acute cholecystitis showing thickened gallbladder wall (*arrows*), gallstones, casting an acoustic shadow. Open arrows are gallbladder boundary. The patient was extremely tender to palpation by the transducer right over the gallbladder (sonographic Murphy's sign).

the cystic duct wall (Fig. 11–56). Sufficient time must be given to fill the gallbladder. This time interval depends on whether or not morphine is administered. Morphine increases the tone of the sphincter of Oddi and increases intraluminal common bile duct pressure to overcome the resistance to bile flow into the gallbladder in chronic cholecystitis, but not in acute cholecystitis when a stone obstructs the duct. Acute cholecystitis is diagnosed when absence of activity is noted either 45 minutes after morphine augmentation or after 4 hours without morphine augmentation. Delayed gallbladder visualization after 1 hour usually reflects chronic cholecystitis. On CT, the morphologic findings in patients with acute cholecystitis are similar to the US findings, including gallstones and thickened and inhomogeneous gallbladder wall. However, CT is not as sensitive as US or NM to the presence of either gallstones or to acute cholecystitis. MR imaging can depict the presence of gallbladder wall inflammation in the absence of wall thickening by demonstrating wall enhancement following Gd infusion (Fig. 11–57). The exact role of MR imaging in cholecystitis has not yet been completely evaluated. Angiography has no role in the diagnosis of cholecystitis.

Many potential complications and conditions are associated with cholecystitis. These include hydrops, porcelain gallbladder, milk-of-calcium bile, and emphysematous cholecystitis.

Hydrops refers to the marked distention of the gallbladder by clear, sterile mucus, usually under conditions of chronic, complete cystic duct obstruction. On imaging studies, the primary finding is enlargement of the gallbladder (Fig. 11–58).

Porcelain gallbladder refers to calcification of the gallbladder wall, as a result of chronic inflammation causing dystrophic calcification and often associated with recurrent acute cholecystitis. Gallbladder stones are usually present, and there is a higher incidence (approximately 10%–20%) of gallbladder carcinoma. On imaging studies, complete or incomplete circular wall calcification is present and is seen as a curvilinear, highly echogenic wall on US or as a curvilinear, high-attenuation wall on CT (Fig. 11–59).

Milk-of-calcium bile refers to a precipitation of calcified material within the lumen of the gallbladder, usually associated with chronic cholecystitis. US shows echogenic sludge-like material, possibly with gallstones. CT demonstrates the distinctive appearance of a horizontal bile-calcium level.

Emphysematous cholecystitis is a distinctive condition. Like acute cholecystitis, it is marked by intense gallbladder wall inflammation, but unlike acute cholecystitis, it is not necessarily associated with gallstones. It may be related to ischemia of the gallbladder wall from small-vessel disease, and it affects an older age

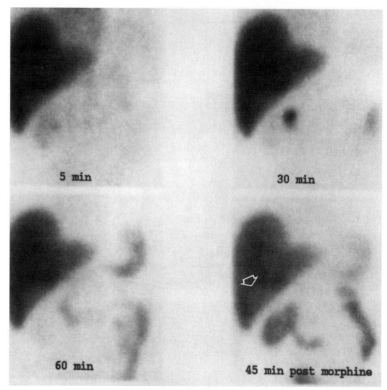

Fig. 11–56. NM hepatobiliary scan in acute cholecystitis showing the absence of gallbladder activity in the gallbladder fossa (*arrow*), after 60 minutes following administration of the agent and even after administration of morphine. (Courtesy of James Ball, M.D., Winston-Salem, NC.)

group than does acute cholecystitis. Gas is released by bacterial invasion and accumulates in the gallbladder wall, lumen, or both. On US, gas is seen as an echogenic focus producing poorly defined or "dirty" shadowing behind it.

The wall is thickened, perhaps focally, with gas. On CT, air-density gas is seen within the lumen or wall (Fig. 11–48). MR imaging and angiography have no current role in evaluation of these complications.

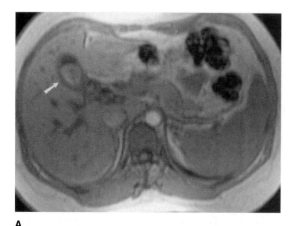
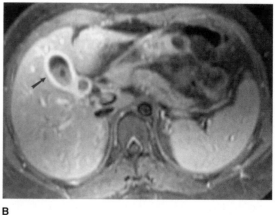

A   B

Fig. 11–57. **A** Preinfused T$_1$-weighted MR imaging scan showing cholelithaisis and a low signal intensity gallbladder wall (*arrow*). **B** Postinfused T$_1$-weighted MR imaging scan demonstrating gallbladder wall enhancement (*arrow*), reflecting the hyperemia of inflammation, signifying acute cholecystitis.

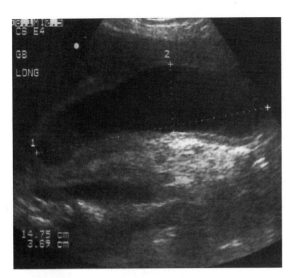

Fig. 11–58. Longitudinal US in hydrops showing a massively enlarged gallbladder due to complete obstruction of the cystic duct and accumulation of clear mucus.

Like inflammation of the gallbladder, inflammation of the biliary ducts, or *cholangitis*, is an important clinical condition. It is less common than cholecystitis. AIDS-associated cholangiopathy, ascending cholangitis, and oriental cholangiohepatitis are three important forms of cholangitis.

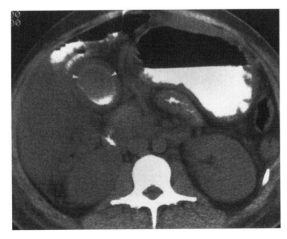

Fig. 11–59. CT in porcelain gallbladder showing the calcification of the gallbladder wall (*arrowheads*) and the dependent accumulation of calcified material in the gallbladder lumen.

AIDS-associated cholangiopathy is marked by the frequent isolation of opportunistic organisms, including *Cryptosporidium* and cytomegalovirus from the bile, and by considerable inflammation of the bile duct wall. On US or CT, the gallbladder or biliary duct walls may be markedly thickened (greater than 4 mm) (Fig. 11–47) and may contain irregular lamina. Inflammation is present, but stones may or may not be present. Cholangiography shows irregular strictures, papillary stenosis, or both.

Ascending cholangitis is a bacterial inflammation of both walls and lumina of the biliary system, including the gallbladder. It is almost always due to obstruction of the biliary tract, especially when caused by choledocholithiasis and distal bile duct stenosis. The presence of grossly purulent material within the duct indicates suppurative cholangitis. Cross-sectional imaging studies are used to define the level and cause of obstruction. Cholangiography can show the abnormal biliary ducts directly. The purulent material of suppurative cholangitis may be seen as echogenic material on US, high-density material on CT, or filling defects on cholangiography.

Oriental cholangiohepatitis is a common illness in endemic areas of Asia and can be seen in Asian immigrants in this country. It may be caused by bile duct wall injury from the parasitic infestation. Ductal stones commonly form, and the ducts are dilated. A characteristic finding is the presence of intraductal (especially intrahepatic ductal) calculi. These findings are readily demonstrated with US, CT, and cholangiography.

EXERCISE 11-5: PANCREATIC INFLAMMATION

Clinical Histories:

Case 11-15. A 54-year-old alcoholic male presents with marked epigastric pain and increased amylase (Fig. 11–60).

Case 11-16. A 45-year-old male presents with marked epigastric pain and a falling hematocrit; he is "crashing" (Fig. 11–61).

Case 11-17. A 65-year-old male presents with chronic epigastric pain (Fig. 11–62).

Questions:

11-15. The most likely diagnosis in Case 11-15 (Fig. 11–60) is

A. acute edematous pancreatitis.

B. pancreatic abscess.

C. pancreatic phlegmon.

D. hemorrhagic pancreatitis.

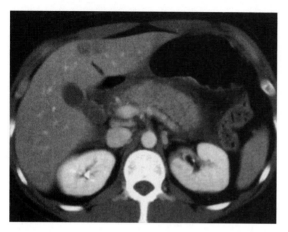

Fig. 11–60.

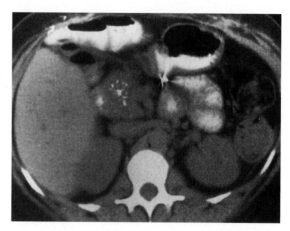

Fig. 11–62.

11-16. The most likely diagnosis in Case 11-16 (Fig. 11–61) is
  A. acute edematous pancreatitis.
  B. hemorrhagic pancreatitis.
  C. gastroduodenal artery pseudoaneurysm.
  D. pancreatic abscess.

11-17. The most likely diagnosis in Case 11-17 (Fig. 11–62) is
  A. acute edematous pancreatitis.
  B. chronic pancreatitis.
  C. pancreatic phlegmon.
  D. hemorrhagic pancreatitis.

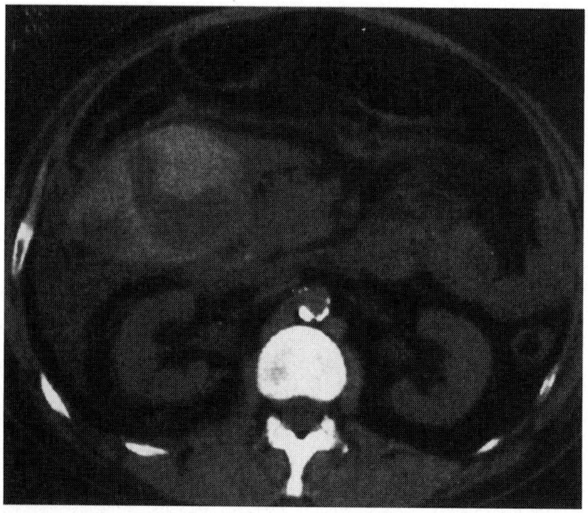

Radiologic Findings:

11-15. In Fig. 11–60, the overall size of the pancreas is enlarged, the tissue around the pancreas is edematous, and the fat planes between the pancreas and the stomach are blurred, findings of acute edematous pancreatitis. (*A* is the correct answer to Question 11-15.)

11-16. In Fig. 11–61, peripancreatic inflammatory changes and a high-density collection are seen adjacent to the pancreatic head, representing a collection of blood created by hemorrhagic pancreatitis. (*B* is the correct answer to Question 11-16.)

11-17. In Fig. 11–62, multiple high-density calcifications are distributed throughout the pancreatic head, and the pancreatic head is mildly enlarged, findings of chronic calcific pancreatitis. (*B* is the correct answer to Question 11-17.)

Discussion:

Pancreatitis, an inflammatory condition of the pancreas, has a number of causes including alcohol abuse, trauma, cholelithiasis, peptic ulcer, hyperlipoproteinemia, hypercalcemia, and infection. Pancreatic inflammation may be acute or chronic. Acute pancreatitis and chronic pancreatitis may not represent different stages of the same disease.

Acute pancreatitis can occur once or repetitively and usually has the potential for healing. It can be associated with mild to severe inflammatory edema (edematous or interstitial pancreatitis) or with hemorrhage (hemorrhagic or necrotizing pancreatitis). These two forms of acute pancreatitis may be distinguishable only by the severity and time course of the disease. Edematous pancreatitis resolves within 2 to 3 days with appropriate therapy, whereas hemorrhagic pancreatitis requires much longer to

Fig. 11–61.

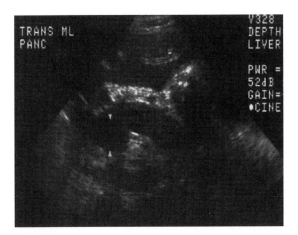

Fig. 11–63. Transverse US in acute pancreatitis showing a diffusely hypoechoic pancreas with more pronounced hypoechogenicity in the pancreatic head (*arrowheads*).

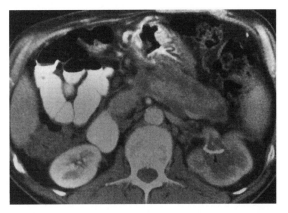

Fig. 11–64. CT in pancreatitis showing the presence of poorly defined soft-tissue planes around the pancreas, obscuring the boundary between the pancreas and the stomach and colon. Note the stent in the renal pelvis (*arrowhead*) of the left kidney, placed to relieve urinary obstruction.

resolve. The diagnosis of simple pancreatitis is usually based on medical history, physical examination, and laboratory results. With this information imaging studies are usually unnecessary, and scans show the pancreas to be normal or only slightly enlarged. The surrounding fat is edematous. The pancreas appears hypoechoic on US (Fig. 11–63). On CT the surrounding fat appears as areas of streaky interstitial soft-tissue density in the transverse mesocolon around the pancreas (Fig. 11–64).

Clinical criteria to predict the severity or likelihood of complications of pancreatitis correlate well with the presence and extent of extrapancreatic abnormalities on imaging studies. Imaging is useful in acute pancreatitis when assessing potential complications. These complications include hemorrhagic pancreatitis, vascular complications, phlegmon, and abscess.

Hemorrhagic pancreatitis is usually due to erosion of small vessels, is often a serious problem, and indicates an acutely and critically ill patient. It appears as a collection of echogenic material on US. On CT it appears as a collection of high-density material, and can be extremely extensive because it is an aggressive process (Fig. 11–65). This material represents the blood.

Large vessels are at risk for developing pseudoaneurysms when the histiolytic enzymes released by the inflamed pancreas erode their walls, leading to a focal, highly vascular structure within the region of the pancreas. The splenic, gastroduodenal, and hepatic arteries are particularly vulnerable. On US and CT, flow within an enlarged rounded vessel can be seen. Angiography establishes the diagnosis by showing a focally enlarged vessel, sometimes with extravasation. However, CTA is also effective for detecting pseudoaneuryms related to pancreatitis.

Phlegmon is an inflammatory, boggy, edematous, soft-tissue mass, distinct from fluid, arising from the pancreas and diffusely spreading away from it. Phlegmon appears as a diffuse soft-tissue echogenicity or density process surrounding the pancreas and contains neither the blood of hemorrhagic pancreatitis nor the fluid of an abscess (Fig. 11–66).

Abscesses are a potentially life-threatening complication of pancreatitis. Infection associated with pancreatitis

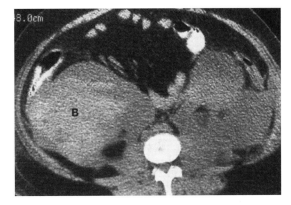

Fig. 11–65. CT in hemorrhagic pancreatitis showing diffusely distributed pancreatic inflammatory exudate containing high-density blood (B) in the right side of the abdomen.

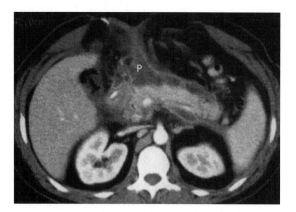

Fig. 11–66. CT in pancreatic phlegmon showing the presence of poorly defined phlegmonous exudate (P) surrounding the entire pancreas and extending from the pancreas toward the anterior abdominal wall.

can be thought of as representing infected necrosis (diffuse infection without pus collection) or pancreatic abscess (collection of pus surrounded by a capsule). Infected necrosis is harder to identify on imaging studies than is pancreatic abscess, since it is less distinct and blends into the surrounding edema. On US, an abscess appears as a poorly defined anechoic or hypoechoic lesion. It enhances sound posteriorly and may contain debris. Gas appears as a poorly defined echogenic focus within the nondependent aspect of the lesion and casts a "dirty" shadow. On CT, the lesion is poorly defined and may contain gas collections (Fig. 11–67). After contrast material infusion, the border enhances. If gas is absent, abscess cannot be differentiated from phlegmon or pseudocyst. In

general, NM and angiography do not have a major role in evaluation of acute pancreatitis.

Unlike acute pancreatitis, chronic pancreatitis is considered to indicate permanent pancreatic damage. Chronic pancreatitis may or may not be preceded by prior attacks of acute pancreatitis. The pancreas will develop calcifications within the ductal system (Fig. 11–62). Mass-like enlargement of the pancreas can periodically occur, but often the gland eventually atrophies. The pancreatic duct may dilate. These findings are visible on both US and CT. NM and angiography do not have a current major role in evaluation of chronic pancreatitis.

EXERCISE 11-6: PANCREATIC NEOPLASM

Clinical Histories:

Case 11-18.   A 62-year-old female presents with vague, deep, and persistent abdominal pain (Fig. 11–68).

Case 11-19.   A 65-year-old male presents with mid-epigastric pain over a long period of time (Fig. 11–69).

Case 11-20.   Consider a 32-year-old healthy, asymptomatic woman (Fig. 11–70).

Questions:

11-18.   The most likely diagnosis in Case 11-18 (Fig. 11–68) is

    A.   pancreatic cyst.
    B.   ductal pancreatic carcinoma.
    C.   pancreatic metastasis.
    D.   peripancreatic lymphadenopathy.

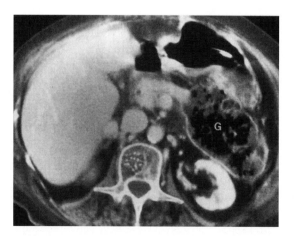

Fig. 11–67. CT in pancreatic abscess showing the presence of gas in the pancreatic tail (G) from a gas-forming organism.

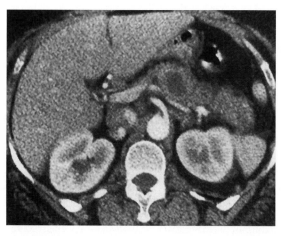

Fig. 11–68.

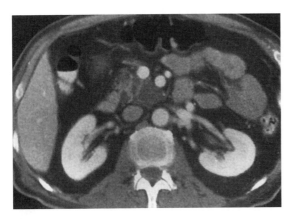

Fig. 11–69.

11-19. The most likely diagnosis in Case 11-19 (Fig. 11–69) is
  A. cholangiocarcinorna.
  B. cystic pancreatic neoplasm.
  C. ductal pancreatic carcinoma.
  D. pancreatic cyst.

11-20. The most likely diagnosis in Case 11-20 (Fig. 11–70) is
  A. acute edematous pancreatitis.
  B. pancreatic pseudocyst.
  C. pancreatic cyst.
  D. cystic pancreatic neoplasm.

Radiologic Findings:

11-18. In this case (Fig. 11–68), there is a low, but not fluid, density lesion in the pancreatic body, expanding the contour of the pancreas, and not associated with any inflammatory changes in the peripancreatic fat,

findings most consistent with a ductal adenocarcinoma. (*B* is the correct answer to Question 11-18.)

11-19. Figure 11–69 shows a fluid density lesion within the pancreatic head and uncinate process of the pancreas, not associated with inflammatory changes in the peripancreatic fat, findings most compatible with a cystic neoplasm of the pancreas. (*B* is the correct answer to Question 11-19.)

11-20. In Fig. 11–70, several small, simple, unilocular cysts are seen in the pancreatic parenchyma, without inflammatory changes or signs of peripancreatic extension of any disease process. (*C* is the correct answer to Question 11-20.)

Discussion:

Pancreatic masses include tumors, tumor-like masses such as cysts and developmental anomalies, and inflammatory lesions. These can overlap in appearance, such as when an inflammatory mass simulates a neoplastic mass on imaging studies. They can be causally related, such as when a neoplastic mass secondarily causes an inflammatory mass. Therefore, differentiation among them is not entirely possible, either clinically or radiographically. However, the prognostic and management implications of the lesions that create pancreatic masses differ considerably and therefore require extensive and often invasive investigation. Although contrast studies of the gastrointestinal tract can be used to infer the presence of a mass, cross-sectional imaging studies are usually employed to establish the diagnosis.

Tumors of the pancreas are important clinical entities; some have an extremely poor prognosis and some produce serious clinical symptoms. They can be classified according to origin as epithelial tumors, endocrine tumors, and miscellaneous lesions. Epithelial tumors can be solid or cystic. Solid ductal adenocarcinoma is the most common overall and carries the worst prognosis (mean survival of 4 months). Cystic tumors can be divided into cystic lesions arising from the pancreatic parenchymal cells, such as cystadenoma or cystadenocarcinoma, and those arising from the pancreatic ductal cells, such as intraductal papillary mucinous tumors. Compared to adenocarcinoma, these tumors have a less serious prognosis. Endocrine, or islet cell, tumors elaborate hormonal substances and can create serious symptoms. The two most common of these are insulinoma, which releases insulin and produces hypoglycemia, and gastrinoma, which releases gastrin and produces Zollinger-Ellison syndrome. There are many other important kinds of hormonally active pancreatic endocrine tumors, and each is designated by the hormone it secretes (e.g., glucagonoma, somatostatinoma). Miscellaneous lesions arise from pancreatic parenchymal tissue (e.g., metastases, especially from melanoma, and lung or

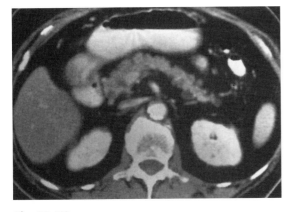

Fig. 11–70.

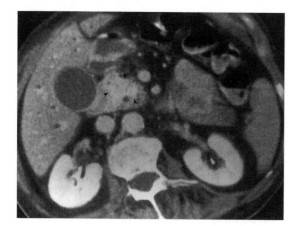

Fig. 11–71. CT in pancreatic ductal adenocarcinoma showing an enhancing tumor in the pancreatic head (*arrowheads*).

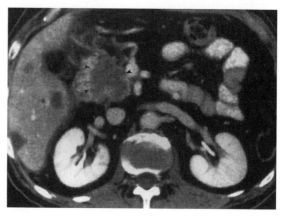

Fig. 11–72. CT in metastatic pancreatic carcinoma showing a pancreatic mass (*arrowheads*) and numerous liver metastases.

breast cancer) or from tissue other than pancreas (e.g., intrapancreatic cholangiocarcinoma or peripancreatic lymph node). These miscellaneous lesions are important because they sometimes strongly simulate true pancreatic neoplasms on imaging studies.

Ductal adenocarcinoma has a variety of appearances on imaging studies. On US, it usually is seen as a focal, hypoechoic, irregular, solid mass. Rarely, it is isoechoic or involves the entire gland. In some pancreatic head masses, the only finding may be that the uncinate process is rounded. The pancreatic or biliary duct may be dilated by the obstructing tumor. *Pseudocysts*, cystic collections in or around the pancreas, may form because of pancreatic duct dilatation and perforation. On CT, the tumor presents as a solid, low-density, irregular mass, perhaps with ductal dilatation, pseudocyst formation, or both (Fig. 11–68). Occasionally, the tumors will enhance brightly (Fig. 11–71). Angiography may be used to demonstrate the vascular anatomy and establish definitively whether certain key vessels (e.g., the superior mesenteric artery or vein) are encased. If so, the lesion is unresectable. NM currently has no established role in evaluation of pancreatic tumors. Associated metastases in the liver establish the fact that a pancreatic mass cannot be simply inflammatory (Fig. 11–72). General pertinent negatives on cross-sectional imaging may help to differentiate adenocarcinoma from other nontumorous masses. Calcification is rarely, if ever, seen in ductal adenocarcinoma, and it is almost never hypervascular.

Ductal adenocarcinoma is simulated by a number of other entities. These include peripancreatic lymphadenopathy, intrapancreatic cholangiocarcinoma, and pancreatic metastases.

Peripancreatic lymphadenopathy from lymphoma, leukemia, or any other primary malignancy can closely resemble a pancreatic mass. On imaging studies it may appear as solid soft tissue in the pancreatic region (Fig. 11–73). Keys to differentiating lymphadenopathy from a primary solid mass include smooth lobulation and pseudoseptations caused by incomplete coalescence of

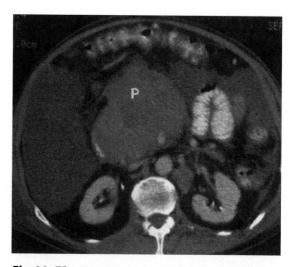

Fig. 11–73. CT in parapancreatic lymphadenopathy showing the presence of a large soft-tissue mass (P), simulating a pancreatic carcinoma, but without the biliary duct obstruction that is normally caused by a lesion this size (normal biliary tree not shown).

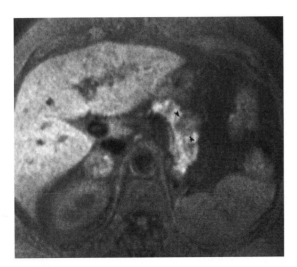

Fig. 11–74. Transverse MR imaging of a pancreatic metastasis from lung carcinoma (*arrowheads*).

dilatation. Metastases appear as solid intrapancreatic lesions, but with necrosis, they appear as fluid masses. Because they may be completely indistinguishable from primary tumors, the diagnosis may be inferred only from the clinical history. Pancreatic metastases are quite uncommon, usually arise from melanoma or lung primary lesions, and mimic a focal mass lesion of any neoplastic origin (Fig. 11–74).

Pancreatic endocrine tumors may also simulate ductal adenocarcinoma and, in fact, no specific features consistently distinguish the two. Occasionally, however, certain imaging features can be helpful, especially when combined with the history. Many islet cell tumors appear simply as solid masses within the pancreas. However, some (especially in insulinoma) may appear hypervascular when studied with fast bolus, or dynamic, CT, and they may appear as extremely dense lesions immediately after enhancement with intravenous contrast material. Calcifications, which sometimes are very dense, are more commonly seen with islet cell tumors. MR imaging may have a role in the evaluation of islet cell tumors, because these tumors have a characteristic appearance on MR studies. Islet cell tumors and their metastases have extremely high signal intensity on T_2-weighted MR imaging, which can be used to characterize the origin of the lesion.

Primary cystic pancreatic malignancies and pancreatic cysts are not readily confused with typical ductal adenocarcinoma. Currently, cystic pancreatic masses are classified according to whether they arise from parenchymal cells or ductal cells. Cystic malignancies arising from pancreatic parenchyma are classified as either microcystic

the lymph nodes. Also, peripancreatic lymphadenopathy is much less likely to obstruct the pancreatic duct, although suprapancreatic lymph nodes obstruct the biliary duct as it passes through the porta hepatis.

Two uncommon neoplastic processes that occur in the pancreas are cholangiocarcinoma and metastases. Cholangiocarcinoma usually does not occur within the pancreas, but when it does, it can exactly mimic a pancreatic head mass to the extent of producing biductal

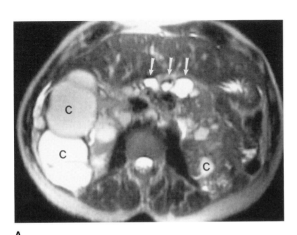

A

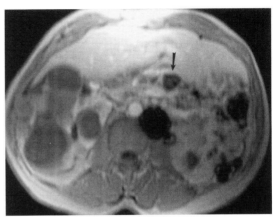

B

Fig. 11–75. **A** T_2-weighted MR imaging of a patient with von Hippel-Lindau disease, showing cystic lesions in the pancreas (*arrows*). Note the presence of multiple cystic masses (C) in both kidneys, right more than left. **B** Postinfused T_1-weighted MR imaging of the same patient as in part *A*, showing the absence of enhancement (*arrow*), differentiating cysts from vascularized cystic masses.

adenomas or mucinous cystic neoplasms. This classification is helpful, because the two lesions are distinguishable from each other and from solid lesions on imaging studies. Microcystic adenomas are composed of innumerable very small cysts (1 mm to 2 cm). Sometimes they contain highly vascularized fibrous septa and a central stellate fibrotic scar, which may calcify. They are not thought to be malignant or premalignant. Mucinous cystic neoplasms are composed of unilocular or multilocular cysts larger than 5 cm and may have large papillary excrescences. They are considered malignant or premalignant lesions. Both microcystic adenomas and mucinous cystic neoplasms are cystic, but differences in the sizes of the cysts can be recognized on US or CT. Cystic malignancies arising from pancreatic ductal epithelial cells are called *intraductal papillary mucinous tumors*. These tumors contain considerable mucus and therefore exhibit complex appearances on MR imaging. Pancreatic cysts can occur as isolated congenital cysts or as part of a more generalized multiorgan process that includes adult polycystic disease or von Hippel-Lindau disease (Fig. 11–75). Regardless, their appearance is similar to that of a cyst in any other organ (Fig. 11–70). US and CT depict a uniloculated or multiloculated cyst. A pancreatic cyst may be difficult to differentiate from a mucinous cystic neoplasm.

BIBLIOGRAPHY

Friedman AC, Dachman AH. *Radiology of the Liver, Biliary Tract, and Pancreas.* St. Louis: Mosby; 1994.

Moss AA, Gamsu G, Genant HK. *Computed Tomography of the Body with Magnetic Resonance Imaging.* 2nd ed. Philadelphia: Saunders; 1993.

Nghiem HV, Jeffrey RB Jr, Mindelzun RE. CT of blunt trauma to the bowel and mesentery. *AJR* 1993;160:53.

Semelka RC. *Abdominal-Pelvic MRI.* New York: Wiley-Liss; 2002.

Takahashi N, Brown JJ. MRI of the pancreas. *Appl Radiol* 2002;31:17–25.

PART 5

Head and Spine

Brain and Its Coverings

12

Michelle S. Bradbury & Daniel W. Williams III

INTRODUCTION

Technologic advances in radiology during the past 30 years have vastly improved our ability to diagnose neurologic diseases. Prior to the introduction of computed tomography in 1974, neuroradiologic examinations of the brain consisted primarily of plain films of the skull, cerebral arteriography, pneumoencephalography, and conventional nuclear medicine studies. Unfortunately, these techniques, for the most part, provided only indirect information about suspected intracranial processes, were insensitive in detecting subtle or early brain lesions, or were potentially harmful to the patient. Computed tomography (CT) revolutionized the radiologic workup of central nervous system abnormalities because for the first time normal and abnormal structures could be directly visualized with minimal risk to the patient.

In the late 1980s, it became apparent that magnetic resonance (MR) imaging would become the procedure of choice for evaluating many neurologic disorders, as well as for demonstrating vascular flow phenomena. Since then, many technologic advances have been associated with this modality. These include improvements in magnet and coil design, decrease in imaging time, and the development of new pulse sequences such as MR angiography (MRA), MR spectroscopy (MRS), diffusion-weighted (DW) and perfusion-weighted (PW) MR imaging, and functional MR imaging (fMRI).

Revolutionary breakthroughs in CT scanning technology during the 1990s facilitated the development of advanced CT applications, namely, dynamic contrast-enhanced CT angiography (CTA) and CT perfusion (CTP). These techniques, which allow high spatial resolution imaging of the cervical and intracranial vasculature, are currently being used in the evaluation of the acute stroke patient in many medical centers. Furthermore, recent technologic advances in CT imaging have markedly decreased scan times and have allowed evaluation of very tiny anatomic structures due to improvements in spatial resolution.

Recent advances in nuclear medicine functional imaging techniques, including single photon emission computed tomography (SPECT) and positron emission tomography (PET); improvements in conventional arteriographic methods; and expansion of catheter-based therapeutic procedures have provided the neuroradiologist today with an even greater variety of strategies for diagnosing and treating neurologic abnormalities.

The main purpose of this chapter is to acquaint the reader with the major radiologic techniques currently being used to evaluate the brain and its coverings. The strengths and weaknesses of these techniques are discussed. Imaging anatomy of the brain and its coverings is briefly reviewed. Basic guidelines pertaining to technique selection for evaluating common neurologic conditions are provided. Finally, examples of common brain abnormalities are presented. It is assumed that readers have a basic understanding of neuroanatomy and neuropathology.

Although this chapter may give some insight into neuroradiologic study interpretation, that is not its primary goal. Rather, readers should expect to become reasonably familiar with the various techniques employed to examine the brain and should gain some idea about the appropriate ordering of examinations in specific clinical situations.

TECHNIQUES

Radiologic modalities useful in evaluating the brain and its coverings can be divided into two major groups: anatomic modalities and functional modalities. Anatomic modalities, which provide information mostly of a structural nature, include plain films of the skull, computed tomography, magnetic resonance imaging, cerebral arteriography, and ultrasonography. On the other hand, SPECT and PET imaging, CTP, DW and PW MR imaging, fMRI, and MRS are primarily functional modalities,

which give information about brain perfusion or metabolism. Some techniques provide both anatomic and functional information. For example, cerebral arteriography depicts blood vessels supplying the brain but also allows us to estimate brain circulation time. Ultrasonography of the carotid bifurcation is another modality that provides both anatomic and functional information. A routine sonogram of the carotid bifurcation gives anatomic data that, when combined with Doppler data, readily provides information about blood flow.

The following discussion of current neuroradiologic techniques emphasizes relative examination cost and patient risk, along with the advantages and disadvantages of each technique. The normal imaging appearance of the brain and its coverings is also illustrated.

Plain Radiographs

Plain radiographs of the skull are obtained by placing a patient's head between an x-ray source and a recording device (i.e., x-ray film). Bones of the skull can block a large number of x-rays and, therefore, cast a white "shadow" on the x-ray film (Fig. 12–1). On the other hand, soft tissues such as scalp or brain cast little, if any, shadow on the film. Because the skull has a spherical shape, bones will be superimposed on one another. As a result, multiple routine views of the skull, including frontal, lateral, and axial projections, may be needed to adequately assess the calvarium and to accurately localize a lesion (Fig. 12–1). Even then, these studies can occasionally be tricky to interpret because of the large number of superimposed structures. The resultant skull radiograph primarily gives information about the bones of the skull, but no direct information about the intracranial contents. Indirect information about intracranial abnormalities can sometimes be obtained from the skull plain radiograph, although this information can be quite subtle, even in the setting of advanced disease. Skull plain radiographs have been largely replaced today by more sensitive techniques such as CT or MR imaging. Even in the setting of suspected skull fracture, plain radiographs are rarely indicated, because CT scans also show the fracture, as well as any intracranial abnormality that might require treatment.

Computed Tomography

CT scans consist of computer-generated cross-sectional images obtained from a rotating x-ray beam and detector system. Recent advances in scanning technology now permit simultaneous acquisition of multiple images during a single rotation of the x-ray tube (e.g., up to 16 as of 2004) during a breath-hold. The resultant images, unlike plain films, exquisitely depict and differentiate between soft tissues, thus allowing direct visualization of

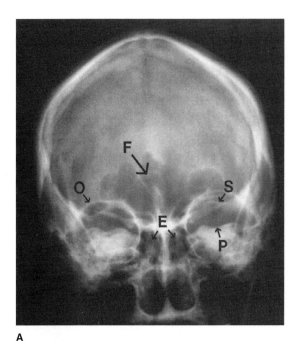
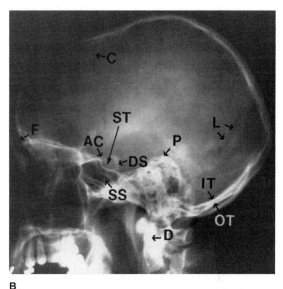

A   **B**

Fig. 12–1. Frontal **A** and lateral **B** plain films of the normal skull. Anatomic landmarks include ethmoid sinuses (E), frontal sinus (F), orbital roof (O), superior surface of the petrous portion of the temporal bone (P), sphenoid ridge (S), coronal suture (C), dens (D), anterior clinoid process (AC), dorsum sella (DS), sella turcica (ST), lambdoid suture (L), inner table of calvarium (IT), outer table of calvarium (OT), and sphenoid sinus (SS).

intracranial contents and abnormalities associated with neurologic diseases. The contrast or brightness ("window" or "level," respectively) of these images can be adjusted to highlight particular tissues.

Typically, a head CT consists of images adjusted to emphasize soft-tissue detail (soft-tissue windows) as well as images adjusted to visualize bony detail (bone windows) (Fig. 12–2). As stated earlier, cortical bone appears white (has a high attenuation value or Hounsfield unit), whereas air within the paranasal sinuses appears black (has a low attenuation value) (Fig. 12–2). Cerebral white matter has a slightly lower Hounsfield number than does cerebral gray matter and consequently appears slightly darker than gray matter on a head CT scan (Fig. 12–2*A*). Intracranial pathologic conditions can be either dark (low attenuation) or bright (high attenuation), depending on the particular abnormality. For example, acute intracranial hemorrhage is typically very bright, whereas an acute cerebral infarction demonstrates low attenuation when compared to the surrounding normal brain because of the presence of edema.

The CT technologist can change the slice thickness and angulation, among other technical factors, to alter the way an image appears. Axial images are most commonly obtained, but coronal images can be obtained with hyperextension of the patient's neck. Because CT images are computer generated, data making up the axial images can be reformatted in the coronal, sagittal, or oblique planes or as a 3-D image, although some resolution may be lost.

CT examinations are often performed after intravenous administration of an iodinated contrast agent. These agents "light up" or enhance normal blood vessels and dural sinuses, as well as intracranial structures that lack a blood–brain barrier (BBB), such as the pituitary gland, choroid plexus, or pineal gland. Pathologic conditions that interrupt the BBB also demonstrate enhancement after contrast material administration. For this reason, lesions that may be invisible on a noncontrast study are often obvious on a contrast-enhanced scan.

Volumetric images of intravenously injected contrast as it passes through the arterial circulation, or CTA, can now be routinely performed. These high spatial resolution 3-D CTA images of the cervical and intracranial vasculature have been implemented into recently developed acute stroke protocol examinations. In particular, CTA accurately identifies the location and extent of large vessel occlusions, which may predict response to reperfusion

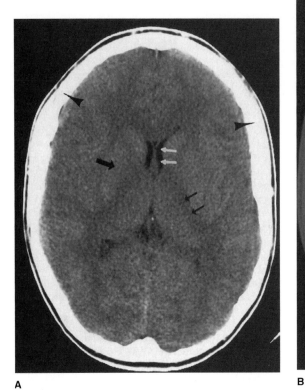
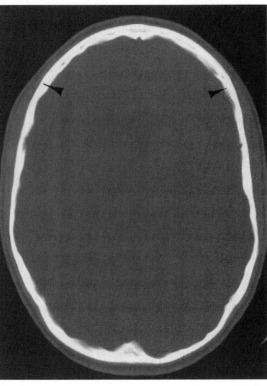

A   **B**

Fig. 12–2. Normal axial head CT images. Appropriate window selection allows visualization of both intracranial contents **A** and bony calvarium **B**. Note differences in attenuation between gray matter (right basal ganglia, *large arrow*), white matter (left internal capsule, *small black arrows*), cerebrospinal fluid (CSF; frontal horn of the left lateral ventricle, *white arrows*), and bone (skull, *arrowheads*).

therapies. Tailored software analysis of CTA data can produce maps of whole-brain perfusion. These permit a physiologic determination of the extent of collateral circulation and volume of brain tissue affected by an ischemic event, as well as a measure of the severity of the insult. This information can additionally be supplemented by a more detailed, quantitative evaluation of the cerebral microvascular hemodynamics (CTP) during the early phase of bolus passage. The potential utility of CTA/CT perfusion imaging in the acute stroke patient is based on the high specificity and accuracy of this functional assessment.

Another recent application of CTA is in the screening evaluation of blunt cerebrovascular injury, including closed head injuries, seat belt abrasion (or other soft tissue injury) of the anterior neck, basilar skull fracture extending through the carotid canal, and cervical vertebral body fracture. It is an accurate technique for detecting internal carotid artery (ICA) dissections and for assessing stenoses, although evaluation is difficult in areas of

surrounding dense bone as a result of associated "streak artifact." However, this noninvasive, relatively short imaging procedure rivals conventional angiographic methods, because it requires no patient transfer, and can sensitively identify vascular injury in relation to other associated brain insults, cervical spine injury, or facial or basilar skull fractures.

High-resolution data acquisition during the venous phase following intravenous contrast administration (CT venography) can be used to identify dural sinuses and cerebral veins, evaluate for dural venous sinus thrombosis, and distinguish partial sinus obstruction from venous occlusion in the setting of adjacent brain masses. CT venography can also differentiate slow flow from thrombosis, which may occasionally be difficult with MR techniques.

The major advantages of CT scanning are that it is inexpensive, widely available, can be used in patients with MR-incompatible hardware, and allows a relatively quick assessment of intracranial contents in the setting

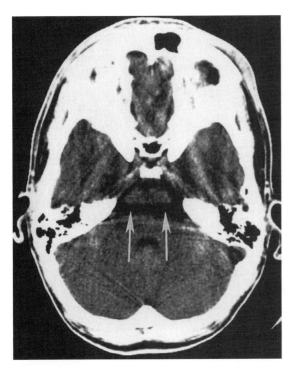

Fig. 12–3. Streak artifacts (*arrows*) commonly obscure portions of the brain stem, posterior fossa, and temporal lobes on routine head CT scans.

of a neurological deficit. The images obtained are very sensitive to the presence of acute hemorrhage and calcification, and images revealing exquisite bony detail of the skull and skull base can be acquired. Because of the configuration of the scanner, patients are reasonably accessible for monitoring during the examination.

CT scanners do have a number of disadvantages, however. Patients are exposed to ionizing radiation and iodine-based contrast agents (although lower doses of contrast are needed with the newer multidetector scanners). Imaging artifacts can interfere with accurate interpretation. In particular, images of the brain stem and posterior fossa are often degraded by "streak artifacts" from dense bone (Fig. 12–3). Streak artifacts from metallic objects (e.g., fillings, braces, surgical clips) can also obscure abnormalities. Images can be severely degraded by patient motion. Fortunately, unlike MR scans, individual CT images degraded by motion can be rapidly reacquired.

Magnetic Resonance Imaging

One of the most exciting developments in radiology during the past 30 years has been the translation of nuclear magnetic resonance phenomena, initially used for probing the physicochemical structure of molecules, to imaging. The product of this application, MR imaging, has profoundly affected the radiologic evaluation of most neurologic disorders. MR examinations, like CT scans, consist of computer-reconstructed cross-sectional images (Fig. 12–4). In MR imaging, however, unlike CT scans or plain radiographs, the information collected is not x-ray beam attenuation. The MR image is a visual display of nuclear magnetic resonance data collected principally from nuclei within body tissues—especially hydrogen nuclei within water and fat molecules. Intrinsic tissue relaxation occurs by two major pathways, called *longitudinal*, or T_1, and *transverse*, or T_2, *decay*. MR imaging sequences that emphasize T_1 decay are commonly referred to as T_1-weighted, images; sequences that accentuate T_2 relaxation properties are called T_2-weighted images (Fig. 12–4). Most MR scans of the brain use both of these sequences, because certain abnormalities may only be obvious on one or the other. T_2-weighted images are usually easy to identify because fluid (e.g., cerebrospinal, globe vitreous) is very bright; fluid on a T_1-weighted scan is usually dark.

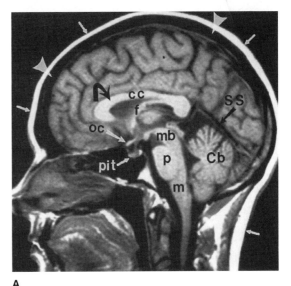

A

Fig. 12–4. Normal head MR images. Sagittal T_1-weighted **A**, axial T_1-weighted **B**, and axial T_2-weighted **C** images. Note differences in signal between gray matter (*large arrows*), white matter (*curved arrows*), CSF (*small arrowheads*), fat (*small arrows*), and cortical bone (*large arrowheads*) on different pulse sequences. Normal structures include the genu (g) and splenium (s) of the corpus callosum (cc), fornix (f), optic chiasm (oc), pituitary gland (pit), midbrain (mb), pons (p), medulla (m), cerebellar vermis (Cb), straight sinus (SS), caudate head (c), putamen (pt), and thalamus (T).

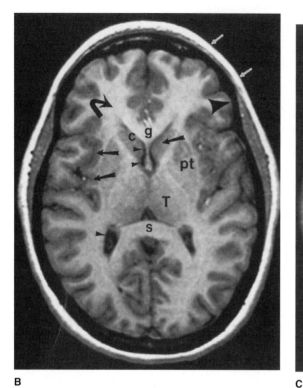

B

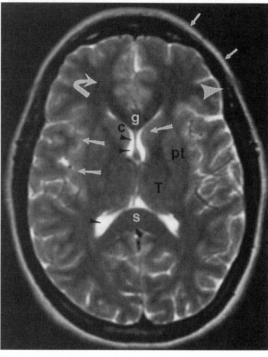

C

***Fig. 12–4.** Cont.*

Fat is bright on T_1-weighted scans, but darker on T_2-weighted images. On the other hand, both cortical bone and air are very dark on all imaging sequences. Brain tissue has intermediate intensity; vessels can have almost any signal, depending on the velocity of flowing blood.

The most commonly used, clinically approved contrast agent for MR imaging is gadopentetate-dimeglumine or Gd-DTPA, which is very well tolerated and extremely safe. Its major use in the central nervous system (CNS) is to improve lesion detectability by "lighting up" pathologic conditions that either lack a BBB or have a disrupted BBB.

Conventional MR imaging depicts excellent soft-tissue contrast. Traditionally, long image acquisition times, image artifacts related to patient motion, and the increased cost of scanning due to limited patient throughput have hampered the clinical utility of MR imaging. During the past 15 years, technical advances in gradient technology, coil design, image reconstruction algorithms, contrast administration protocols, and data acquisition strategies have accelerated the development and implementation of fast imaging methods. These techniques, including fast gradient echo imaging, fast spin echo imaging, FLAIR (fluid-attenuated inversion recovery), and echo planar imaging, have enabled substantial reductions in imaging time. Images may be acquired during a single

breath-hold on a clinical scanner, eliminating respiratory and motion artifacts. Vessel conspicuity can be enhanced by application of fat-suppression sequences, which eliminate unwanted signal from background tissues. These improvements have led to a vast range of applications that were previously impractical, including high-resolution MRA, DW and PW MR imaging, MRS, fMRI, and real-time monitoring of interventional procedures.

Since its first clinical application nearly 15 years ago, MRA has proven to be a useful tool for evaluation of the cervical or intracranial carotid vasculature. MRA represents a class of techniques that utilize the MR scanner to noninvasively generate three-dimensional images of the carotid or vertebral-basilar circulations (Fig. 12–5). While a detailed discussion of these techniques is beyond the scope of this chapter, several comments are noteworthy. These methods permit distinction between blood flow and adjacent soft tissue, with or without administration of intravenous contrast. As noted above, revolutionary developments have permitted MRA images to be rapidly acquired with ever-improving temporal and spatial resolution.

Presently, MRA serves as one of the first-line studies for evaluation of arterial occlusive disease and for screening of intracranial aneurysms. These methods have largely replaced conventional arteriographic studies for

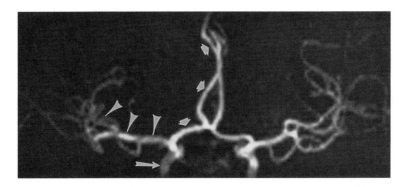

Fig. 12–5. Normal frontal view of intracranial MR angiogram at the level of the circle of Willis. Note the internal carotid artery (*large arrow*), anterior cerebral artery (*small arrows*), and middle cerebral artery (*arrowheads*).

evaluation of atherosclerotic disease, except in cases of critical stenosis (> 70%). In these instances, the degree of luminal narrowing may be overestimated by MRA, and may require verification with a catheter-based study or Doppler ultrasound. Moreover, aneurysms detected on an intracranial MRA typically require a catheter-based study for detailing aneurysm size and orientation, for establishing the location of adjacent vessels and collateral flow, for confirming suspicious vascular dilation, and for detecting the presence of vasospasm or additional aneurysms that may not be readily apparent on the MRA study. In an increasing number of cases, catheter-based studies will additionally be performed for coil embolization (obliteration) of detected aneurysms, rather than surgical clipping.

Molecular diffusion, the random translational movement of water and other small molecules in tissue, is ther-mally driven, and referred to as *Brownian motion.* Over a given time period, these random motions, expressed as molecular displacements, can be detected using specifically designed diffusion-sensitive MR sequences. A common application of diffusion imaging is the detection of early ischemic infarction, where the infarcted tissue "lights up" due to the "restricted diffusion" state within the intracellular compartment. Other applications of diffusion-sensitive sequences include differentiating cysts from solid tumors, as well as evaluating inflammatory/infectious conditions (encephalitis, abscess) or white matter abnormalities (hypertensive encephalopathy).

Perfusion MR imaging measures cerebral blood flow (CBF) at the capillary level of an organ or tissue region. Perfusion-weighted MR imaging has applications in the evaluation of a number of disease states, including cerebral ischemia and reperfusion, brain tumors (Fig. 12–6),

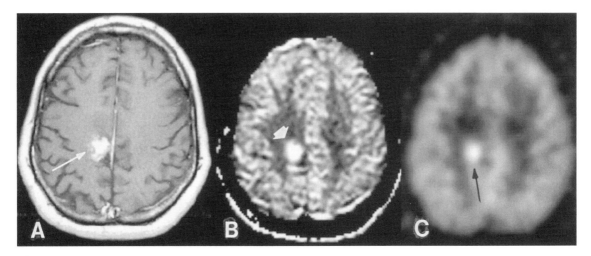

Fig. 12–6. Perfusion (cerebral blood volume) mapping of a high-grade glioma in a patient who had previously undergone radiotherapy. **A** Axial postcontrast T₁ image shows an enhancing lesion (*arrow*) present within the right posterior frontal deep white matter. **B** Axial cerebral blood volume map shows a corresponding high cerebral blood volume area measured (*arrow*). **C** PET image using radiolabeled glucose. High glucose uptake is demonstrated at the site of the lesion (*arrow*). (Courtesy of Dr. Hannu Aronen, Helsinki, Finland.)

epilepsy, and blood flow deficits in Alzheimer's disease. In addition, the close spatial coupling between brain activity and CBF permits the application of perfusion MR techniques to imaging brain function.

Functional MR imaging is an important brain mapping technique that uses fast imaging techniques to depict regional cortical blood flow changes in space and time during performance of a particular task (e.g., flexion of the index finger). The utilization of this technique to localize brain activity is historically based on measurable increases in cerebral blood flow (and blood volume) with increased neural activity, referred to as *neurovascular coupling*. The hemodynamic response to a stimulus is not instantaneous, but on the order of a few seconds. Consequently, fMRI techniques are considered an indirect approach to imaging brain function, but provide excellent spatial resolution and can be precisely matched with anatomic structures. Changes in blood oxygenation and perfusion can be imaged using the fMRI technique, which has become the most widely used modality for depicting regional brain activation in response to sensorimotor or cognitive tasks.

An important clinical application of fMRI is presurgical mapping, whereby eloquent brain cortex can be defined in relation to mass lesions (Fig. 12–7). This allows for the judicious selection of an appropriate management strategy (surgical versus nonsurgical) according to the functional nature of the adjacent brain tissue. A second application involves determination of the cerebral hemisphere responsible for language and memory tasks in a patient with complex partial seizures, prior to undergoing temporal lobectomy. Additionally, several groups have reported successful functional activation studies for lateralizing language preoperatively utilizing fMRI.

MR spectroscopy provides qualitative and quantitative information about brain metabolism and tissue composition. This functional analysis is based on detecting variations in the precession frequencies of spinning protons in a magnetic field. One factor influencing the precession or resonance frequency is the chemical environment of the individual proton. Protons in different cerebral metabolites can be sensitively discriminated on this basis, and the position of these metabolites can be displayed as a spectrum. The x-axis position of a given metabolite reflects the degree of "chemical shift" of the metabolite with respect to a designated reference metabolite, and it is expressed in units of parts per million (ppm). The area under the peak is determined by the number of protons that contribute to the MR signal.

The major metabolites detected in the CNS are *N*-acetyl aspartate (NAA), a neuronal marker; choline, a marker for cellularity and cell membrane turnover; creatine, a marker for energy metabolism; and lactate, a marker for anaerobic metabolism. In addition to these metabolites, others have been assessed, including alanine, glutamine, myoinositol, and succinate, using various MR strategies. Presently, MRS is being used in clinical practice to provide functional information regarding many CNS abnormalities, and it complements the conventional MR imaging study. A common application relates to the pre- and post-treatment evaluation of brain tumors, with MRS playing an important role in assessing for residual or recurrent tumor following surgical resection.

MR imaging offers a number of advantages over CT in the workup of patients with neurologic disease. Its soft-tissue contrast resolution is superior to that of CT, and lesions that may be subtle or invisible on CT are frequently obvious on MR imaging. MR imaging also allows acquisition of multiplanar views in the sagittal, axial, coronal, and oblique projections that may be impossible to obtain with CT. Furthermore, MR imaging gives information about blood flow without the need for a contrast agent, and bony streak artifacts that obscure lesions of the brain stem and cerebellum on CT scans are not present on MR images. Finally, MR imaging does not expose the patient to ionizing radiation.

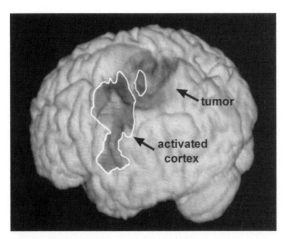

Fig. 12–7. Volume-rendered 3-D fMRI for presurgical brain tumor mapping. Note that the area of motor cortex activation partially overlaps the tumor volume within the left cerebral hemisphere. (Courtesy of Dr. Joseph Maldjian, Winston-Salem, NC.)

Cerebral Arteriography

Cerebral arteriography involves the injection of water-soluble contrast material into a carotid or vertebral artery. Contrast material is injected into the desired vessel via a small catheter, which has been introduced into the body through the femoral or brachial artery. Information about the arterial, capillary, or venous circulation of the brain is recorded on serial plain films or digitized for viewing on a TV monitor or for storage within a computer (Fig. 12–8).

Cerebral arteriograms are expensive (two to three times as much as MR examinations) and are relatively more risky procedures than other neuroradiologic studies. The major risk of the procedure is stroke, which may occur in 1 of every 1000 patients. Stroke during cerebral arteriography occurs either from an embolic event (e.g., inadvertent injection of air, thrombus formation on catheter tip, atherosclerotic plaque dislodged by catheter manipulation) or from catheter-related local vessel trauma (e.g., dissections, occlusions).

Although CA is an invasive study with well-known risks, it is invaluable in the workup of vascular diseases affecting the CNS. It is the gold standard for assessing vascular stenosis and atherosclerosis or vasculitis, and it is indispensable in identifying and evaluating cerebral aneurysms and certain intracranial vascular malformations or fistulae. It is useful in assessing carotid or vertebral artery integrity after trauma to the neck, especially in the setting of acute neurologic deficit. Finally, it is unsurpassed for showing vascular anatomy of the brain and is, therefore, useful as a preoperative road map. CT and MR imaging have replaced cerebral arteriography in the workup of most other neurologic diseases and, as previously mentioned, rival cerebral arteriography in the detection of arterial occlusive disease, aneurysms, and vascular injury following blunt trauma to the neck.

The field of interventional neuroradiology continues to grow and exert considerable impact on the diagnosis and treatment of certain CNS diseases. New catheter designs and materials, recently developed endovascular

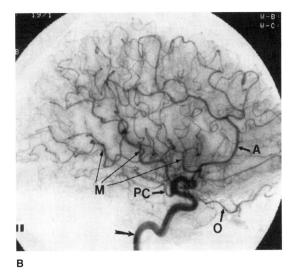

A   **B**

Fig. 12–8. Normal cerebral arteriogram. **A** Lateral view of the cervical carotid artery. Catheter is located within the common carotid artery, and contrast material fills internal (*arrows*) and external (*arrowheads*) carotid arteries. **B** Lateral view of the head after injection of the carotid artery (*arrow*). Note anterior cerebral (A), ophthalmic (O), posterior communicating (PC), and middle cerebral (M) branches.

devices (extracranial/intracranial stents), and an increasing number of trained specialists performing endovascular procedures have led to novel therapeutic applications and approaches for managing previously untreatable conditions. Endovascular diagnostic and therapeutic procedures, based on fundamental cerebral arteriography principles, have gained widespread acceptance and, in some cases, rival traditional neurosurgical approaches in terms of complication rates, clinical outcomes, and long-term survival benefit. Although a full discussion of these techniques is beyond the scope of this chapter, they include thrombolysis of intracranial clot in the setting of acute infarction or dural sinus thrombosis, embolization (obliteration) of intracranial aneurysms using thrombosing material (i.e., coils), carotid artery angioplasty and/or stent placement for critical stenotic narrowing or radiation-induced arterial stricture, preoperative or definitive devascularization of a hypervascular mass or arteriovenous malformation, embolization of small, bleeding external carotid artery branches in epistaxis, balloon occlusion tests of the carotid artery, and endovascular treatment of vasospasm. Embolization materials include particulate emboli, liquid adhesive glues, and various coils.

Ultrasonography

Ultrasonography is the diagnostic application of ultrasound to the human body. Major applications of ultrasonography in CNS disease include gray-scale imaging and Doppler evaluation of carotid artery patency and flow in the setting of atherosclerosis, assessssment of vasospasm in the setting of subarachnoid hemorrhage using transcranial Doppler, screening evaluation of intracranial abnormalities in the newborn and young infant (Fig. 12–9), and detection of intracranial hemorrhage in premature infants prior to extracorporeal membrane oxygenation therapy. Ultrasonography has also been used intraoperatively to demonstrate the spinal cord and surrounding structures during spine surgery and to define tumor and cyst margins during craniotomies.

Transcranial Doppler is a recently developed tool in the evaluation of cerebrovascular disorders. It uses low-frequency sound waves to adequately penetrate the skull, and produces spectral waveforms of the major intracranial vessels for evaluation of flow velocity, direction, amplitude, and pulsatility. Present clinical applications include diagnosis of cerebral vasospasm, evaluation of stroke and transient ischemic attack, detection of intracranial emboli, serial monitoring of vasculitis in children with sickle cell disease, and assessment of intracranial pressure and cerebral blood flow changes in patients with head injury or mass lesions.

Ultrasound examinations, although moderately expensive, are virtually risk free to the patient, involve no ionizing radiation, and are portable (i.e., can be performed at the bedside). However, examination quality and therefore diagnostic accuracy are operator dependent. Also, the heavy reliance of ultrasonography on the presence of an adequate "acoustic window" through which an examination can be performed diminishes its usefulness in examining the brain after the fontanelles close in infancy. Finally, to the untrained eye, anatomic structures and pathologic processes as depicted by US

Fig. 12–9. Coronal **A** and sagittal **B** head ultrasound images of a neonate. Normal structures include the corpus callosum (CC), lateral ventricle (LV), cavum septum pellucidum (CS), sylvian fissure (SF), third ventricle (3V), fourth ventricle (4V), temporal lobe (T), frontal lobe (FR), occipital lobe (OCC), cerebellum (CER), and thalamus (TH).

A

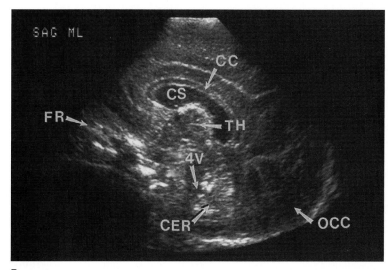

B

Fig. 12–9. *Cont.*

are not as readily apparent as they are on CT or MR images.

Single Photon Emission Computed Tomography

SPECT uses a rotating gamma camera to reconstruct cross-sectional images of the distribution of a radioactive pharmaceutical that has been administered to a patient (usually intravenously). For brain imaging, radioactive iodine (^{123}I) or technetium (^{99m}Tc) is combined with a compound that rapidly crosses the BBB and localizes within brain tissue in proportion to regional blood flow. The rotating gamma camera detects gamma rays emitted by the radiopharmaceutical and produces cross-sectional images of the brain that are really a map of brain perfusion (Fig. 12–10). SPECT imaging also gives indirect information about brain metabolism, because perfusion is usually highest to parts of the brain with high metabolic activity and lowest to areas with low metabolic demand. Normal SPECT examinations demonstrate activity concentrated primarily in areas of high perfusion/metabolism, such as the cortical and deep gray matter (Fig. 12–10).

SPECT studies are moderately expensive (as much as or more than brain MR imaging), and, as expected, they provide limited anatomic information. SPECT also exposes patients to ionizing radiation. Because patients rarely have allergic reactions to the radiopharmaceuticals used, the examination is of low risk. While SPECT provides critical information regarding regional

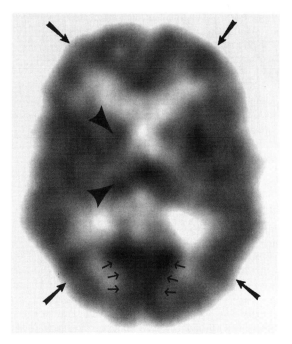

Fig. 12–10. Axial SPECT image of normal cerebral perfusion. Note that perfusion is greatest to gray matter structures, including the cerebral cortex (*large arrows*) and deep gray nuclei (*arrowheads*). White matter and ventricles are nearly invisible because of low or no perfusion. The greatest perfusion is to the visual cortex area (*small arrows*).

cerebral perfusion, particularly in the setting of stroke, this information can be more readily obtained during CTA/CT perfusion or MR perfusion acquisitions. SPECT has also been used with varying degrees of success in the workup of patients with epilepsy or dementia.

Positron Emission Tomography

PET scans consist of computer-generated cross-sectional images of the distribution and local concentration of a radiopharmaceutical. This technique is very similar to SPECT imaging. The main difference is that PET studies use radiopharmaceuticals labeled with a cyclotron-produced positron emitter. These agents are very expensive to produce and have a very short half-life (on the order of seconds to minutes). The most widely used radiotracer is ^{18}F-deoxyglucose. PET scanning with this agent gives a measurement of brain glucose metabolism. Other agents are useful in assessing regional cerebral blood flow, neuroreceptor function, and the like.

At first glance, PET scans resemble CT scans. Images can be viewed on a TV monitor or on x-ray film. Areas of high metabolic activity (i.e., cerebral cortex, deep gray

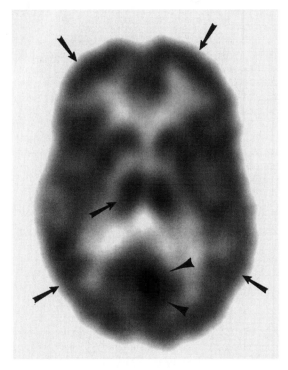

Fig. 12–11. Normal axial image of brain PET scan. As in the SPECT study (Fig. 12–10), areas of high activity correspond to metabolically active gray matter (*arrows*), especially the visual cortex (*arrowheads*).

nuclei) demonstrate greater radiopharmaceutical uptake than do areas of low metabolic activity, such as white matter or cerebrospinal fluid (Fig. 12–11). The bones of the skull and scalp soft tissues are, for the most part, invisible.

PET scans are very expensive, costing approximately twice as much as an MR scan. This expense is directly related to the high cost of operating the PET facility, which requires on-site physicists as well as an on-site cyclotron for radiotracer production. Therefore, PET scanning is not generally available in community hospitals. Although patients undergoing PET examinations are exposed to ionizing radiation, the overall risk to the patient is low. Anatomic resolution, although not as good as with CT or MR imaging, is better than with SPECT imaging. The major advantage of PET imaging is that it is extremely versatile, providing *in vivo* information about brain perfusion, glucose metabolism, receptor density, and, ultimately, brain function.

PET provides useful information in the setting of stroke, epilepsy, dementia, and tumors. At present, the two main indications are in the workup of patients with complex partial seizures and in identifying tumor recurrence in patients who have undergone surgery, radiation therapy, or both, for brain tumors.

TECHNIQUE SELECTION

The primary goal of a radiologic examination is to provide useful information for disease management. Radiologic studies can provide a diagnosis or can give information about disease extent or response to treatment. In the present medical climate, it has also become imperative that radiologic workups be performed efficiently and in a cost-effective manner. This requirement presents a problem for clinicians trying to decide which test to order in a given clinical situation.

The major strengths and weaknesses of neuroradiologic examinations were discussed earlier in this chapter. The following brief discussion concerns the appropriate ordering of examinations in clinical situations. Several points should be emphasized. First, although a recommended modality may clearly be superior to another in evaluating a particular neurologic condition, the choice of examination is not always obvious before the diagnosis is established. For example, in patients with nonfocal headache, MR scans are more sensitive than CT scans for detecting most intracranial abnormalities. However, if the headache is produced by subarachnoid hemorrhage, CT would be a much better examination than MR imaging, since subarachnoid hemorrhage is nearly invisible on MR images.

Choice of examinations may also be limited by what is locally available. If MR imaging is unavailable or if the

MR scanner is of poor quality or if the interpreting radiologist is inadequately trained in MR image interpretation, then CT would be an excellent examination for evaluating most neurologic disorders.

Next, it is important to realize that the least expensive examination is not always the best first choice, even in this cost-conscious age. For example, most suspected skull fractures should be evaluated with CT scanning and not with plain films, despite the significant cost differential, because what is really important in management decisions is not the fracture itself but the potential underlying brain injury. Some neurologic diseases require multiple radiologic studies for accurate evaluation. Complex partial seizures refractory to medical management frequently require multiple examinations to localize the seizure focus prior to temporal lobectomy. Such a workup normally includes MR imaging and, ictal/interictal SPECT and/or PET scanning of the brain, as well as a cerebral arteriogram to identify cerebral dominance.

Finally, certain examinations are contraindicated in certain patients, and an alternative test must suffice. Patients with ferromagnetic cerebral aneurysm clips or pacemakers should not undergo MR imaging. Patients with a strong history of allergic reaction to iodinated contrast media should not routinely undergo contrast-enhanced CT scanning, unless they are pretreated with anti-inflammatory agents (i.e., steroids). MR scanning is frequently unsuccessful in claustrophobic or uncooperative patients unless they are sedated.

Congenital Anomalies

Congenital anomalies of the brain are best evaluated by MR imaging. MR imaging is the very best examination for demonstrating intracranial anatomy. It provides excellent discrimination between gray matter and white matter, superb views of the posterior fossa and craniocervical junction, and, most importantly, the ability to view the brain in any plane. MR imaging has, for all practical purposes, completely replaced CT for this indication. The one exception is in evaluation of skull abnormalities such as suspected fusion of the sutures.

Craniocerebral Trauma

CT is the preferred modality for studying practically all acute head injuries. Examination times are short, intracranial hemorrhage is well demonstrated, and skull fractures are readily apparent. Unstable patients can also be easily monitored. Intravenous administration of contrast agents is unnecessary in this setting. Occasionally cerebral arteriography is performed to look for carotid or vertebral artery injury when there has been penetrating trauma to the neck. Similarly, a CTA, MRA, or catheter-based study may be required to evaluate suspected carotid artery dissection associated with blunt head trauma or to assess carotid laceration in skull-base fractures.

While MR imaging is not routinely performed in the acute trauma setting, it may sometimes be helpful in patients with neurologic deficits unexplained by a head CT examination. For example, traumatic brain stem hemorrhages are often difficult to see on CT scans but are usually quite obvious on MR images. MR imaging is also useful in demonstrating tiny shear lesions within the brain in diffuse axonal injury and in assessing the brain in remote head trauma.

Intracranial Hemorrhage

The best examination to perform in most cases of suspected acute intracranial hemorrhage is a head CT scan. CT scans can be obtained quickly, allowing rapid initiation of treatment, and they are very good at demonstrating all types of intracranial hemorrhage, including subarachnoid blood. MR imaging takes much longer to perform in a potentially unstable patient, and subarachnoid hemorrhage may be difficult to see. MR imaging is more useful in the subacute or chronic setting, especially since it gives information about when a hemorrhagic event occurred. This information might be useful in such settings as nonaccidental head trauma (e.g., child abuse). MR imaging is also very sensitive to petechial hemorrhage that frequently accompanies a cerebral infarction and could potentially help to identify an underlying cause for an intracranial hemorrhage (e.g., tumor, arteriovenous malformation, occluded dural sinus). Finally, because most nontraumatic subarachnoid hemorrhage occurs secondary to a ruptured intracranial aneurysm, cerebral arteriography is routinely performed after detection of subarachnoid hemorrhage. More recently, obtaining a CTA study following the acquisition of a conventional head CT in the emergency department has promoted the concept of "one-stop shopping" for aneurysm detection and characterization prior to determining the appropriate management.

Aneurysms

The vast majority of intracranial aneurysms in which surgical intervention is planned require evaluation by cerebral arteriography. Cerebral arteriography not only allows aneurysm identification, but also provides other critical preoperative information such as aneurysm orientation, presence of vasospasm, location of adjacent vessels, and collateral intracranial circulation. Arteriography also helps to determine which aneurysm has bled when more than one aneurysm is present. As mentioned earlier, interventional neuroradiologists can treat aneurysms, usually in nonsurgical patients, by placing thrombosing material (i.e., coils) within the aneurysm itself via an endovascular approach.

Although most patients with symptomatic cerebral aneurysms present with subarachnoid hemorrhage, some aneurysms act like intracranial masses. These situations usually warrant evaluation by MR imaging as a first examination. The same is sometimes true with posterior communicating artery aneurysms (which can produce symptoms related to the adjacent third cranial nerve) or with aneurysms arising from the ICA as it courses through the cavernous sinus (which can affect any of the cranial nerves that lie within this structure, including cranial nerves III, IV, V, or VI).

Vascular Malformations

Patients with a vascular malformation (e.g., arteriovenous malformation, cavernous angioma, venous angioma, capillary telangiectasia) often seek medical attention after an intracranial hemorrhage or a seizure. In this setting, the first test that should be performed is either a CT examination (to look for intracranial hemorrhage) or MR imaging. Although an intracranial hemorrhage is usually very obvious on a CT scan, the vascular malformation itself may be difficult, if not impossible, to see unless intravenous contrast material is administered. MR imaging, on the other hand, is quite sensitive for detecting vascular malformations, whether they have bled or not. As can be seen, the choice of the initial examination for evaluation of a vascular malformation can be difficult. Usually, patients undergo noncontrast head CT scanning to look for intracranial hemorrhage when they come to the emergency department. Head CT is followed by gadolinium-enhanced MR imaging to further characterize the CT findings. If a high-flow true arteriovenous malformation is suspected, either clinically or from a cross-sectional imaging study, then cerebral arteriography is performed prior to initiation of treatment. MR angiography may someday replace conventional arteriography in the workup of these lesions, as with aneurysms.

Infarction

Most patients today with suspected cerebral infarction undergo CT scanning in the acute setting, even though infarctions are demonstrated earlier and are more obvious on MR imaging. So why is CT usually performed first? The answer is that clinicians who manage stroke patients are not so interested in seeing the infarct itself. Infarct location is usually suspected from the physical examination and acute infarcts may not even be visible on CT scans for 12 to 24 hours after onset of stroke symptoms. Clinicians are very interested, though, to know if a stroke is secondary to something besides an infarct (e.g., intracranial hemorrhage, brain tumor), or if an infarct is hemorrhagic, since thrombolytic agents would be contraindicated in this setting. CT can quickly answer both of these questions. MR imaging, specifically diffusion-weighted imaging, can sensitively detect acute infarctions and is typically ordered in cases of high clinical suspicion, when the initial CT study is nondiagnostic or when brain stem or posterior fossa infarcts are suspected.

The underlying cause of most cerebral infarctions is thromboembolism related to atherosclerosis. A CT/CTA or MR/MRA (including DW and PW MR imaging) study may provide a positive imaging diagnosis of brain infarction, reveal the extent and location of vessel occlusion, demonstrate the volume and severity of ischemic tissue, predict final infarct size and clinical prognosis, and, in the case of MR, potentially identify poorly perfused tissue at risk of infarction. Ultrasonography and cerebral arteriography can also be performed in the setting of stroke or transient ischemic attack to identify vascular stenoses or occlusions; these examinations are usually reserved for patients who might be candidates for carotid endarterectomy. Functional examinations (SPECT and PET) have also been used in patients with stroke-like symptoms to identify regions of the brain at risk for infarction. These studies are not widely available, and therefore do not enter into the imaging algorithm for most stroke patients.

Brain Tumors and Tumor-like Conditions

The best examination to order in the setting of suspected brain tumor is a contrast-enhanced MR scan. This is true for primary neoplasms as well as for metastatic disease. MR imaging is especially useful in identifying tumors of the pituitary region, brain stem, and posterior fossa, including the cerebellopontine angle.

Although MR imaging is the preferred examination for intracranial neoplasms, it is occasionally supplemented by a CT scan, which can give important pretreatment information not provided by MR images. For example, CT can demonstrate tumor calcification, occasionally a useful factor in differentiating between types of neoplasms. Also, CT is very useful in identifying bone destruction in skull base lesions.

In most medical centers, MR imaging and often MRS are performed to assess brain tumor response to treatment. PET scanning has also been used for this purpose. MRS and PET scanning can frequently differentiate recurrent tumor from postradiation tissue necrosis, which can mimic tumor on an MR or a CT scan.

Cerebral arteriography is rarely performed for brain tumor evaluation today except to map the blood supply of very vascular tumors (i.e., juvenile angiofibromas, paragangliomas) preoperatively. Such lesions can also be devascularized prior to surgery to minimize blood loss by injecting various materials into feeding vessels to occlude them.

Infection

Intracranial infections are best evaluated by contrast-enhanced MR imaging. Abscesses, cerebritis, subdural empyemas, and other infectious or inflammatory processes are all very well demonstrated. MR imaging is especially useful in assessing patients with the acquired immune deficiency syndrome (AIDS). Not only does it allow identification of secondary infections (e.g., toxoplasmosis, cryptococcosis, progressive multifocal leukoencephalopathy), but it is also exquisitely sensitive to the white matter changes produced by the human immunodeficiency virus (HIV) itself. CT scanning is less sensitive than MR imaging in the detection of intracranial infections and should be reserved for patients in whom MR imaging is contraindicated. Cerebral arteriography is only useful in one particular situation, suspected vasculitis. Involvement of brain arteries and arterioles in this condition requires arteriography for diagnostic confirmation.

Inherited and Acquired Metabolic, White Matter, and Neurodegenerative Diseases

As with suspected intracranial infections, this large and diverse group of diseases is best evaluated with MR imaging, which sensitively detects white matter abnormalities. In fact, one of the very first clear indications for MR imaging was in the workup of suspected multiple sclerosis. Although brain abnormalities in these conditions may be quite obvious on MR imaging, there is one problem: Many of these conditions appear very similar and an exact diagnosis may not be possible. In patients with dementia and suspected neurodegenerative disease, PET imaging is currently the procedure of choice for diagnostic evaluation.

EXERCISES

EXERCISE 12-1: CONGENITAL ANOMALIES

Clinical Histories:

Case 12-1.   A 2-day-old male infant presents with multiple craniofacial deformities, including frontal bossing, microcephaly, and a fleshy mass on the bridge of the nose. Sagittal and coronal T$_1$-weighted MR images of the brain are shown in Fig. 12–12A,B.

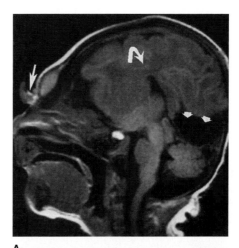

A

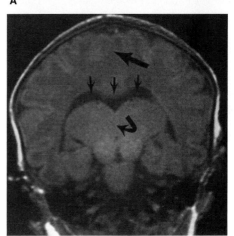

B

Fig. 12–12.

Case 12-2.   A 15-month-old female infant presents with new onset of seizures. Axial T$_1$- and T$_2$-weighted MR images are shown in Fig. 12–13A,B.

Questions:

12-1.   In Case 12-1, what is the major abnormality?
   A.   Enlarged ventricles
   B.   Cyst in the posterior fossa
   C.   Lack of brain cleavage into two hemispheres
   D.   Herniation of intracranial contents through a skull defect
   E.   Abnormal migration of gray matter

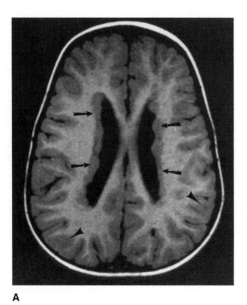

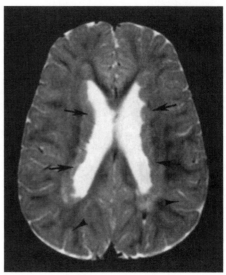

A   **B**

Fig. 12–13.

12-2. In Case 12-2, what is the etiology of the patient's seizures?

    A. Brain tumor
    B. Gray matter in the wrong place (i.e., heterotopic gray matter)
    C. Congenital infection
    D. Nodules along ventricles in a patient with tuberous sclerosis
    E. Infarction of periventricular white matter

Radiologic Findings:

12-1. In this case, the corpus callosum (*curved arrow*) is absent on the sagittal T$_1$-weighted MR image (Fig. 12–12A). Also note other midline abnormalities, including abnormal tissue at the bridge of the nose (*large arrow*) and a posterior cyst (*small arrows*). The coronal T$_1$-weighted MR image (Fig. 12–12B) demonstrates a monoventricle (*small arrows*) and thalamic fusion (*curved arrow*). Also note the lack of separation of the two hemispheres (*large arrow*). (*C* is the correct answer to Question 12-1.)

12-2. In this case, T$_1$-weighted (Fig. 12–13A) and T$_2$-weighted (Fig. 12–13B) MR images show abnormal tissue lining the lateral ventricle (*arrows*). Signal of this tissue follows that of normal gray matter (*arrowheads*) on both T$_1$- and T$_2$-weighted images. (*B* is the correct answer to Question 12-2.)

Discussion:

Two common reasons for performing MR scans in young infants are illustrated by the cases in this section. Infants with craniofacial anomalies frequently have underlying congenital malformations of the CNS. Seizures, too, may be the first sign of an underlying brain malformation. As discussed in the section on technique selection, whenever a congenital brain anomaly is suspected, MR imaging is the best examination to perform.

Insults to the developing brain lead to predictable alterations of brain morphology. By analyzing patterns of altered brain morphology, we can often determine which stage of CNS development has been disrupted. This analysis, combined with a knowledge of neuroembryology, has allowed for the development of systems to classify congenital anomalies of the CNS. One simplified classification system divides congenital malformations into disorders of organogenesis (which include abnormalities of neural tube closure, diverticulation/cleavage, sulcation/cellular migration, and size, as well as destructive lesions acquired *in utero*), disorders of histogenesis (i.e., neurocutaneous syndromes), and disorders of cytogenesis (i.e., congenital neoplasms). Readers are referred to the Bibliography at the end of this chapter for further information on this topic.

The patient in Case 12-1 has alobar holoprosencephaly, a classic example of disordered ventral induction. In this condition, there is complete (alobar) or partial (semilobar, lobar) failure of separation of the forebrain (prosencephalon) into two hemispheres. In alobar holoprosencephaly, the most severe form of this disorder, there is no separation of the two hemispheres at all. The thalami are fused, a central monoventricle is present, and there is no corpus callosum. Infants with this form of holoprosencephaly frequently have severe facial anomalies.

In Case 12-2, the patient has heterotopic gray matter lining the lateral ventricles. This congenital anomaly is one type of disordered cellular migration. Neurons that make up the gray matter of the cerebral cortex actually develop along the edges of the lateral and third ventricles within the so-called germinal matrix zone. They then migrate outward to their final cortical location. If this

normal neuronal migration is disrupted, a normal cortex may not develop, and clumps of gray matter may be present in abnormal locations along the migration route. Collections of these normal neurons in abnormal locations are called *gray matter heterotopias.*

Several different types of heterotopias have been described. The case presented in this section demonstrates a focal nodular gray matter heterotopia involving the subependymal region at the edge of the lateral ventricles. Seizures frequently occur in patients with this condition, as in the patient in Case 12-2. Because MR imaging usually provides an exact diagnosis of this condition, biopsies of CNS tissue are unnecessary.

In contrast to focal nodular heterotopias, diffuse (or laminar) heterotopias are commonly seen within or adjacent to the cortex, while "band"-type heterotopias are located deep to the normal cortex, in a subcortical location, separated by a thin interface of white matter (Fig. 12–14). Band-type heterotopias are well defined, with smooth margins, demonstrating signal intensities identical to normal gray matter. Mass effect on the underlying white matter or deep gray structures may be seen, and the sulcation pattern of the brain superficial to the heterotopia may be abnormal. Associated CNS anomalies may be present, such as agenesis of the corpus callosum, holoprosencephaly, or herniation of brain tissue (encephaloceles). While, at first glance, the cortex may appear to be markedly thickened, closer examination will reveal an additional band of gray matter in a subcortical location, that may or may not demonstrate increased 18F-FDG activity on a PET scan. This band of heterotopia is known to be associated with intractable seizures, occurring earlier than in the focal type, as well as severe developmental delay.

Several types of Chiari malformations were initially described by the German pathologist Hans Chiari, who classified these congenital hindbrain anomalies into

A

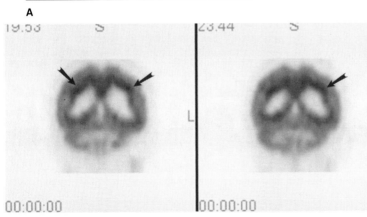

B

Fig. 12–14. A Postcontrast coronal T$_1$-weighted image of the brain in a 32-year-old patient with intractable seizures. An additional circumferential band of gray matter is seen (*arrows*) deep to the normal gray matter within the occipital region. This finding was noted to be diffusely present throughout the remaining brain parenchyma (not shown). **B** The corresponding PET image in the same patient reveals increased activity of the band heterotopia relative to the adjacent normal cortex (*arrows*), of unclear significance.

three types. In each case, abnormal descent of cerebellar tissue into the cervical canal is demonstrated. A Chiari I malformation consists of elongated peg-like cerebellar tonsils below the foramen magnum, while the brain stem is normal in location. In cases where the tonsils, vermis, pons, medulla, and an elongated fourth ventricle are displaced inferiorly into the upper cervical canal, a Chiari II malformation is diagnosed (Fig. 12–15). Chiari III malformations are associated with occipital or high cervical encephaloceles, containing cerebellar tissue, with or without brain stem.

In a Chiari II malformation, displacement of the fourth ventricle may elongate the aqueduct and compress the fourth ventricle, with resulting hydrocephalus. Because the whole posterior fossa is smaller than expected, the posterior fossa structures have a distorted appearance, and also assume abnormal locations. The superior cerebellum towers superiorly through a widened tentorium incisura, with the remainder of the cerebellum wrapping around the brain stem. The tectum of the midbrain is beaked, and the massa intermedia is enlarged. A kink may be present at the cervicomedullary junction. Complete agenesis of the corpus callosum may be present in up to one-third of cases, and partial agenesis may be seen in 75% to 90% of cases, predominantly involving the splenium.

Disorders of histogenesis include the neurocutaneous syndromes, which are a heterogeneous group of disorders with CNS and, for the most part, cutaneous manifestations. Visceral and connective tissue abnormalities may be prominent. Common disorders within this group include neurofibromatosis types I and II, tuberous sclerosis, von Hippel-Lindau disease, and Sturge-Weber syndrome, where the abnormal lesions corresponding to these entities are neurogenic tumors, tubers, hemangioblastomas, and angiomas, respectively.

Neurofibromatosis type 1 is the most common of all the neurocutaneous syndromes, accounting for 90% of all neurofibromatosis cases, and is the only such entity discussed here. It is transmitted on the long arm of chromosome 17 and is a disease of childhood. Autosomal dominant transmission occurs in 50%, while the remainder sporadically appear as new mutations in a patient with no known family history of the disease. The diagnosis is established when two or more of the following criteria are

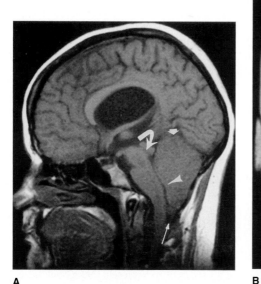

A

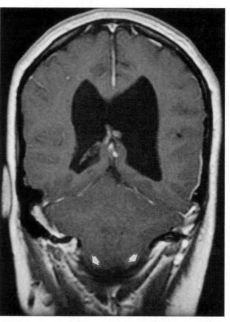

B

Fig. 12–15. Uninfused sagittal T$_1$-weighted **A** and coronal FLAIR **B** imaging in a 30-year-old patient with a Chiari II malformation. **A** A small posterior fossa is present, resulting in cerebellar tonsillar ectopia (*long arrow*), towering of the cerebellum (*short arrow*), beaking of the tectum (*curved arrow*), and compression of the fourth ventricle (*arrowhead*) with resulting hydrocephalus. Partial agenesis of the rostrum and splenium of the corpus callosum is noted. **B** Cerebellar tonsillar ectopia into the foramen magnum is demonstrated (*arrows*).

present: (1) six or more café-au-lait spots (brown skin pigmentation), (2) two or more Lisch nodules (hamartomas) of the iris, (3) two or more neurofibromas, (4) one or more plexiform neurofibromas, (5) axillary freckling, (6) one or more bone dysplasias (i.e., dysplasia of the greater sphenoid wing), (7) optic nerve glioma, or (8) first-degree relative with neurofibromatosis type 1.

The optic pathway gliomas are generally nonaggressive (low-grade) pilocytic astrocytomas that present in childhood and may not affect vision until greatly increased in size (Fig. 12–16A). Cerebellar, brainstem, and cerebral astrocytomas may additionally be seen. High T_2 signal intensity foci may be identified within the peduncles or deep gray matter of the cerebellum, brainstem, basal ganglia (particularly, globus pallidus), and supratentorial white matter (Fig. 12–16B). The nature of these lesions remains unresolved.

EXERCISE 12-2: STROKE

Clinical Histories:

Case 12-3. A 47-year-old female presents with diabetes mellitus and recent development of left-sided hemiplegia. Axial images from an uninfused head CT examination are shown in Fig. 12–17A,B.

Case 12-4. A 66-year-old woman presents with gradual onset of nausea, dizziness, and ataxia. The patient became comatose 24 hours after the onset of symptoms. Axial T_2-weighted and sagittal T_1-weighted images are shown in Fig. 12–18A,B.

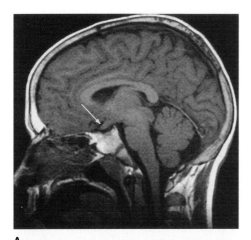

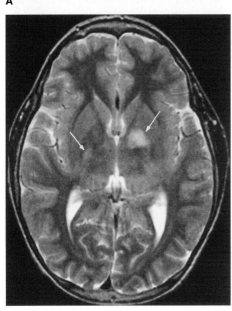

Fig. 12–16. Noncontrast T_1-weighted **A** and T_2-weighted **B** images in a 10-year-old male with neurofibromatosis. **A** Bulbous enlargement of the optic chiasm is present (*arrow*), suggesting an optic glioma. **B** Foci of increased T_2 signal abnormality are demonstrated within the globus palladi (*arrows*).

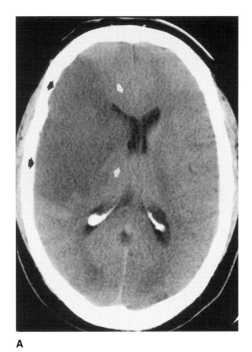

A

Fig. 12–17.

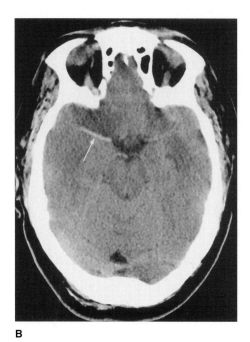

B

Fig. 12–17. *Cont.*

Case 12-5. A 42-year-old female hypertensive renal transplant patient presents with acute mental status changes and left hemiparesis. A single axial image from a noncontrast head CT scan is shown in Fig. 12–19.

Questions:

12-3. In Case 12-3, what is the most likely diagnosis?
    A. Intracranial abscess
    B. Arachnoid cyst
    C. Metastatic brain tumor
    D. Primary brain tumor
    E. Cerebral infarction

12-4. In Case 12-4, what is the likely cause of the patient's problem?
    A. Brain stem infarction
    B. Brain stem compression from cerebellar infarction
    C. Brain stem tumor
    D. Cerebellar astrocytoma
    E. Posterior fossa hemorrhage

12-5. In Case 12-5, what is the most likely diagnosis?
    A. Thalamic glioma
    B. Subarachnoid hemorrhage
    C. Metastatic disease
    D. Hypertensive hemorrhage in the basal ganglia
    E. Cerebral contusion

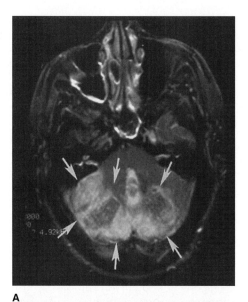

A

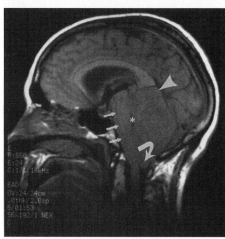

B

Fig. 12–18.

Radiologic Findings:

12-3. In this case, the axial CT image (Fig. 12–17*A*) demonstrates a well-defined area of hypodensity (*arrows*) in the right middle cerebral artery (MCA) territory. There is associated mass effect on the surrounding brain parenchyma with a corresponding shift of the midline structures to the left. In a more inferior axial image (Fig. 12–17*B*), note the bright right MCA (*arrow*) corresponding to an acute thrombus in the main trunk of this vessel. (*E* is the correct answer to Question 12-3.)

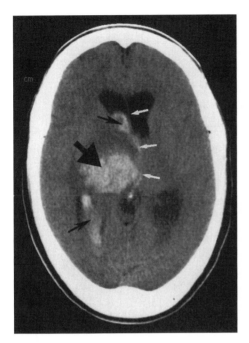

Fig. 12–19.

12-4. In this case, the axial T_2-weighted MR image (Fig. 12–18A) shows areas of increased T_2 signal (arrows) corresponding to edema within the cerebellum. A sagittal T_1-weighted image (Fig. 12–18B) shows a swollen cerebellum, as well as upward transtentorial (*arrowhead*) and downward tonsillar (*curved arrow*) herniation of cerebellar tissue. Also note compression of the brain stem (*small arrows*) and fourth ventricle (*asterisk*). These changes are compatible with a recent cerebellar infarction with brain stem compression caused by the swollen cerebellum. (*B* is the correct answer to Question 12-4.)

12-5. In this case, an axial CT scan (Fig. 12–19) demonstrates a right basal ganglia hematoma (*large black arrow*) with intraventricular extension (*small black arrows*). Note the shift of midline structures (*white arrows*). This is most likely secondary to the patient's known hypertension. (*D* is the correct answer to Question 12-5.)

Discussion:

Stroke is a lay term for acute neurologic disfunction. The usual image of a stroke patient is that of an elderly individual with a hemiparesis, often associated with abnormal speech. There are actually many different causes of stroke. These include cerebral infarction, intracerebral hemorrhage, subarachnoid hemorrhage, and miscellaneous causes such as dural sinus occlusion with associated venous infarction. Although these conditions

may have similar clinical presentations, they have different treatments and prognoses.

The vast majority of strokes are cerebral infarctions associated with atherosclerosis. The radiologic manifestations of cerebral infarction vary with time. The head CT scan of the patient in Case 12-3 was obtained several days after the onset of symptoms and shows typical findings of a subacute infarct in a major vascular territory, in this case the right middle cerebral artery region. By this time, the infarct is a very well-defined area of low attenuation compared to normal surrounding brain. There is associated mass effect from the edematous tissue. Acute infarcts (less than 24 hours since onset of symptoms) may be invisible on head CT scans, although diffusion-weighted MR imaging often demonstrates brain abnormalities within several hours (or less) of symptom onset. Subtle changes on head CT scans in acute infarction can sometimes be seen, but may be overlooked if the examination is not closely scrutinized. Sometimes the only apparent change on CT scans is a subtle loss of gray matter white matter differentiation in the area of infarction. CT scanning is performed in acute cerebral infarction because scans can be quickly obtained, and CT is a very good test for identifying intracranial hemorrhage, an important finding for management considerations. If the infarct is not obvious on the initial CT scan, an MR scan is usually obtained to verify high clinical suspicion.

An acute or subacute infarction will exhibit a diffusion signal abnormality that reflects the restricted movement of water molecules, and it typically persists for 1 to 2 weeks within infarcted tissue. Leptomeningeal enhancement that extends into the cortical sulci may be seen within several days of a cerebral infarction (Fig. 12–20). Parenchymal enhancement is commonly identified within the gray matter, which usually has a band-like, tubular, or gyriform appearance. Solid or ring-enhancing areas, as well as more amorphous-appearing patterns of enhancement, can occasionally occur.

Case 12-4 illustrates an important point to consider when deciding which test to order in the setting of acute stroke. In this case, the patient's symptoms were worrisome for a brain stem process. CT scanning of the brain stem and posterior fossa is frequently degraded by streak artifacts emanating from the dense bone of the skull base. Subtle (and sometimes not so subtle) abnormalities may not be apparent. Therefore, for most neurologic conditions that involve the brain stem or posterior fossa, MR scans are much better at depicting an abnormality. Notice that the patient in Case 12-4 did not in fact have a brain stem infarct, as was suspected clinically, but rather had brain stem compression from a large cerebellar infarct.

Case 12-5 illustrates how essential an imaging examination is in managing stroke. The patient had signs and

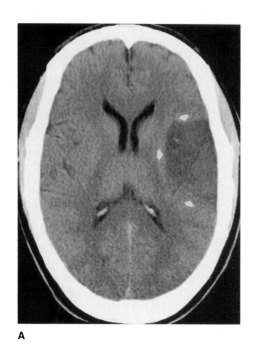

A

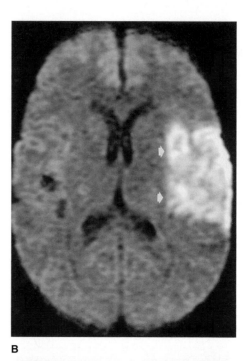

B

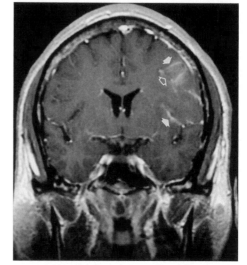

C

Fig. 12–20. **A** Noncontrast axial CT image of a subacute left MCA infarction in a middle-aged man with right-sided hemiparesis. A well-defined area of decreased attenuation is seen within the left MCA distribution (*arrows*). **B** The subsequent diffusion-weighted MR image demonstrates a well-circumscribed, wedge-shaped area of increased signal (*arrows*) corresponding to this CT signal abnormality. **C** Postcontrast coronal T$_1$-weighted MR image reveals linear enhancement along several cortical sulci (*closed arrows*), with associated band-like enhancement involving the adjacent cortex (*open arrow*).

symptoms of an acute cerebral infarction. The CT scan demonstrated an obvious basal ganglia hemorrhage, probably secondary to the patient's hypertension. Management of these two conditions is considerably different. Hypertension is the main cause of nontraumatic intracranial hemorrhage. In adults, these hemorrhages typically occur in the putamen/external capsule. Other locations for hypertensive hemorrhage include the thalamus, pons, cerebellum, and, rarely, subcortical white matter. Acute parenchymal hematomas, as in this case, are usually hyperdense on CT scans. With time these lesions become darker and eventually appear as round or slit-like cavities. The MR imaging appearance of a parenchymal hematoma is complex and depends largely on the presence of hemoglobin breakdown products within the clot.

EXERCISE 12-3: BRAIN TUMORS

Clinical Histories:

Case 12-6. A 33-year-old Hispanic man presents with a syncopal episode and involuntary tremors. Noncontrast sagittal T_1-weighted and axial T_2-weighted images, as well as postcontrast axial T_1-weighted images are shown in Fig. 12–21*A–C*.

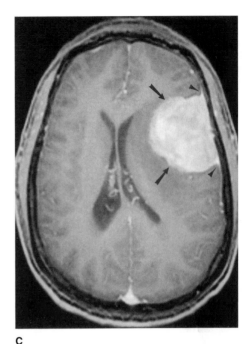

C

Fig. 12–21. *Cont.*

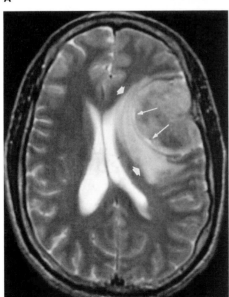

A

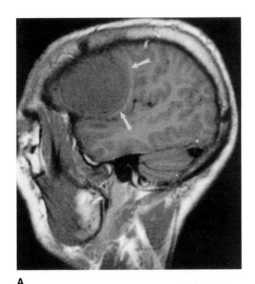

B

Fig. 12–21.

Case 12-7. A 48-year-old woman presents with a history of headaches and seizures. Initial coronal T_2-weighted FLAIR and axial contrast-enhanced T_1-weighted images were obtained (Fig. 12–22*A,B*).

Case 12-8. A 58-year-old man presents with a history of lung cancer and mental status changes. A contrast-enhanced axial CT scan and a gadolinium-enhanced axial T_1-weighted MR image are shown in Fig. 12–23 *A,B*.

Questions:

12-6. In Case 12-6, what is the most likely diagnosis?
    A. Extra-axial brain tumor
    B. Intra-axial brain tumor
    C. Frontal contusion
    D. Subdural hematoma
    E. Encephalocele

12-7. In Case 12-7, what is the most likely cause of the patient's symptoms?
    A. Multiple sclerosis
    B. Inner ear abnormality
    C. Intraventricular meningioma
    D. Hematoma
    E. Malignant brain tumor

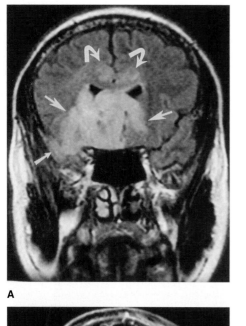

A

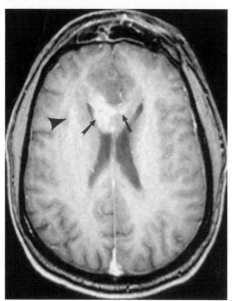

B

Fig. 12–22.

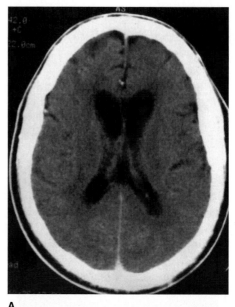

A

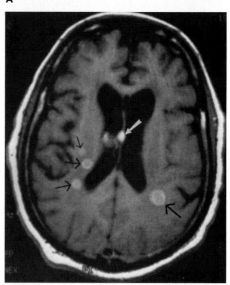

B

Fig. 12–23.

12-8. In Case 12-8, what is the most likely explanation for the patient's mental status changes?
A. Metastatic disease
B. Intracranial hemorrhage
C. Small infarcts
D. Sarcoidosis
E. Arteriovenous malformation

Radiologic Findings:

12-6. In this case, the sagittal T_1-weighted image before contrast administration (Fig. 12–21*A*) shows an extra-axial, left frontal convexity mass (*arrows*). This homogeneous-appearing, smoothly marginated mass is isointense to the normal gray matter, and is sometimes difficult to differentiate from normal brain tissue on unenhanced T_1 images. On T_2-weighted imaging (Fig. 12–21B), the mass has a heterogeneous appearance, but is predominantly isointense to gray matter. The mass is circumscribed by a thin rim (pseudocapsule) of increased T_2 signal (*long arrows*), as well as marginated by a more peripherally located band of T_2 signal hyperintensity along its medial and posterior borders (*short arrows*). There is distortion of the adjacent brain parenchyma, with compression of the left lateral ventricle, and a mild shift of the midline structures to the right. Following intravenous Gd-DTPA administration (Fig. 12–21C), the mass enhances uniformly (*arrows*), and dural tails are observed (*arrowheads*), allowing easy identification. These features are fairly typical of a meningioma. (*A* is the correct answer to Question 12-6.)

12-7. In this case, a coronal T_2-weighted FLAIR MR image (Fig. 12–22A) demonstrates a large area of T_2 signal hyperintensity involving the inferior frontal regions (*large white arrows*) and right temporal lobe (*small white arrow*), with extension into the corpus callosum (*curved arrows*). On the infused axial view, at the level of the body of the corpus callosum (Fig. 12–22B), subtle, ill-defined enhancement is present within the right cerebral hemisphere (*arrowhead*) with patchy enhancement (*arrows*) extending into the body of the corpus callosum. This is one appearance of a malignant brain tumor, in this case, an anaplastic oligodendroglioma. (*E* is the correct answer to Question 12-7.)

12-8. In this case, a contrast-enhanced axial CT scan (Fig. 12–23A) shows no definite abnormality. A gadolinium-enhanced axial T_1-weighted MR image (Fig. 12–23B) shows multiple enhancing lesions (*arrows*) within the brain parenchyma. In a patient with known lung cancer, metastatic disease is the most likely explanation for multiple intracranial enhancing lesions (A is the correct answer to Question 12-8.)

Discussion:

Brain tumors can be classified in a variety of ways. The traditional classification of intracranial neoplasms is based on histology. In this system, brain tumors are either primary (they arise from the brain and its linings) or secondary (they arise from somewhere outside the CNS, i.e., metastases). Primary tumors, which account for approximately two-thirds of all brain neoplasms, can be subdivided into glial and nonglial tumors. Secondary tumors, especially from lung and breast cancer, account for the remaining one-third of brain neoplasms. Metastases are most commonly parenchymal, but can also involve the skull and meninges.

Brain tumors can also be classified according to patient age and general tumor location (i.e., adult or child, supratentorial or infratentorial). Finally, brain tumors can be classified according to the specific anatomic region involved. For example, we can generate lists of brain tumors that specifically affect the pineal or the pituitary regions.

Case 12-6 illustrates a useful principle for interpreting studies of patients with suspected brain tumors. It is very important to first decide whether a mass is within the brain parenchyma (intra-axial) or outside the brain (extra-axial). Extra-axial masses usually turn out to be meningiomas, many of which can be removed surgically with a very low incidence of recurrence. Intra-axial masses frequently turn out to be astrocytomas, and the prognosis is less favorable.

The patient in Case 12-6 has an extra-axial, dural-based, frontal convexity mass that markedly enhances with Gd-DTPA. Meningiomas comprise 15% to 20% of intracranial tumors, occur predominantly in females, and exhibit a peak age incidence of 45 years. They are the most common nonglial primary CNS tumors. They can occur anywhere within the head but typically occur along the dural venous sinuses. The parasagittal region and cerebral convexities are the most common locations. Anterior basal or olfactory groove meningiomas account for 5% to 10% of intracranial meningiomas. Anosmia results from involvement of the olfactory tracts by the tumor. These expansile lesions are slow growing, and the ensuing mass effect on the adjacent brain parenchyma is gradual. The absence of reactive edema in a subset of these lesions can be seen as a result of their slow growth. These masses usually demonstrate intense and uniform enhancement, independent of tumor size. A layer of thickened dural enhancement ("dural tail") is commonly seen extending away from the base of the meningioma. In many cases, this finding represents reactive thickening without tumor involvement.

Case 12-7 demonstrates a large, infiltrating (aggressive or high-grade) glioma involving the majority of the right frontotemporal lobe, with extension into the corpus callosum. While there is some overlap of the MR imaging features characteristically seen with these invasive neoplasms and their less aggressive (lower grade) counterparts, the imaging features of higher grade neoplasms, on the whole, are distinctly different from those seen with lower grade lesions. High-grade gliomas, namely, anaplastic astrocytomas and oligodendrogliomas (as in this case), as well as glioblastoma multiforme (the most highly malignant glioma), demonstrate heterogeneous signal characteristics, generally a reflection of the variable cellularity, in addition to the presence of necrosis, hemorrhage, and cystic foci. Calcification and hemorrhage are more common in oligodendrogliomas, often accompanied by cyst formation and necrosis. The spectroscopic findings of decreased NAA and increased choline suggest decreased neuronal/axonal

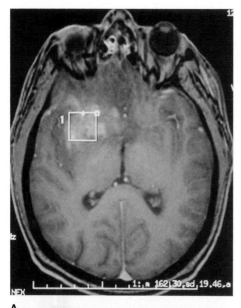

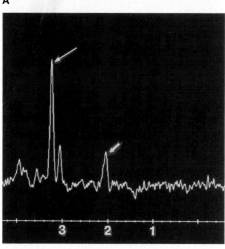

B

Fig. 12–24. The same patient as in Figure 12-22.
A At a more inferior level, the patchy, heterogeneous
enhancement of this mass within the right inferior
frontal/temporal regions is better appreciated. A
region-of-interest or volume element (i.e., voxel) was
centered within the enhancing tumor volume, and
an MR spectrum was obtained. **B** MR spectrum. The
NAA peak is abnormally decreased (*short arrow at
2.0*), and the choline signal is elevated (*long arrow at
3.2*), supporting the diagnosis of a malignant brain
tumor.

density and increased breakdown of cell membranes
(Fig. 12–24*A,B*).

Oligodendrogliomas account for about 5% of primary gliomas, occurring most frequently within the
frontal lobe and often involving the cortex. The majority
of patients present with seizures. On the other hand,
glioblastoma multiforme is the most common primary
malignant brain neoplasm and occurs most frequently in
patients older than 50 years of age. Patients with glioblastoma multiforme present with neurologic deficits or
new-onset seizures. The prognosis in these latter cases is
dismal; postoperative survival averages 8 months.

On T_2-weighted scans, these high-grade masses usually
exhibit heterogeneous signal characteristics, with areas of
high T_2 signal attributable to tumor tissue, necrosis, cysts,
and reactive edema, while regions of low signal may reflect
hemorrhage or calcification. The corresponding tissue
pathology of this region often shows tumor cells residing
within and extending beyond the surrounding edema.
Enhancement is highly variable within anaplastic oligodendrogliomas. Other types of malignant gliomas, such as
glioblastoma multiforme, typically demonstrate intense
enhancement. The corpus callosum is often involved by a
high-grade glial tumor, which may grow medially from an
adjacent hemispheric source or may arise independently
within this structure. "Wings" may extend symmetrically
or asymmetrically into both cerebral hemispheres, exhibit-
ing a butterfly-type appearance (Fig. 12–25), appropriately termed *butterfly glioma*.

Case 12-8 illustrates a very important point to remember when working up patients with suspected metastatic

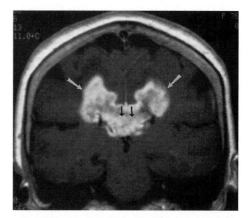

Fig. 12–25. Coronal contrast-enhanced T_1-weighted
MR image of a glioblastoma multiforme in a 76-year-old
woman with a 6-month history of progressive gait
ataxia and frequent falling is shown. An enhancing
mass (*white arrows*) extends through the corpus callosum (*black arrows*) into both hemispheres.

disease to the brain: MR imaging is considerably more sensitive than CT in detecting metastases. This is not a trivial point, since surgical resection of single, not multiple, brain lesions is sometimes performed. Conversely, the successful application of radiotherapy protocols relies on sensitively and accurately detecting the entire metastatic tumor burden. Metastatic disease to the brain has a variety of manifestations, the most common being parenchymal involvement. Typical hematogenous brain metastases demonstrate solid or ring-like enhancement on CT or MR scans, occur near gray matter white matter junctions, and are usually surrounded by a marked amount of edema. They most commonly metastasize from lung or breast primaries.

EXERCISE 12-4: INTRACRANIAL INFECTIONS

Clinical Histories:

Case 12-9.   A 75-year-old man presents with a history of recurrent lymphoma complicated by multiple infections and new mental status changes. Postcontrast axial T_1-weighted and diffusion-weighted MR images are shown in Fig. 12–26A,B.

Case 12-10.   A 4-year-old girl presents with lethargy and seizure activity. An axial T_2-weighted MR image of the brain is shown in Fig. 12–27.

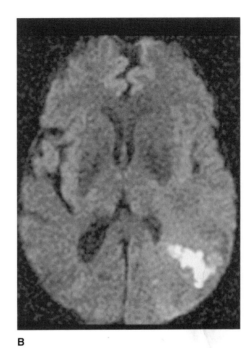

B

Fig. 12–26. *Cont.*

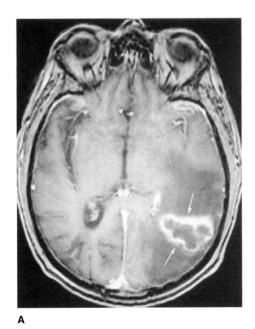

A

Fig. 12–26.

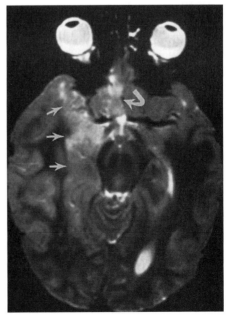

Fig. 12–27.

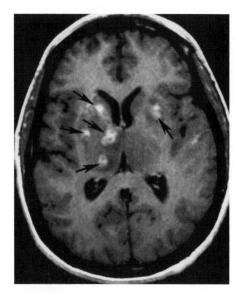

Fig. 12–28.

Case 12-11. A 43-year-old man presents with head-ache and weakness. An axial contrast-enhanced T$_1$-weighted MR image is shown in Fig. 12–28.

Questions:

12-9. In Case 12-9, what is the most likely diagnosis?
  A. Frontal contusion
  B. Aneurysm with intraventricular hemor-rhage
  C. Parietal lobe abscess
  D. Intracranial lymphoma
  E. Cerebritis

12-10. In Case 12-10, the location of the abnormal-ity is pathognomonic for which type of infection?
  A. Toxoplasmosis
  B. Tuberculosis
  C. Cryptococcus
  D. Herpes
  E. Staphylococcus

12-11. In Case 12-11, the major differential diagnosis for this lesion is toxoplasmosis versus
  A. cryptococcus.
  B. intracranial lymphoma.
  C. sarcoidosis.
  D. metastatic disease.
  E. cytomegalovirus (CMV).

Radiologic Findings:

12-9. In this case, the contrast-enhanced MR scan (Fig. 12–26A) shows a ring-enhancing lesion (*arrows*) in the left parietal lobe with decreased surrounding T$_1$ sig-nal. A diffusion signal abnormality is present on the cor-responding diffusion-weighted image (Fig. 12–26B) within the central aspect of the lesion, found to be compatible with an area of restricted water motion. The patient's history is compatible with an intracranial infec-tion, and the demonstrated MR imaging findings favor an abscess. (*C* is the correct answer to Question 12-9.)

12-10. In this case, the T$_2$-weighted MR image (Fig. 12–27) shows high-signal abnormality in the medial aspect of the right temporal lobe (*arrows*) and within the inferior right frontal lobe (*curved arrow*). These changes are commonly seen in patients with herpes encephalitis. (*D* is the correct answer to Question 12-10.)

12-11. In this case, multiple enhancing lesions are present within the basal ganglia, especially on the right (*arrows*), on the gadolinium-enhanced T$_1$-weighted MR image (Fig. 12–28). The most common lesions with this appearance in an HIV-positive patient are toxoplasmosis and intracranial lymphoma. (*B* is the correct answer to Question 12-11.) The patient markedly improved after antitoxoplasmosis therapy, and the lesions shown on the MR image disappeared.

Discussion:

A host of infectious diseases can involve the brain and its coverings. Because the CNS has a limited number of ways of responding to an infectious agent, many in-tracranial infections appear identical on neuroimaging studies. It is, therefore, very important to closely corre-late the imaging findings with the clinical presentation and other diagnostic tests, such as lumbar puncture or stereotactic brain aspiration.

For our purposes, it is useful to classify CNS infec-tions according to the intracranial compartment in-volved, especially since this has treatment implications. Intracranial infections can be either parenchymal or extraparenchymal. Parenchymal manifestations include cerebritis/abscess and encephalitis. Extraparenchymal disease includes epidural abscess, subdural empyema, and leptomeningitis. Bacterial, viral, fungal, and para-sitic agents can all affect the CNS. Although a few infec-tious agents preferentially involve a particular anatomic compartment of the CNS, most are not site specific.

Case 12-9 demonstrates the classic ring-enhancing lesion of an abscess, in this case, due to nocardia. No specific features of this abscess distinguish it from a typ-ical pyogenic abscess. The diffusion signal abnormality has been postulated to arise from restricted water mo-tion in the presence of viscous, prurulent material within the abscess cavity, and it can mimic an area of acute ischemia. Cerebral infection by nocardia usually arises from a pulmonary focus in an immunocompromised host. Similarly, most pyogenic abscesses are the result of hematogenous dissemination from a non-CNS source. Pyogenic brain abscesses can also result from direct extension of an infectious process from an adjacent area (e.g., sinusitis or mastoiditis) or from trauma (e.g., penetrating wound or surgery).

Abscesses usually occur at gray matter white matter junctions, although they can occur anywhere in the brain. Patients frequently present with seizures or symptoms related to intracranial mass effect. If abscesses develop near the brain surface, they may rupture into the subarachnoid space, producing a meningitis; they may also produce a ventriculitis if they rupture into the ventricular system. Most abscesses are treated surgically.

Herpes encephalitis (Case 12-10) is caused by the herpes simplex virus (HSV). Older children and adults are usually infected by HSV-1, either primarily or as a result of reactivation of a latent virus. The ensuing necrotizing encephalitis in this condition typically involves the temporal and inferior frontal lobes, insular cortex, and cingulate gyrus. Focal abnormalities of attenuation (on CT) or signal (on MR) in these characteristic locations, often with enhancement after contrast administration, are practically pathognomonic of HSV-1 encephalitis. Early diagnosis of this condition is extremely important, because antiviral therapy can significantly affect patient outcome.

Neonatal herpes simplex infection differs from infection in the older child and adult. The offending organism is usually HSV-2, which may be acquired *in utero* or during birth from mothers with genital herpes. HSV-2 infection can produce severe destructive changes within the developing brain. Unlike HSV-1 infection in older children and adults, neonatal herpes encephalitis can involve any area of the brain, having no predilection for the temporal lobe.

Patients with AIDS (Case 12-11) commonly develop intracranial infections during the course of their disease. HIV itself can directly infect the CNS, producing encephalopathy in up to 60% of AIDS patients. The most common neuroimaging finding in HIV encephalopathy is cerebral atrophy, often with patchy white matter hypointensity (on CT) or increased T_2 signal (on MR imaging) from demyelination and gliosis (Fig. 12–29). Other common CNS infections in the immunocompromised AIDS patient include toxoplasmosis, cryptococcosis, and progressive multifocal leukoencephalopathy (from a papovavirus infection).

Toxoplasmosis usually presents as multiple lesions of varying size, and demonstrates ring enhancement with surrounding edema on CT or MR imaging (Fig. 12–28). Lesions commonly occur in the basal ganglia or at the

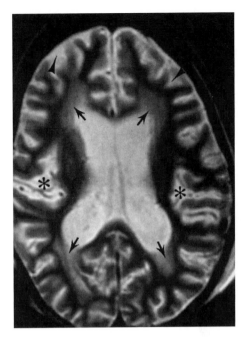

Fig. 12–29. An 8-year-old girl with AIDS and new onset of seizures. Axial T_2-weighted image shows white matter high signal (*arrows*). Also note the diffuse prominence of gyri and sulci (*arrowheads*) and sylvian fissures (*asterisks*), compatible with cerebral atrophy.

gray matter white matter junction within the cerebral hemispheres. Individual masses may have a solid appearance or demonstrate central necrosis or hemorrhage. The enhancement pattern is variable; both rim-enhancing and more solidly enhancing lesions can be seen. Their appearance is almost identical to that of primary intracranial lymphoma, another common intracranial condition in AIDS. Metabolic studies, such as PET or SPECT scans (no increase in ^{18}F-FDG activity with toxoplasmosis, increased with lymphoma), MR spectroscopy (no choline elevation in toxoplasmosis, elevated in lymphoma), and perfusion-weighted sequences (lower cerebral blood volume in toxoplasmosis) may assist in distinguishing these pathologies.

Meningitis is the most frequent manifestation of cryptococcosis in AIDS, although parenchymal lesions, termed *cryptococcomas*, are occasionally encountered. In progressive multifocal leukoencephalopathy, extensive areas of white matter demyelination are shown on MR imaging. A number of other intracranial infections can occur in AIDS patients and the reader is referred to the Bibliography at the end of this chapter for sources of further information.

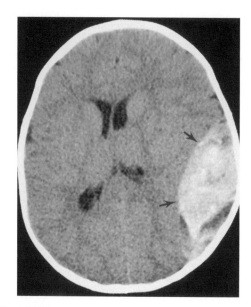

Fig. 12–30.

EXERCISE 12-5: HEAD TRAUMA

Clinical Histories:

Case 12-12. A young man who has been in a motor vehicle accident presents with a head injury. Soft-tissue window from an axial non-contrast head CT scan is shown in Fig. 12–30.

Case 12-13. A 24-year-old man presents with multiple facial fractures and frontal scalp soft-tissue swelling resulting from a motor vehicle accident. Axial noncontrast head CT images are shown in Fig. 12–31.

Questions:

12-12. In Case 12-12, what is the diagnosis?
A. Subdural hematoma
B. Cerebral contusion
C. Epidural hematoma
D. Meningioma
E. Subdural hygroma

12-13. In Case 12-13, what is the main radiologic finding?
A. Subdural hematoma
B. Epidural hematoma
C. Duret hemorrhage
D. Cerebral contusions
E. Shearing injuries

Radiologic Findings:

12-12. In this case (Fig. 12–30), a predominantly high-density, extra-axial, hemorrhagic collection (*arrows*) is producing mass effect on the left temporoparietal lobe on an unenhanced head CT scan. The biconvex appearance of this lesion is typical of an epidural hematoma, which is an acute finding in this case. (*C* is the correct answer to Question 12-12.)

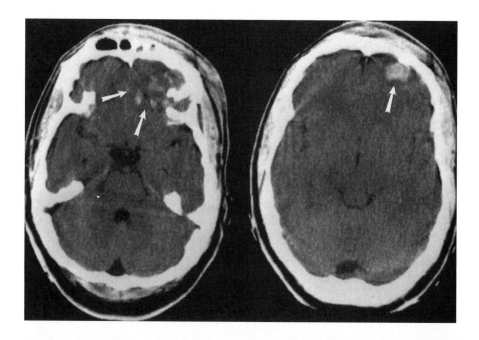

Fig. 12–31.

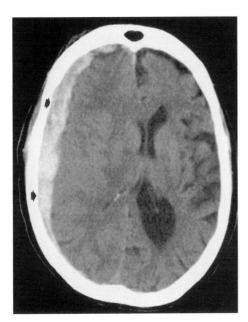

Fig. 12–32. Uninfused axial CT image in a middle-aged patient following a fall. A large, crescentic, extra-axial hemorrhagic collection layers over the right lateral convexity (*arrows*), consistent with an acute subdural hematoma. There is associated mass effect on the adjacent brain parenchyma, with effacement of the cortical gyri, compression of the right lateral ventricle, and shift of the midline structures to the left.

12-13. In this case, multiple areas of increased attenuation within the frontal lobes, especially on the left (*arrows*), are seen in Fig. 12–31. These areas correspond to multiple hemorrhagic contusions involving the brain parenchyma. (*D* is the correct answer to Question 12-13.)

Discussion:

Intracranial abnormalities in head trauma can be classified as either primary or secondary. Primary lesions occur at the moment of injury and include skull fractures, extra-cerebral hemorrhage (e.g., epidural or subdural hematomas, subarachnoid hemorrhage), and intracerebral hemorrhage (e.g., brain contusion, brain stem injury, diffuse axonal injury).

The secondary effects of head trauma are actually complications of the primary intracranial injury. Elevated intracranial pressure and cerebral herniations are responsible for most of the secondary effects of head trauma, which in many cases may be more devastating to the patients than the initial injury.

Epidural hematoma is usually associated with skull fractures that lacerate the middle meningeal artery or a dural sinus. Up to one-half of patients with epidural hematomas have a lucid interval after the head trauma occurs. On CT, epidural hematomas usually appear as biconvex, high-attenuation, extra-axial masses. Most are located in the temporoparietal area. Underlying skull fractures are common. Intracranial brain herniation may also be a prominent feature in this condition. One important imaging feature in epidural hematomas is that they do not cross skull sutures.

Subdural hematoma, on the other hand, is usually a crescent-shaped extra-axial collection that may cross suture lines (Fig. 12–32). These lesions are more lethal than are epidural hematomas; the subdural hematoma mortality rate is greater than 50%. CT can usually, but not always, distinguish between epidural hematomas and subdural hematomas. Subdural hematomas are a commonly identified abnormality in the abused child (nonaccidental trauma). CT scans are obtained to detect the presence of subdural hematomas (Fig. 12–33). Brain MR imaging, however, can more sensitively delineate

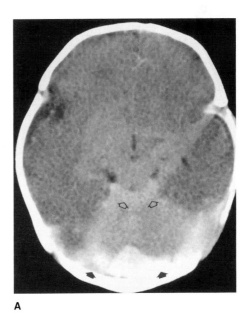

A

Fig. 12–33. Noncontrast axial CT images **A, B** in a 21-day-old male following nonaccidental trauma. Large, bilateral subdural hematomas layer over the tentorium cerebelli in **A** (*closed arrows*) and within the interhemispheric fissure in **B** (*arrow*). In addition, a small amount of subarachnoid hemorrhage is seen within the quadrigeminal plate cistern in **A** (*open arrows*), as well as within the left lateral ventricle (not shown). Loss of the normal cerebral gray white differentiation is demonstrated. These features are pathognomonic for nonaccidental trauma with diffuse anoxic insult.

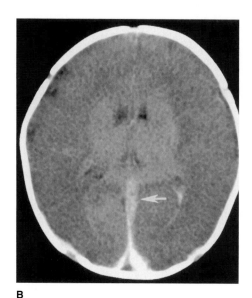

B

Fig. 12–33. Cont.

EXERCISE 12-6: INTRACRANIAL VASCULAR ABNORMALITIES

Clinical Histories:

Case 12-14. A 59-year-old woman presents with a severe headache. An axial head CT image and a cerebral arteriogram are shown in Fig. 12–34*A,B*).

Case 12-15. An 11-year-old boy presents with an acute decline in mental status. Axial head CT image and cerebral arteriogram are shown in Fig. 12–35*A,B*).

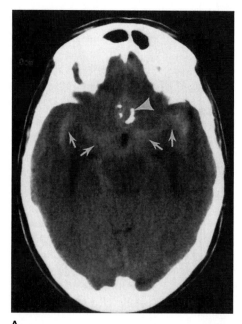

A

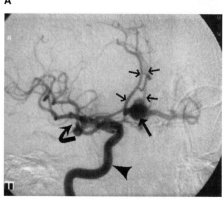

B

Fig. 12–34.

small extra-axial hematomas, subdural hematomas of varying ages, and coexisting cortical contusions or shearing injuries. A shearing injury (or diffuse axonal injury) is associated with an overall poor prognosis, and it is recognized as small petechial hemorrhages at the gray white junction and in the corpus callosum. Interhemispheric (para- and intrafalcial) subdural hematomas may arise from tearing of bridging veins along the falx cerebri in shaking injuries and is nearly pathognomic for nonaccidental trauma (Fig. 12–33*B*). Retinal hemorrhages may be present and are also suspicious, especially if bilateral. In addition, cerebral ischemia/infarction and multiple, complex, unexplained skull fractures may be associated findings.

Cerebral contusions (Case 12-13) are the second most common form of brain parenchymal injury in primary head trauma. (Diffuse axonal injury is the most common parenchymal injury.) Cerebral contusions can be thought of as brain bruises. They result either from the brain striking a bony ridge inside the skull during rapid acceleration/deceleration, as occurs in a motor vehicle accident, or from a depressed skull fracture. These lesions tend to occur in particular anatomic locations, especially the undersurfaces and poles of the frontal and temporal lobes. CT scans show areas of low attenuation (edema) and hemorrhage at the site of injury. Delayed hemorrhage, 1 to 2 days after a head injury, is common with contusions.

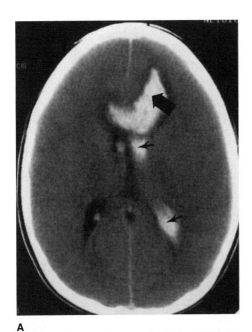

A

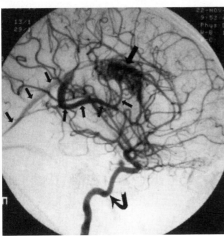

B

Fig. 12–35.

Questions:

12-14. In Case 12-14, what is the reason for the abnormality on the CT scan?

    A.   Cerebral aneurysm
    B.   Arteriovenous malformation
    C.   Head trauma
    D.   Carotid dissection
    E.   Vasculitis

12-15. In Case 12-15, what is the reason for the abnormality on the CT scan?

    A.   Cerebral aneurysm
    B.   Arteriovenous malformation
    C.   Head trauma
    D.   Carotid dissection
    E.   Vasculitis

Radiologic Findings:

12-14. In this case, the CT scan (Fig. 12–34A) shows extensive subarachnoid hemorrhage filling the basal cisterns (*arrows*). Curvilinear calcifications (*arrowhead*) are present in the region of the anterior communicating artery. Oblique frontal view from a carotid arteriogram (Fig. 12–34B) demonstrates the source of this bleeding: a large aneurysm (*large arrow*) between the anterior cerebral arteries (*small arrows*). Also note the internal carotid (*arrowhead*) and middle cerebral (*curved arrow*) arteries. (*A* is the correct answer to Question 12-14.)

12-15. In this case, the CT scan (Fig. 12–35A), shows intraparenchymal (*large arrow*) and intraventricular hemorrhage (*small arrows*). The lateral view of a carotid arteriogram (Fig. 12–35B) demonstrates a tangle of blood vessels typical of an arteriovenous malformation (*large arrow*) with early draining veins (*small arrows*). Note the internal carotid artery (*curved arrow*). (*B* is the correct answer to Question 12-15.)

Discussion:

Cerebrovascular disorders (strokes) were discussed in Exercise 12-2, which dealt mainly with cerebral infarction secondary to atherosclerosis. For information on other causes of cerebral infarction, the reader is referred to the bibliography at the end of this chapter. This section addresses two other common vascular conditions affecting the CNS: aneurysms and vascular malformations.

Most cerebral aneurysms, like Case 12-14, are saccular or "berry" aneurysms. These focal arterial dilatations tend to occur at cerebral arterial branch points. They have traditionally been thought to develop at congenitally weak areas of a blood vessel wall. Recent evidence, however, has questioned this view, and many now believe that saccular aneurysms are probably acquired lesions from abnormal hemodynamic stresses that damage the arterial wall.

Intracranial aneurysms are usually asymptomatic until they rupture, at which time the patient typically presents with a severe headache resulting from subarachnoid hemorrhage (SAH). The vast majority of nontraumatic SAHs occur as a result of aneurysm rupture. CT is very good at demonstrating SAH. Patients usually undergo cerebral arteriography whenever nontraumatic SAH is detected.

Common locations for intracranial aneurysms include the anterior communicating artery, the internal carotid artery at the origin of the posterior communicating artery, and the middle cerebral artery trifurcation.

Posterior fossa aneurysms are less common; they make up only around 10% of all intracranial aneurysms.

Vascular malformations can be divided into four major types: true arteriovenous malformations (as demonstrated in Case 12-15), cavernous hemangiomas, venous angiomas, and capillary telangiectasias. Arteriovenous malformations (AVMs) are congenital lesions consisting of a tangle of abnormal blood vessels, usually within the brain parenchyma, that are fed by enlarged cerebral arteries and drained by dilated, tortuous veins. Because there is no normal intervening brain parenchyma for the blood to flow through, blood is rapidly shunted from the arterial to the venous side. This shunting is dramatically demonstrated on cerebral arteriography. Patients with AVMs usually present with intracranial hemorrhage or seizures. MR imaging or contrast-enhanced CT can demonstrate the tortuous vascular channels of most AVMs, although cerebral arteriography is the definitive study in this condition.

The other intracranial vascular malformations have very characteristic appearances on MR imaging, although they are frequently invisible on cerebral arteriography. Patients with these "low-pressure" malformations can present with headaches, seizures, or, rarely, intracranial hemorrhage. Many of these lesions, however, are incidentally discovered on MR scans performed for other reasons.

EXERCISE 12-7: WHITE MATTER DISEASES

Clinical Histories:

Case 12-16. A 23-year-old woman presents with numbness, weakness, and blurred vision. Axial T_2-weighted and coronal FLAIR MR images of the brain are shown in Fig. 12–36A,B.

Case 12-17. A 77-year-old woman presents with a long history of hypertension and recent onset of dementia. An axial T_2-weighted MR image is shown in Fig. 12–37.

Questions:

12-16. In Case 12-16, what is the most likely diagnosis?
  A. Pseudotumor cerebri
  B. Metastatic disease
  C. Septic emboli
  D. Radiation necrosis
  E. Multiple sclerosis

12-17. In Case 12-17, what is most likely responsible for the abnormalities seen on the MR image?
  A. Cardiac arrhythmia
  B. Chronic hypertension

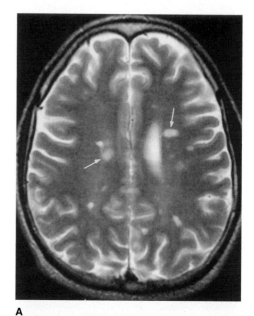

A

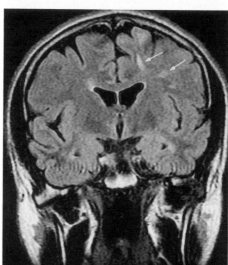

B

Fig. 12–36.

  C. Remote trauma
  D. Hepatic failure
  E. Carbon monoxide poisoning

Radiologic Findings:

12-16. In this case, the axial T_2-weighted and coronal FLAIR MR images (Fig. 12–36A,B) show multiple foci of increased T_2 signal within the white matter (*ar-*

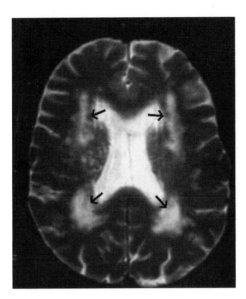

Fig. 12–37.

rows). These lesions are quite characteristic of multiple sclerosis. (*E* is the correct answer to Question 12-16.) The patient's visual difficulties were due to optic neuritis, a common abnormality in multiple sclerosis.

12-17. In this case (Fig. 12–37), there are patchy areas of increased T_2 signal (*arrows*) within the periventricular white matter. Usually seen in elderly hypertensive patients, these lesions correspond to focal areas of demyelination secondary to deep white matter ischemia. (*B* is the correct answer to Question 12-17.)

Discussion:

Diseases that primarily affect the cerebral white matter have a host of causes. Unfortunately, very few of these conditions have specific appearances on CT or MR scans. Neuroimaging is usually performed to determine whether there are changes within the brain that are compatible with one of the white matter diseases and to rule out other conditions that might mimic white matter disease.

White matter diseases include both inherited and acquired conditions. They can be further subdivided into demyelinating conditions (destruction or injury of normally formed myelin) and dysmyelinating conditions (abnormal formation or maintenance of myelin, usually because of an enzyme deficiency). The dysmyelinating conditions are rare and, for the most part, include the leukodystrophies, such as adrenoleukodystrophy and metachromatic leukodystrophy. Although the MR appearance can be striking in some of these diseases, it is often nonspecific. These conditions are not discussed here.

Multiple sclerosis (MS) (Case 12-16) is the most common demyelinating disease. Because there is no generally accepted etiology for MS, it is also referred to as a primary demyelinating disease. Secondary demyelinating conditions are those caused by a known agent or event. MS usually occurs in young adults and more often in women than men (approximately 2:1). The disease is characterized by a relapsing and remitting course and by varying neurologic symptoms, depending on the location of the lesion within the CNS. Although diagnosis of MS is usually based on clinical criteria, MR imaging can be a very helpful confirmatory test. Typical MS plaques appear as ovoid, T_2 signal hyperintensities within the periventricular and deep white matter. Lesions are also common within the corpus callosum, brain stem, cerebellar peduncles, spinal cord, and optic nerves. MS plaque enhancement on gadolinium-infused MR images suggests active disease (i.e., breakdown of the BBB). Confluent areas of T_2 signal abnormality in the periventricular white matter are common in severe cases.

Ischemic demyelination (Case 12-17) is usually seen in patients with small-vessel disease (such as from longstanding hypertension). This condition, also called *leukaraiosis* (white matter softening), occurs because of hypertension-induced arteriolar sclerosis of penetrating medullary arteries that supply the deep white matter of the brain. This leads to a reduction in white matter blood flow with accompanying ischemic demyelination. This condition occurs most commonly in older patients and is associated with small-vessel brain infarcts (lacunar infarcts). MR imaging usually demonstrates patchy areas of increased T_2 signal in the deep white matter. The lesions are often bilaterally symmetric and periventricular in distribution.

BIBLIOGRAPHY

Aksoy FG et al. Dynamic contrast-enhanced brain perfusion imaging: technique and clinical applications. *Semin Ultrasound CT MRI*. 2000;21:462–467.

Atlas SW, ed. *Magnetic Resonance Imaging of the Brain and Spine*. New York: Raven Press; 2002.

Cullen SP et al. Dynamic contrast-enhanced computed tomography of acute ischemic stroke: CTA and CT perfusion. *Semin Roentgenol*. 2002;37:192–205.

Grossman RI, Yousem DM. *Neuroradiology: The Requisites*. St. Louis; Mosby; 2003.

Liu H et al. MR-guided and MR-monitored neurosurgical procedures at 1.5T. *JCAT*. 2000;24:909–918.

Philips CD et al. CTA and MRA in the evaluation of extracranial carotid vascular disease. *Radiol Clin N Am*. 2002;40:783–798.

Orrison WW et al. *Functional Brain Imaging*. St. Louis: Mosby; 1995.

Osborn AG. *Diagnostic Neuroradiology*. St. Louis: Mosby; 1994.

Yock DH. *Magnetic Resonance Imaging of CNS Disease*. St. Louis: Mosby; 2002.

Imaging of the Spine

Lawrence E. Ginsberg

INTRODUCTION

It goes without saying that the spine is critical for normal human function. The spine provides height and mobility for turning and bending and protects the spinal cord and spinal nerves. Given the wide range of pathologic conditions that may affect the spine, radiologists are frequently called on for spine imaging. Recognition of normal anatomy and variants, differentiation from abnormal anatomy, and diagnosis of different pathologic conditions are the goals of spine imaging.

It is assumed in this chapter that the reader is already familiar with basic spine anatomy learned early in medical school. With such a foundation, this presentation of the imaging appearance of the spine will serve to solidify and perhaps even enhance this knowledge base.

The purpose of this chapter is to review the different techniques employed in spine imaging and to emphasize normal anatomy as depicted with these techniques. The imaging appearance of certain common lesions will also be presented. Relative advantages and disadvantages of the various imaging modalities will be reviewed within the context of an overall imaging strategy. It is not intended that the reader will be an accomplished spine radiologist after reading this chapter. Rather, it is hoped that the reader will gain basic familiarity with normal imaging anatomy and the imaging appearance of certain types of abnormalities, as well as a sense of which test might be the best to order for a given clinical circumstance.

TECHNIQUES

Prior to the advent of computed tomography (CT) in the 1970s, spine imaging consisted primarily of plain-film radiography and an adjunct test, myelography, to be discussed below. Spine imaging was revolutionized by CT and, subsequently, magnetic resonance (MR) imaging, which for the first time allowed direct acquisition of axial and sagittal (multiplanar) images. Not until the era of CT could the spinal cord itself be directly visualized. Refinements of these cross-sectional imaging techniques are ongoing, with exciting progress undoubtedly still to come. These imaging modalities have so changed the face of spine diagnosis and treatment that virtually no neurosurgeon today would undertake spine surgery without first obtaining a CT or MR imaging study. Unfortunately, however, the widespread availability of this technology, combined with unscrupulous entrepreneurs and an adversarial legal climate, has resulted in the performance of many unnecessary scans. Perhaps health care changes, malpractice reform, or both will help to reduce the number of unnecessary examinations.

This section reviews the major modalities currently employed to image the spine. The highly specialized technique of spinal arteriography, which is used principally to detect vascular malformations, is beyond the scope of this review. Nuclear medicine scanning also will not be discussed, because it is seldom used as a primary diagnostic study in the evaluation of spinal disease (though spinal metastases are frequently diagnosed with whole-body isotope bone scanning).

Plain Film

Plain films are conventional radiographs, which are commonly referred to as x-rays. They may be obtained in a frontal projection [anteroposterior (AP) or posteroanterior (PA)—the difference is insignificant in the spine], a lateral projection (side view), or an oblique projection (Figs. 13–1, 13–2, and 13–3). Plain films are most useful for the visualization of bony structures. Soft-tissue structures (everything but bone) are largely radiolucent and cannot be seen clearly on plain films unless abnormal density such as calcification is present. Although plain films depict bone anatomy quite well, certain structures may be obscured by other structures in front of or behind them. For instance, on a lateral projection, both pedicles would be superimposed on one another (Figs. 13–1*B* and 13–3*B*). For this reason, multiple views are always obtained as part of a routine examination.

On conventional radiographs, bony structures appear white. This appearance is referred to as *radiodense* or simply *dense*. Normally mineralized bones have a recognizable radiodensity, which should always be assessed when viewing x-rays. Certain pathologic conditions (e.g., osteopenia and osteolytic metastases) can result in decreased bone density, and other conditions (e.g., osteoblastic metastases and some exotic diseases) may result in abnormally increased bone density.

After bone density is assessed, the next observation should be the alignment of the spine. A normal spine should show cervical and lumbar lordosis (anterior convexity) (Figs. 13–1 and 13–3) and thoracic kyphosis

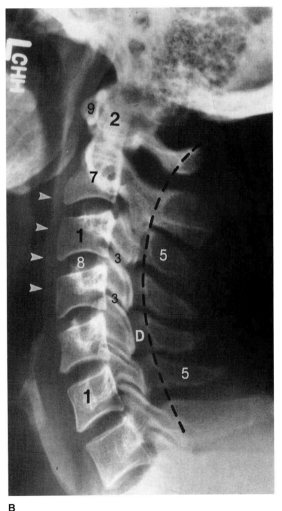

A   **B**

Fig. 13–1. Plain film of normal cervical spine. **A** Anteroposterior view. **B** Lateral view. Arrowheads indicate prevertebral soft-tissue stripe. Note normal lordosis and continuity of spinolaminar line (*dashed line*).

(posterior convexity). Abnormalities in alignment may result from incorrect positioning of the patient but often reflect an underlying problem. Such abnormalities may be minor such as straightening or reversal of normal cervical lordosis in the case of muscle spasm. More significant misalignments, such as scoliosis, may be either idiopathic or secondary to an underlying lesion. Major alterations in alignment, such as subluxation, may result from trauma. In assessing alignment it is important to determine whether the vertebral bodies, as well as the posterior elements (i.e., spinous processes, pedicles, and laminae), are appropriately aligned. Remember that the spinal cord rests within the spinal canal formed by the vertebral

foramen of each vertebra and that the spinal cord is invisible on plain films. One must therefore evaluate where the spinal cord should be. The anterior margin of the spinal canal is the posterior aspect of the vertebral body. The posterior limit of the spinal canal can be approximated by locating on a lateral radiograph the junction of the spinous process and the laminae. Identification of the spinolaminar line also helps in the evaluation of alignment (Fig. 13–1*B*).

Most anatomic features of the spine are readily identifiable on plain radiographs (Figs. 13–1, 13–2, and 13–3). Vertebral bodies, facet joints, disc spaces, pedicles, laminae, transverse and spinous processes, and the neural foramen can all be visualized. Certain anatomic areas can be seen only on specialized views. For instance, the open-mouth view facilitates visualization of the atlantoaxial (C1–2) articulation and provides an additional view of the dens (Fig. 13–1*D*). This view is an essential component of a trauma workup. Oblique views allow visualization of the neural foramen in the cervical spine (lateral views are used for this purpose in the thoracolumbar spine), which transmit the paired spinal nerves (Fig. 13–1*C*). As you recall, there are 8 pairs of cervical spinal nerves, 12 pairs of thoracic spinal nerves, and

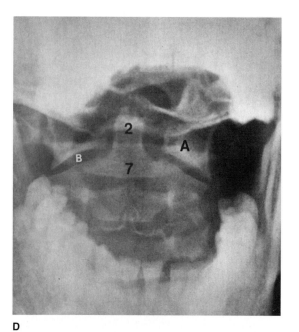

C

D

Fig. 13–1. **C** Oblique view. **D** Open mouth. (Courtesy of Stanley P. Bohrer, M.D., Wake Forest University School of Medicine.) *Key* (for Figs. 13–1, 13–2 and 13–3): 1 = vertebral body; 2 = odontoid process (dens); 3 = articular facet joint; 4 = intervertebral (neural) foramen; 5 = spinous process; 6 = transverse process; 7 = body of axis (C2); 8 = intervertebral disc space; 9 = anterior arch of atlas (Cl); A = lateral mass of atlas; B = atlantoaxial joint; C = uncinate process; D = lamina; E = pedicle; F = pars interarticularis; S = sacrum; I = sacroiliac joint.

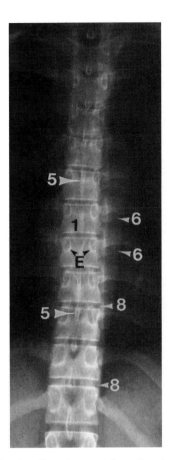

Fig. 13–2. Plain film of normal thoracic spine, anteroposterior view. (See key in Fig. 13–1 caption.)

gest atherosclerotic vascular narrowing. In the evaluation of cervical trauma, one should always include assessment of the width of the normal soft-tissue stripe, which is anterior to the vertebral bodies (Fig. 13–1*B*). This prevertebral soft-tissue stripe may become widened in cervical spine trauma (prompting a closer search for fracture) and also in certain inflammatory conditions. When reviewing thoracic or lumbar spine films, attention to the soft tissues may facilitate diagnosis of a host of conditions ranging from pneumonia and lung cancer to retroperitoneal diseases and abdominal aortic aneurysms. Therefore, it is important not to focus only on the spine when interpreting spine radiographs.

Myelography

Contrast myelography has been around since its accidental discovery in 1922, when Sicard and Forestier, intending to administer extradural Lipiodol to treat sciatica, inadvertently introduced the material into the subarachnoid space. This radiopaque oil was noted to move freely, and it was immediately recognized that with the use of fluoroscopy (real-time radiography) and conventional radiography, this procedure would be useful

5 pairs of lumbar spinal nerves. To allow for spinal nerve exit, these neural foramina are formed by the pedicles above and below (Figs. 13–1*C* and 13–3*B*). Abnormal bony projections, known as *osteophytes,* are a common manifestation of degenerative spine disease and, if present within the neural foramen, may be a cause of nerve root compression. Spinal nerves also can be compressed by disc herniations, but this type of neural compression cannot be diagnosed by means of plain film alone.

Certain small bony structures, such as the cervical transverse foramen (for the vertebral artery) and the small facets for rib articulation in the thoracic spine, are not well visualized on plain radiographs. Because "soft-tissue" structures also are poorly demonstrated on plain radiographs, the intervertebral disc is not well seen with x-ray unless calcified (and therefore dense). However, the soft tissues should not be ignored. In the cervical spine, for instance, one may identify calcification in the region of the carotid artery bifurcation, which may sug-

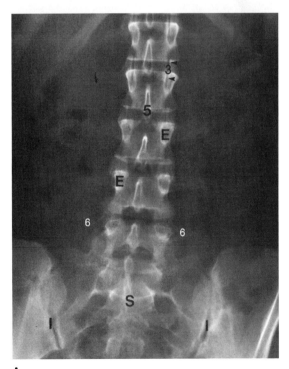

A

Fig. 13–3. Plain film of normal lumbar spine. **A** Anteroposterior view.

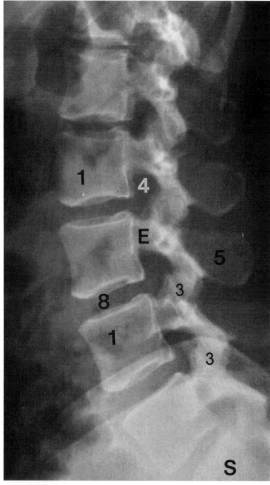

B

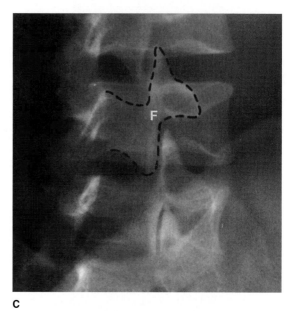

C

Fig. 13–3. **B** Lateral view. **C** Oblique view. Notice "Scottie dog" configuration formed by facet joints and pedicle in this projection (*dashed line*). The "neck" of the Scottie dog represents the pars interarticularis. (See key in Fig. 13–1 caption.) (Part *C* courtesy of Stanley P. Bohrer, M.D., Wake Forest University School of Medicine.)

for diagnosing intraspinal tumors. Lipiodol quickly replaced air as the medium of choice for myelography. [Air is lucent and is therefore a "negative" contrast agent; iodinized oils such as Lipiodol and, later, the popular Pantopaque (iophendylate) are dense and therefore "positive" contrast agents.] Following Mixter and Barr's 1934 report on the syndrome of herniated intervertebral disc, myelography became a widely used test. In the 1980s, the wide availability of less toxic water-soluble agents and, finally, nonionic contrast agents such as iopamidol and iohexol made myelography a readily tolerated procedure.

Myelography is employed most commonly to evaluate for disk herniations and to rule out spinal cord compression caused by tumor or trauma. In many parts of the United States, CT and MR imaging have all but replaced myelography. However, in many locations, myel-

ography is still commonly performed. A myelogram is often followed by a postmyelogram CT examination, which is addressed later in this chapter.

The technique for performing myelography is simple. The patient is placed in the prone position on a fluoroscopy table. Under fluoroscopic guidance, a lumbar puncture (LP) is made with an 18- to 22-gauge spinal needle. (A fluoroscopically guided LP is much easier than an LP performed on a sick patient on the ward in the decubitus position.) Cerebrospinal fluid (CSF) is then drawn for laboratory tests, if needed, and contrast material is placed into the subarachnoid space. Once instillation of the contrast agent is fluoroscopically confirmed, the needle can be withdrawn and the patient studied. Depending on the spinal level to be examined, the patient can be standing, flat, or in Trendelenburg position. Typically, multiple views including lateral, AP,

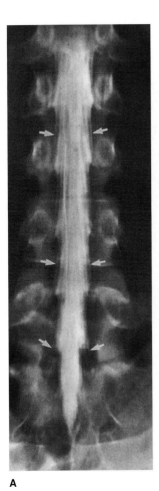
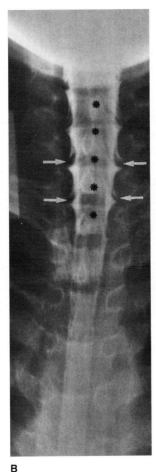

A   B

Fig. 13–4. A Normal lumbar myelogram, AP view. Note dense white contrast within the thecal sac. The nerve roots are readily identified as a "negative defect" within the dense contrast (*arrows*). **B** Cervical myelogram, AP view. The spinal cord (asterisks) can be seen as a lower density "defect" within the contrast column. Exiting nerve roots can also be seen (*arrows*).

and oblique views are obtained. In the lumbar region, the cauda equina nerve roots are well visualized (Fig. 13–4*A*). The conus medullaris, usually at L1–2, also can be seen. In the thoracic and cervical levels, the spinal cord can be seen as a "negative" shadow within the dense contrast, and its size and shape can therefore be evaluated (Fig. 13–4*B*). Cervical spinal nerves are also well seen (Fig. 13–4*B*). The presence of any lesions and their precise location relative to the dura usually can be determined on the basis of the myelographic appearance. For instance, lesions may be extradural, intradural but extramedullary (not in the spinal cord), or intramedullary (within the spinal cord).

Computed Tomography

CT utilizes x-rays to obtain images by means of multiple sources and detectors surrounding the patient in a radial fashion. This is why the patient appears to be en-

tering a large doughnut-shaped device during the CT examination. The data obtained are processed by a computer, which then generates an image. Though sagittal reconstructions can be generated and are occasionally useful in spine imaging, the axial plane offers the highest image resolution. Once the raw data are obtained, images can be displayed with different "windows" and "level" values that take advantage of density ("attenuation" in CT lingo) differences between tissues. For instance, filming a set of soft-tissue windows allows differentiation of soft-tissue structures that are very similar in attenuation to adjacent structures (e.g., muscle and fluid). This is one of the key features of CT: whereas plain films usually cannot discriminate between different kinds of soft tissue, CT, with its superior resolution, can do just that. In the spine, CT makes it possible to discriminate between CSF, nerve roots, and ligaments, for instance. Without the administration of contrast agents, therefore, a CT examination

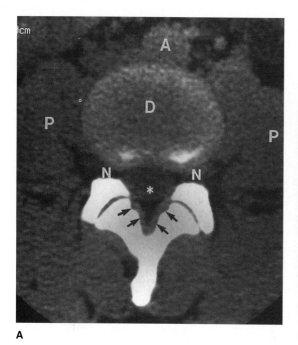

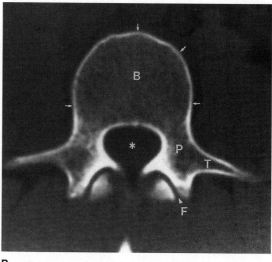

A **B**

Fig. 13–5. CT of normal spine. **A** Soft-tissue windows. A = aorta; D = intervertebral disc; N = neural foramen; P = psoas muscles; *arrows* = ligamentum flavum; *asterisk* = thecal sac. **B** Bone window. Asterisk = spinal canal; P = pedicle; B = vertebral body; T = transverse process; F = facet joint. Notice the excellent bony detail and thin rim of normal dense cortical bone (*arrows*).

can demonstrate the ligamentum flavum, nerve roots, epidural fat, and other structures that cannot be identified discretely on plain films (Fig. 13–5*A*). We also typically film a set of bone windows, whose window and level settings are adjusted to give detailed information on bony structures (Fig. 13–5*B*). On such images, little soft-tissue information is available.

CT is widely used to image the spine in the evaluation of almost all types of pathologic conditions. Most common indications include degenerative disc disease (i.e., to rule out disc herniation in patients with myelopathy or radiculopathy), suspected spinal tumors, and trauma. Assuming a normal appearance on plain films, CT is often the first study ordered in the evaluation of patients with back pain.

CT Myelography

As mentioned earlier, in patients who have undergone myelography, CT is often obtained immediately afterward (Fig. 13–6). It has been shown that a post-myelogram CT is more sensitive in the detection of pathologic conditions than is either test alone. This is particularly true for lesions within the spinal canal, such as disc herniations or tumors unassociated with a bony

component. The presence of subarachnoid contrast allows dramatic visualization of the cauda equina nerve roots and spinal cord in a way that cannot be achieved with regular CT. In our institution, the vast majority of myelograms are immediately followed by CT.

MR Imaging

Since the early 1980s, MR imaging has gained widespread acceptance as the most sensitive imaging modality in the study of spine disease. Though not necessarily the first study performed, MR imaging undeniably allows visualization of intraspinal anatomy with much higher resolution than does any other modality. The ability to image directly in the sagittal plane contributes a great deal to the evaluation of the diseased spine. A description of the physics of MR imaging is beyond the scope of this chapter, and the reader is referred elsewhere for this information.

Because dense cortical bone has few mobile protons (which are necessary to create an MR signal), MR imaging is sometimes limited in its ability to demonstrate either osteophytes that may be a source of clinical symptoms or calcific components of other lesions. In such cases, CT with its superb depiction of bony detail may be useful as

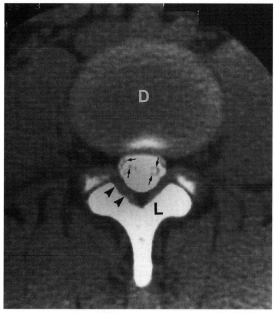

A

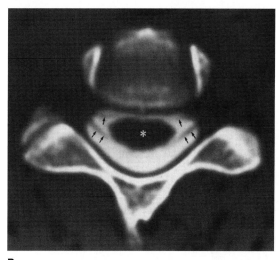

B

Fig. 13–6. Postmyelographic CT. **A** Lumbar spine, soft-tissue window through L4–5 disc space. Dense contrast can be seen surrounding the small cauda equina nerve roots (*arrows*). D = disc; L = lamina; *arrowheads* = ligamentum flavum. **B** Cervical spine, bone window, disc space level. Spinal cord is easily seen (*). Dorsal and ventral nerve roots can be seen as they leave the cord and join to form spinal nerve (*arrows*).

an adjunct examination. On the other hand, MR imaging is very sensitive in its ability to detect abnormalities in bone marrow. The vertebral bodies normally contain a large amount of bone marrow, and an abnormal appearance may be seen in a variety of disorders, such as anemia, infection, and metastatic disease.

MR images can be obtained with a variety of "sequences." The most commonly utilized are called *spin-echo*, and these can be "weighted" for either T_1 or T_2. (A thorough explanation of these parameters can be found elsewhere.) On a T_1-weighted image, normal adult (yellow/fatty) bone marrow has a "high signal" (i.e., it is hyperintense, or whitish in color), and CSF has a "low signal" (i.e., it is hypointense, or black in color). Neural tissue, such as the spinal cord or nerve roots, is intermediate in signal intensity (Fig. 13–7*A*). Cortical bone, lacking mobile protons to produce a signal, is hypointense on all pulse sequences. On T_2-weighted images, marrow becomes lower in signal intensity, CSF becomes hyperintense, and neural tissue maintains an intermediate signal intensity. However, the spinal cord appears relatively lower in signal intensity, surrounded as it is by CSF with its very high signal intensity (Fig. 13–7*B*). The intervertebral discs in normal individuals are typically of intermediate signal on T_1-weighted images and, because of

their water content, appear hyperintense on T_2-weighted images.

Any alterations in the expected normal signal intensity for an anatomic structure should prompt a search for either a technical or a pathologic explanation for the abnormal signal. In some clinical applications, scanning after administration of intravenous gadolinium (gadopentetate dimeglumine) or other paramagnetic contrast agents can add valuable information, which may either clarify questions raised by the precontrast imaging results or permit detection of lesions that were invisible without contrast. In recent years, the use of fat suppression has increased the utility of contrast-enhanced imaging of the spine, particularly in the evaluation of lesions within the spinal canal (Fig. 13–8).

TECHNIQUE SELECTION

A great many clinical circumstances may necessitate spine imaging. The purpose of this section is to convey a sense of which techniques would be most appropriate for the given clinical setting. In some instances, the choice is clear. In others, the test to be performed is determined by the technology available, and often the decision is influenced by the preferences of the person

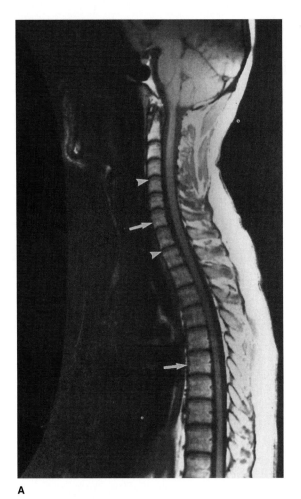

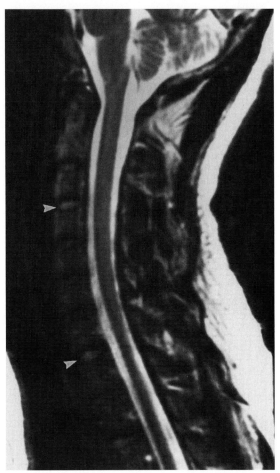

A

B

Fig. 13–7. Normal MR images. **A** T_1-weighted sagittal, cervicothoracic spine. The spinal cord is very easily seen. Note CSF anterior and posterior to the cord is hypointense, or of low signal intensity. The high signal arising from the vertebral body bone marrow (*arrows*) is due to the fat content. The disc spaces are readily visualized and are of lower signal intensity (*arrowheads*). This is the normal relative appearance of bone marrow and disc on T_1-weighted images. Any reversal (i.e., disc is brighter or higher in signal intensity than marrow) should raise the suspicion of marrow disease. **B** T_2-weighted sagittal cervical spine. CSF is now very hyperintense, and spinal cord appears to have relatively low signal intensity. The discs (*arrowheads*), because of their water content (when normal), appear higher in signal intensity when compared with the T_1-weighted image. The bone marrow, on the other hand, is lower in signal intensity (fat fades on T_2).

ordering the test. In some clinical settings more than one imaging modality is acceptable as a first test. If the clinician consults with the radiologist before deciding on the initial test, unnecessary examinations may be avoided. Perhaps most importantly, however, if the clinician consults with the radiologist and conveys to him or her the clinical information, imaging often can be tailored to home in on the most likely site or type

of abnormality. Still, general guidelines can be established to help decide which imaging test is appropriate. What follows is a brief outline providing general imaging recommendations for common clinical problems related to the spine. Only rarely is a particular test the only useful one for a suspected abnormality. In many cases, any of several tests would be useful as a baseline examination, with the understanding that

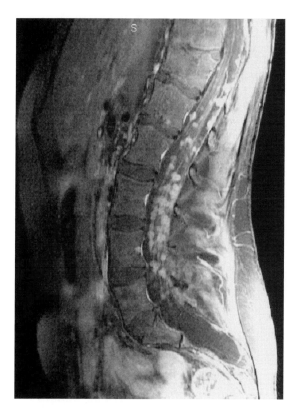

Fig. 13–8. Sagittal fat-suppressed, contrast-enhanced, T$_1$-weighted MR image. A 22-year-old female with metastatic Ewing's sarcoma presented with back and leg pain and lower extremity paresthesias. Numerous brightly enhancing nodules indicate subarachnoid tumor deposits. Contrast-enhanced MR imaging may be the only way to confirm this diagnosis, because CSF cytology is often falsely negative.

additional imaging might be required to answer all clinical questions.

Trauma

Plain films provide the best initial examination for the evaluation of spine trauma. In a potentially unstable patient, they are obtained readily and often yield an immediate diagnosis. For further characterization of complex fractures, for conditions in which plain films would be inadequate (e.g., the cervical thoracic junction), or when additional information is required (e.g., to rule out canal compromise by a bone fragment), CT is frequently performed. CT is the best imaging study to evaluate complex spine fractures. In certain circumstances, such as suspected spinal cord contusion or transection or hemorrhage

within the spinal canal, MR imaging is indicated. It is also useful in evaluating the patient with delayed onset of neurologic dysfunction after trauma to rule out myelomalacia (softening) of the spinal cord or post-traumatic syrinx.

Back Pain

Back pain is one of the most common medical complaints. Though most cases are caused by muscle strains and the like, persistent severe pain, pain associated with sciatica (a shooting pain down the leg), or neurologic findings such as weakness, decreased sensation, or abnormal reflexes should prompt a search for an underlying structural abnormality. The most common pathologic conditions are related to bony degenerative disease (osteoarthritis) or intervertebral disc abnormalities. As with trauma, plain films are a good place to start. Though disc herniations (extrusion of the nucleus pulposus beyond the annulus fibrosus) are not visible on plain films, degenerative changes are generally quite apparent, and any unsuspected lesions such as compression fractures or metastatic disease (both of which are common in older patients) may be detected.

For patients with a suspected herniated disc, MR imaging is generally considered the most sensitive examination. CT is still a good examination for the detection of disc herniation and, when combined with intrathecal contrast (CT myelography), it is still a widely used imaging modality. Although MR imaging is not essential for detecting disc abnormalities, it is more sensitive and is especially useful for detecting other pathologic conditions that might mimic disc herniation, such as lesions of the conus medullaris or metastatic disease. A possible exception to the use of MR imaging as a first-line cross-sectional imaging procedure in degenerative spine disease is for patients suspected of having foraminal nerve impingement by an osteophyte. Osteophytes are small, sharp projections of bone that occur in patients with osteoarthritis and they may impinge on the spinal cord or nerve roots. Such osteophytes in the cervical spine may be difficult to detect with MR imaging. However, it is not always possible to differentiate clinically between patients who have disc herniations and those whose nerves are compressed by osteophytes. All in all, MR imaging is the best test to order for these patients. Occasionally, a CT examination may be needed in addition to answer specific questions.

Myelopathy

In patients who are suspected of having a myelopathy (a true cord syndrome as opposed to radicular symptoms), MR imaging is unequivocally the first study to be employed. MR imaging is the only imaging procedure that allows direct visualization of the spinal cord and it is effective for diagnosing or excluding primary spinal cord lesions such as infarct, tumor, hemorrhage, or inflammatory conditions (e.g., multiple sclerosis or transverse myelitis).

Congenital Spine Lesions

A variety of congenital lesions may affect the spine. Plain films may be useful to survey the spine, but ultimately MR imaging is the modality of choice. Though bony defects may be imaged suboptimally, disorders of the spinal cord or nerve roots can be readily identified on MR images.

Metastatic Disease

If metastatic disease in the spine is suspected, plain films are an economical, easy way to rule out bony metastases. Unfortunately, plain films do not demonstrate such abnormalities until a significant amount of destruction has taken place. MR imaging, on the other hand, is quite sensitive to replacement of normal bone marrow by tumor and can establish the diagnosis much earlier. Gadolinium-enhanced MR imaging is also the best choice if spread of tumor to the subarachnoid space (carcinomatous meningitis or leptomeningeal carcinomatosis) is suspected clinically.

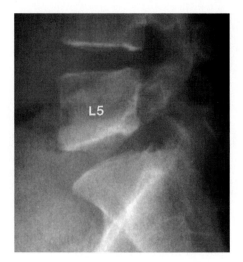

Fig. 13–9.

EXERCISES

EXERCISE 13-1: DEGENERATIVE SPINE DISEASE

Clinical Histories:

Case 13-1. A whiny 45-year-old neuroradiologist presents with low-back pain. A coneddown lateral plain film of the lumbar spine is shown in (Fig. 13–9).

Case 13-2. A 58-year-old man presents with rightsided L5 radiculopathy. A myelogram was performed, and an oblique view demonstrating the right-sided nerve roots is displayed in (Fig. 13–10).

Case 13-3. A 53-year-old woman presents with neck and right arm pain. Plain films of the cervical spine were ordered, and a lateral film is shown in (Fig. 13–11).

Questions:

13-1. In Case 13-1, what is the abnormality seen in Fig. 13–9?
A. The bones are too dense.
B. The bones are not dense enough (osteopenia).

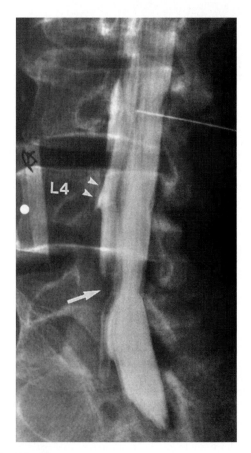

Fig. 13–10.

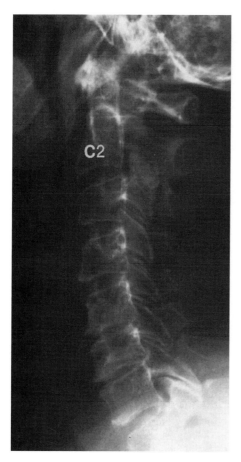

Fig. 13–11.

C. Degenerative disc disease at C5–6 and C6–7

D. Traumatic injury

E. Disc space infection at C5–6 and C6–7

Radiologic Findings:

13-1. In this case, Fig. 13–9 shows a subtle anterior displacement of the L5 vertebral body relative to S1, known as *spondylolisthesis.* (*D* is the correct answer to Question 13-1.)

13-2. In this case, in Fig. 13–10 an extradural defect is seen at and below the L4–5 disc space and the right L5 nerve root does not fill. These changes are most likely caused by a disc herniation. (*A* is the correct answer to Question 13-2.) Note normal filling of the right L4 nerve root (*arrowheads*).

13-3. In this case, Fig. 13–11 shows disc space narrowing and osteophytes are seen at the C5–6 and C6–7 disc spaces. (*C* is the correct answer to Question 13-3.)

Discussion:

Degenerative osteoarthropathy may affect different parts of the spine. When the facet joints are involved, the result is often bony osteophytes, which may project into the neural foramen or spinal canal and compress neural structures. When the disc space is affected, bony changes in the vertebral body endplate can occur. In addition, the intervertebral disc itself may be affected, and disc herniation can occur as a result. Differentiation between disc bulge (less clinically important, usually in the midline, with no significant compression of cord or thecal sac) and actual herniation (larger, off-midline, with possible compression of nerves or thecal sac) is not always possible. Treatment decisions must be based on clinical as well as radiologic data.

In Case 13-1 (author's spine), the spondylolisthesis of L5 over S1 is a result of a defect in the pars interarticularis. This is the place between the superior and inferior articular facet of a given vertebra (Figs. 13–3*C* and 13–12*A*). Spondylolysis, as this defect is known, is usually caused by a chronic stress fracture, though rarely it can be congenital or acute. If, as is commonly the case, the spondylolysis is bilateral, the vertebral body is essentially disconnected from the posterior elements and this allows the anterior slipping, or spondylolisthesis, shown in Fig. 13–9. This entity is included here because it is quite common, and because it predisposes to premature degenerative disease. In older patients, spondylolisthesis can be secondary to degenerative disease in the absence of a pars defect, and this "nonlytic" form is known as *pseudospondylolisthesis* or *degenerative spondylolisthesis.* When present, the spondylolysis defect is readily identified on oblique

C. There is a destructive bony lesion.

D. There is an abnormality of alignment.

E. There is a soft-tissue abnormality.

13-2. In Case 13-2, the lesion represented by an arrow in Fig. 13–10 is most likely to be

A. a right-sided L4–5 herniated nucleus pulposus.

B. an extradural tumor.

C. an epidural abscess.

D. an intradural mass.

E. a bony lesion.

13-3. In Case 13-3, the lateral cervical spine plain film (Fig. 13–11) suggests what as the MOST likely diagnosis?

A. Degenerative disc disease at C2–3 and C3–4

B. Neoplastic disease at C4

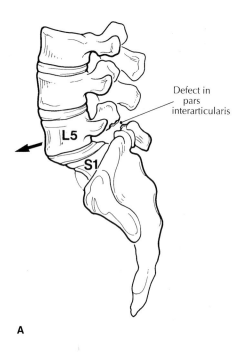

A

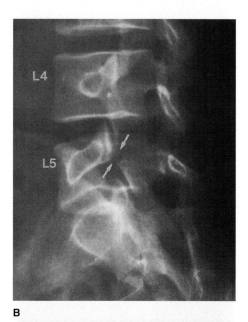

B

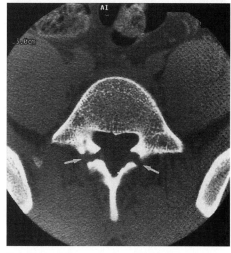

C

lumbar plain films, as a "broken neck on the Scottie dog" (Fig. 13–12B). The lysis defect is also readily detected on CT (Fig. 13–12C) though it may superficially resemble a facet joint.

Disc herniations are a common medical problem. Though they can usually be diagnosed with noninvasive CT or MR imaging, myelography is still employed in some places to diagnose disc herniations. In Case 13-2, Figure 13–10 shows an extradural defect, seen as an area of low density distorting the lateral aspect of the thecal sac, deviating the nerve roots. This is the typical appearance of a herniated nucleus pulposus (HNP) on myelography. We see the effect of the disc rather than the actual disc. On a CT study, the actual herniated disc can be visualized (Fig. 13–13A). Most of the myelographic filling defect can be seen to be below the L4–5 disc space, secondary to inferior migration of disc material. This helps explain why the patient had an L5 radiculopathy. The right L4 nerve root (*arrowheads* in Fig. 13–10) had already exited and would be unaffected by an L4–5 HNP unless it was far lateral (Fig. 13–13B). As previously mentioned, MR imaging is excellent in detecting disc herniations and eliminates the need for painful, invasive procedures such as myelography (Fig. 13–13B, C).

Osteophytic ridging is a common manifestation of degenerative bone disease and in the cervical spine may cause myelopathy (if the cord is compressed) or radicu-

Fig. 13–12. **A** Diagram of spondylolisthesis of L5 over S1 caused by spondylolysis of L5. **B** Oblique plain film of lumbar spine (same patient as in Fig. 13–9) demonstrates a spondylolysis or pars defect on the right side at L5 (*arrows*). Note intact pars at L4 (*). **C** CT bone window of different patient shows spondylolysis defects (*arrows*). Though these resemble facet joints, they are more horizontal in orientation and more irregular, lacking a smooth cortical margin.

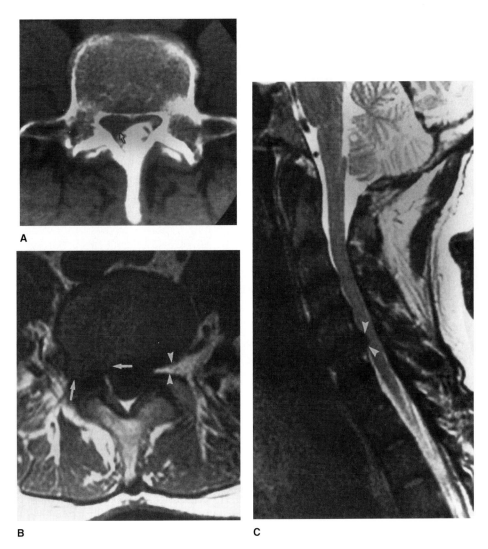

Fig. 13–13. **A** Axial CT (same patient as in Fig. 13–10) just below the L4–5 disc space, shows compression of the right anterolateral aspect of the thecal sac by the HNP (*arrow*). The image was obtained below the L4-5 disc space, indicating inferior migration of herniated disc material. **B** Axial T₁-weighted MR image of a different patient shows a far lateral right-sided HNP (*arrows*) with replacement of normal foraminal fat by intermediate signal representing the disc. Note normal perineural fat (*arrowheads*) in the left neural foramen. A far lateral HNP such as this would probably be missed if only myelography were performed. **C** Sagittal T₂-weighted image shows a midline disc herniation at C5–6 that is compressing the spinal cord (*arrowheads*).

lopathy (if a nerve root is compressed). In Case 13-3, Fig. 13–11 shows marked narrowing and osteophyte formation at C5–6 and C6–7. An oblique radiograph is useful in demonstrating the foraminal compromise that can result if osteophytes occur in that location (Fig. 13–14A). Myelography can demonstrate effacement of nerve roots (Fig. 13–14B). CT, with or without in-

trathecal contrast material, is excellent in depicting foraminal stenosis caused by osteophytes (Fig. 13–14C). As mentioned earlier, MR imaging may be limited in its ability to depict subtle bony abnormalities such as foraminal compromise, though utilization of specialized techniques has resulted in improved detection with MR imaging.

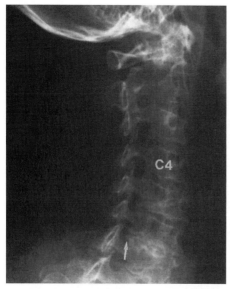

A

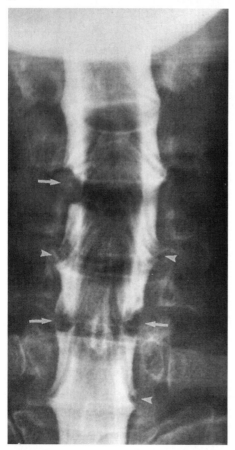

B

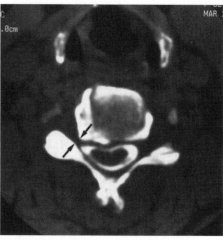

C

***Fig. 13–14.* A** Oblique radiograph shows compromise of the right C6–7 neural foramen by osteophytes (*arrow*). Note that the other foramina are patent. **B** AP view, cervical myelogram of a different patient. Effaced nerve roots (*arrows*) can be seen as defects larger than would be expected for a normal nerve root. Compare with normal nerve roots (*arrowheads*). **C** Axial post-myelographic CT of same patient shows narrowing of the right neural foramen (*arrows*). The contralateral neural foramen is normal.

EXERCISE 13-2: NEOPLASTIC SPINE DISEASE

Clinical Histories:

Case 13-4. A 39-year-old man presents with leg pain and weakness. A prior lumbar spine MR examination was normal. A thoracic myelogram is shown in Fig. 13–15.

Case 13-5. A 70-year-old woman presents with a 5-year history of back pain and recent onset of paresthesia in the groin and inner thighs (saddle distribution) (Fig. 13–16).

Case 13-6. A 63-year-old man presents with severe upper neck pain not responding to anti-inflammatory medication (Fig. 13–17).

Case 13-7. A 65-year-old man presents with back pain. A CT bone window is shown in Fig. 13–18.

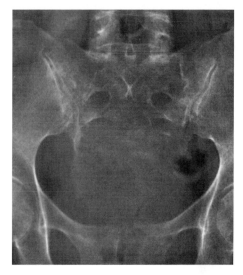

Fig. 13–16.

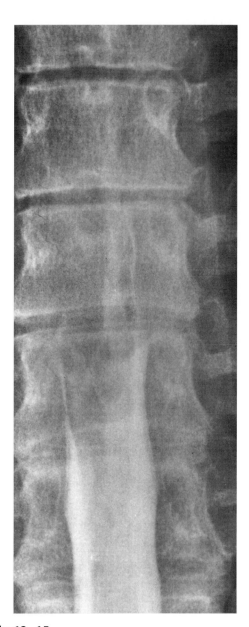

Fig. 13–15.

13-5. In Case 13-5 (Fig. 13–16), what is the most likely diagnosis?
   A. Sacroiliitis
   B. A sacral tumor
   C. Constipation
   D. Osteoporosis
   E. Uterine malignancy

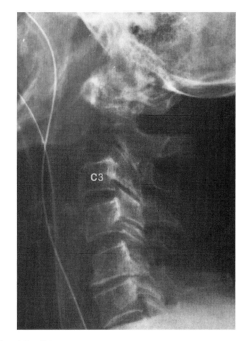

Fig. 13–17.

Questions:

13-4. In Case 13-4, what does this AP view from a thoracic myelogram (Fig. 13–15) show?
   A. A bony abnormality
   B. An extradural mass
   C. An intradural-extramedullary mass
   D. An intramedullary mass
   E. A really big disc herniation

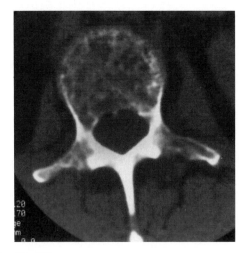

Fig. 13–18.

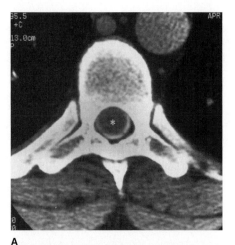

A

13-6. In Case 13-6 (Fig. 13–17), what is the main radiologic finding?
 A. A lesion of the C7 spinous process
 B. An osteoblastic bony lesion
 C. An abnormality of alignment
 D. A destructive lesion at C2
 E. A fracture

13-7. In Case 13-7 (Fig. 13–18), what diagnostic possibilities should be most seriously considered?
 A. Congenital or traumatic lesions
 B. Metabolic or endocrine disease
 C. Myeloma or metastatic disease
 D. Infectious or inflammatory disease
 E. Degenerative or inflammatory disease

Radiologic Findings:

13-4. In this case, the patient has a lower thoracic primary spinal cord astrocytoma. (*D* is the correct answer to Question 13-4.) The cord is normal inferiorly but is seen (in Fig. 13–15) to get wider toward the middle of the image. The contrast column on either side of the lesion is narrowed, most noticeably on the patient's right. This lesion has caused a "block" to the flow of contrast. Subsequent postmyelography CT (Fig. 13–19*A*) confirmed the spinal cord enlargement. An MR image demonstrated the tumor (Fig. 13–19*B*) within the spinal cord.

13-5. In this case, the plain film (Fig. 13–16) shows a large destructive mass replacing most of the lower sacrum. (*B* is the correct answer to Question 13-5.) Notice how normal bone disappears below the midsacrum. A CT showed a large destructive mass with areas of calcification (Fig. 13–20).

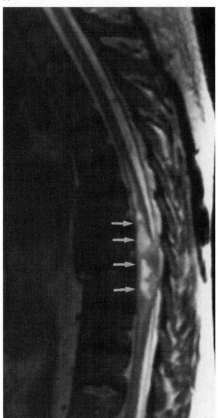

B

Fig. 13–19. **A** Axial postmyelographic CT demonstrates enlargement of the spinal cord (asterisk), representing tumor, with narrowing of the subarachnoid/contrast space surrounding the cord. **B** Sagittal T_2-weighted MR image shows the tumor and resulting enlargement of the thoracic spinal cord, with areas of central hyperintense signal (*arrows*) probably representing necrosis.

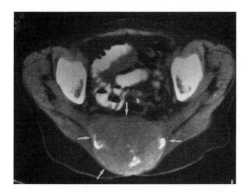

Fig. 13–20. CT study (without intravenous contrast) shows a large mass replacing the lower sacrum (*arrows*). Internal areas of high density represent either tumor calcification or remnants of destroyed bone.

13-6. In this case, the plain film (Fig. 13–17) shows that the body of C2 has been destroyed (lytic destruction). (D is the correct answer to Question 13-6.)

13-7. In this case, the CT image (Fig. 13–18) shows multiple small areas of lytic bony destruction. This is characteristic of either multiple myeloma or metastatic disease. (*C* is the correct answer to Question 13-7.)

Discussion:

Unfortunately, the spine may be involved by tumors of various types. In Case 13-4, the diagnosis was primary spinal cord glioma. Most of these are either astrocytomas or ependymomas. As with this patient, the diagnosis may be elusive for some time while other diseases such as disc herniation are ruled out. This patient even had a normal lumbar MR examination several months prior to the myelogram. While the thoracolumbar junction is usually visualized on a lumbar MR imaging study, this tumor (at T10) was just missed. A thoracic MR examination would certainly have made the diagnosis, but the patient's doctor ordered a myelogram. Spinal cord tumors are generally very difficult to treat. The more malignant ones, usually astocytomas, are associated with a poor prognosis. Ependymomas, because they are less infiltrative and more readily resectable, are associated with a much better prognosis.

Primary bony tumors also may affect the spine. A variety of benign bone tumors and cysts may be encountered. In the sacrum, giant cell tumor is the most common benign tumor. The most common primary sacral malignancy is chordoma. This is the diagnosis in Case 13-5. Chordomas develop from remnants of the embryonic notochord and represent 2% to 4% of primary malignant bone tumors. The sacrum is the most common site for chordoma, accounting for 50% of these lesions. The skull

base accounts for 35% and other vertebrae account for 15%. Typical presentation of sacral chordoma is low-back pain, paresthesias, or rectal dysfunction. Figure 13–16 shows the typical radiographic appearance of expansile, lytic destruction. On CT (Fig. 13–20), a large soft-tissue mass with internal calcifications is characteristic.

By far the most common type of spinal tumor is metastatic disease, with lung and breast being the most frequent primary sites. Virtually any tumor may metastasize to the spine. In general, certain tumors tend to result in osteoblastic or dense metastases, and prostate adenocarcinoma falls in this category. Other primary malignancies, such as those in the lung and breast, tend to have osteolytic, destructive spine metastases. The patient in Case 13-6 had lung carcinoma, and Figure 13–17 represents a hematogenous spread of tumor to the C2 vertebral body. Metastatic disease may affect the spine by other mechanisms. Tumors adjacent to the spine may grow directly into it (Fig. 13–21 *A, B*). This

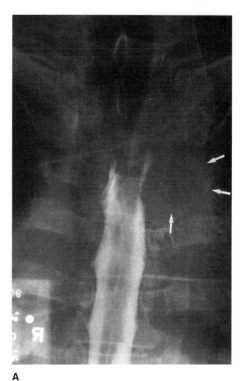

A

Fig. 13–21. **A** A 49-year-old man with lung carcinoma and direct contiguous spread into the spine. AP view, thoracic myelogram shows a mass in the left upper lung with bone destruction (*arrows*). The contrast column was blocked and there was no flow cephalad to the lesion despite steep Trendelenburg positioning. The appearance of this block is typical for an extradural process.

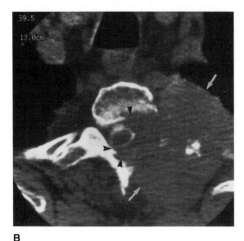

B

Fig. 13–21. **B** Postmyelographic CT of same patient at the level of the block demonstrates the large lung mass (*arrows*) extending into the spine, destroying bone and involving the epidural space (*arrowheads*).

may occur in lung carcinoma and lesions such as neuroblastoma or lymphoma (with retroperitoneal/paraspinal lymphadenopathy). Finally, the spinal canal may be affected by spread of malignant neoplasm. Rarely, a metastatic lesion may occur in the spinal cord itself, usually as a terminal event. Metastatic disease may occur in the subarachnoid space by two methods. First, an intracranial malignancy (i.e., glioma, medulloblastoma) can seed the subarachnoid space and "fall" into the spine. These are known as "drop" metastases. Hematogenous spread to the subarachnoid space may occur in non-CNS primary tumors. Such involvement is known as *leptomeningeal carcinomatosis* or *carcinomatous meningitis* (see Fig. 13–8), and is associated with a very poor prognosis.

Multiple myeloma is a disseminated malignancy caused by a proliferation of plasmacytes, typically occurring in the middle-aged and elderly, with a slight male predominance. The spine may be affected primarily or secondarily, and bone pain caused by pathologic compression fracture is the most common symptom. Plain films may be normal early in the course of the disease or show only mild osteopenia. Later, multiple, small, lytic, "punched-out" lesions may be seen. CT is very sensitive, and Figure 13–18 shows the typical CT appearance of multiple myeloma. The findings, however, would be indistinguishable from those of small lytic metastases of other origin, and for this reason, metastases and myeloma are often mentioned together in the context of multiple small lytic bony lesions. MR imaging of multiple myeloma may have different ap-

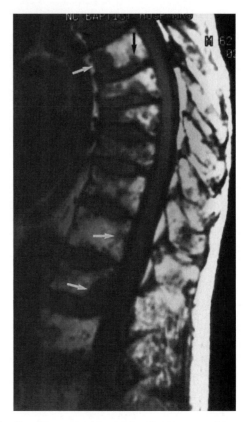

Fig. 13–22. Sagittal T_1-weighted MR image of the thoracic spine shows multiple small hypointense foci of myeloma (*arrows*) replacing normal bone marrow. Compression fractures are also seen, indicated by loss of height of several upper thoracic vertebral bodies. The spinal cord is intact, but spread of tumor or retropulsion of fractured bone could result in cord compression. Note that metastatic tumor other than myeloma could have an identical appearance.

pearances, but the typical pattern would be multiple, small foci of decreased signal intensity replacing the normal hyperintense bone marrow on T_1-weighted images (Fig. 13–22).

EXERCISE 13-3: SPINE TRAUMA

Clinical Histories:

Case 13-8. A 23-year-old woman was involved in a motor vehicle accident (Fig. 13–23).

Case 13-9. A 21-year-old quadriplegic woman had a motor vehicle accident 4 weeks ago (Fig. 13–24).

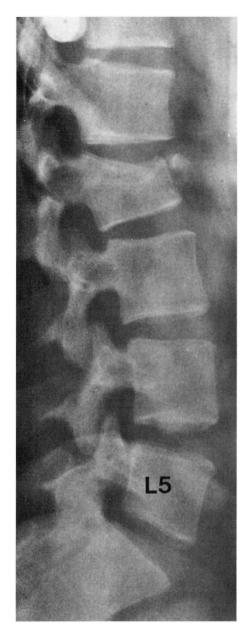

Fig. 13–23.

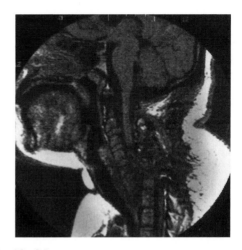

Fig. 13–24.

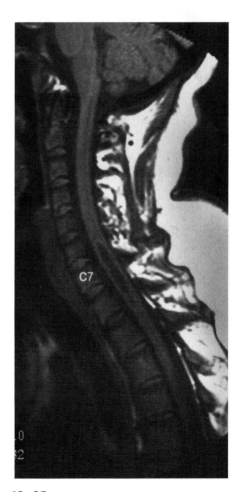

Case 13-10. A 38-year-old woman presents with slowly progressive upper extremity and upper trunk sensory deficits 3 years after a motor vehicle accident (Fig. 13–25).

Fig. 13–25.

Questions:

13-8. In Case 13-8 (Fig. 13–23), what is the most likely diagnosis?

    A. Spinal tumor, aggravated by trauma

    B. Abnormality of bone density

    C. Disruption of facet joints at multiple levels

    D. Subluxation of L4 over L5

    E. L2 compression fracture with kyphotic angulation

13-9. Regarding the patient in Case 13-9 (Fig. 13–24), which of the following is true?

    A. The condition probably predated the trauma.

    B. The prospects for a full recovery are good.

    C. Surgical repair will likely be successful.

    D. The patient will probably never have normal neurologic function below C6.

    E. The spinal cord is intact.

13-10. In Case 13-10 (Fig. 13–25), what is the most likely diagnosis?

    A. Delayed post-traumatic syrinx

    B. Subluxation

    C. Spinal cord tumor

    D. Abnormal bone marrow

    E. Disc abnormality

Radiologic Findings:

13-8. In this case, Fig. 13–23 shows a compression fracture of the L2 vertebral body with kyphotic angulation. (*E* is the correct answer to Question 13-8.)

13-9. In this case, the sagittal T₁-weighted MR image (Fig. 13–29) shows a complete subluxation of C6 on C7 and a complete transection of the cervical spinal cord at that level. In all likelihood this patient will never regain use of her legs or have any normal neurologic function below C6. (*D* is the correct answer to Question 13-9.)

13-10. In this case, the sagittal T₁-weighted MR image shows a low signal abnormality within the cervical spinal cord from C6 to T1. This is a typical appearance of syringomyelia or syrinx. (*A* is the correct answer to Question 13-10.)

Discussion:

Spinal trauma is a major medical problem, usually caused by motor vehicle and occupational accidents. Accurate and complete diagnosis is essential to maintain spine stability and ensure preservation of neurologic function. As mentioned previously, plain films should be obtained initially, and this often makes the diagnosis. However, additional imaging tests are often necessary to fully evaluate a case of spine trauma. For instance, in Case 13-8, there was clinical concern that the spinal canal was compromised. Small bony fragments within the spinal canal may not be visible with plain film alone. For this reason, CT was performed (Fig. 13–26 *A,B*).

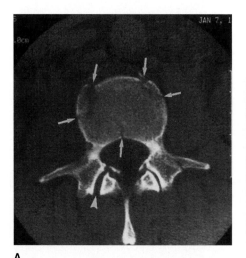

A

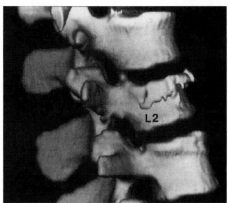

B

Fig. 13–26. **A** Axial CT bone window shows different components of the fracture (*arrows*). The spinal canal was intact. Note the separation of the facet joint on the right (*arrowhead*). **B** Three-dimensional reconstruction shows compression of L2 and fracture sites. Such reconstructions are sometimes useful in cases of spine trauma.

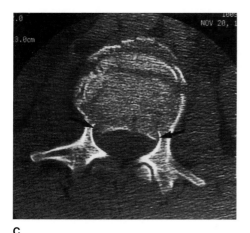

C

Fig. 13–26. **C** Axial CT bone window of a different patient demonstrates multiple fractures and retropulsion of a bone fragment, causing narrowing of the spinal canal (*arrows*).

This allowed a better appreciation of the extent of the fractures and ruled out neural compression. An example of spinal canal compromise is shown in Fig. 13–26C.

In severe trauma, the spinal cord may be affected. Contusions may occur with or without fracture/subluxation, and MR imaging would be required for diagnosis. In a severe fracture/subluxation, the spinal cord can be completely transected. In Case 13-9, the patient was known to have a severe C6–7 subluxation, but because of obesity, plain film and CT imaging were very limited. In this case, only MR imaging was able to demonstrate the full extent of her spinal cord injury.

Rarely, patients who have recovered from an acute spinal injury experience a delayed onset of neurologic symptoms, occurring 1 to 15 years after the trauma. This suggests the possibility of delayed post-traumatic syrinx (Case 13-10). Symptoms include pain upon coughing or exertion, sensory disturbances, or motor deficits. MR imaging is essential for diagnosis. The condition is sometimes amenable to surgical shunting. Syringomyelia can also be idiopathic or can be secondary to certain congenital or inflammatory conditions. Imaging often cannot distinguish among different possible etiologies, and history is important.

BIBLIOGRAPHY

Atlas SW. *Magnetic Resonance Imaging of the Brain and Spine.* 3rd ed. Baltimore: Lippincott, Williams & Wilkins; 2002.

Greenspan A, Montesano P. *Imaging of the Spine in Clinical Practice.* New York: Raven Press; 1993.

Harris JH Jr, Mirvis SE. *The Radiology of Acute Cervical Spine Trauma.* 3rd ed. Baltimore: Williams & Wilkins; 1996.

Manelfe C, ed. *Imaging of the Spine and Spinal Cord.* New York: Raven Press; 1992.

INDEX

Note: Page numbers in italics refer to figures; page numbers followed by *t* indicate tables.